MEDIEVAL HERBAL REMEDIES

Featured here is a modern translation of a medieval herbal, with a study showing how this technical treatise on herbs was turned into a literary curiosity in the nineteenth century. The contours of this second edition replicate the first; however, it has been revised and updated throughout to reflect new scholarship and new findings. New information is presented on Oswald Cockayne, the nineteenth-century philologist who first translated the Old English medical texts for the modern world.

Here the medieval text is read as an example of technical writing (i.e., intended to convey instructions/information), not as literature. The audience it was originally aimed at would know how to diagnose and treat medical conditions and knew or was learning how to follow its instructions. For that reason, while working on the translation, specialists in relevant fields were asked to shed light on its terse wording, for example, herbalists and physicians. Unlike many current studies, this work discusses the *Herbarium* and other medical texts in Old English as part of a tradition developed throughout early-medieval Europe associated with monasteries and their libraries.

The book is intended for scholars in cross-cultural fields; that is, with roots in one field and branches in several, such as nineteenth-century or medieval studies, for historians of herbalism, medicine, pharmacy, botany, and of the Western Middle Ages, broadly and inclusively defined, and for readers interested in the history of herbalism and medicine.

Anne Van Arsdall, Ph.D. (ret.) Publications include papers, book chapters; and (ed.) *Herbs and Healers from the Ancient Mediterranean through the Medieval West* (2012) and *The Old French Chronicle of Morea* (2015), a translation of a crusade chronicle set in Greece.

Praise for the second edition

"I was delighted to see a revised edition of Anne Van Arsdall's *Medieval Herbal Remedies*. For two decades, her book has served as an example of how to make medieval herbalism accessible to readers beyond just specialists in the field, through a much-needed modern translation of the *Old English Herbarium*, a study of the nineteenth-century antiquarian Oswald Cockayne and his own, curious 1864 translation of the *Herbarium*, and a fascinating comparison of early medieval herbalists to modern folk-healers. A welcome update to this edition is Van Arsdall's placement of the *Old English Herbarium* in a broader European context, as an heir to Galenic, monastic, and vernacular medical traditions."

Winston Black, *St. Francis Xavier University, Nova Scotia*

"In the nineteenth century T. Oswald Cockayne introduced Old English medical texts to the modern world. In her 2002 edition Anne Van Arsdall reintroduced Cockayne and his work to the twenty-first century. Now, a valuable second edition dramatically expands the story of the man whose tragic life reads like a 'bittersweet Victorian novel' and whose scholarly work has gone largely unrecognized. More, it dramatically re-envisions the Old English medical texts Cockayne valued only for the vocabulary they contributed to the Old English lexicon. By resituating them, not in an 'Anglo-Saxon' context, but in the larger early medieval European tradition and by reading them as technical medical texts based on herbalism, Van Arsdall charts a promising new path for the study of *The Old English Herbarium* and its textual kin."

Dabney A. Bankert, *Professor Emerita of Medieval Literature,*
James Madison University

"This significantly revised text offers a thought-provoking introduction to medieval medicine through the Old English *Herbarium*. Van Arsdall vividly shows how early medical texts were long thought to be of little value except for studying Germanic philology or folklore. The substantial introductory chapters and notes to the translation presented here show how we need to rethink such texts as technical literature – and indeed a literature that grew out of rich cultures of medical knowledge and practice across Christendom rather than just among the English. The crisp translation of the *Herbarium* makes this fascinating and complex world of learning further accessible. *Medieval Herbal Remedies* will be a valuable resource for teaching new histories of premodern medicine and encouraging new research in the field."

James T. Palmer, *Professor of History, University of St Andrews*

MEDIEVAL HERBAL REMEDIES

The *Old English Herbarium* and Early-Medieval Medicine

Second edition

Anne Van Arsdall

Illustrated by Robby Poore

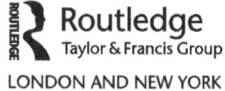
Routledge
Taylor & Francis Group

LONDON AND NEW YORK

Designed cover image: Robby Poore

Second edition published 2023
by Routledge
4 Park Square, Milton Park, Abingdon, Oxon OX14 4RN

and by Routledge
605 Third Avenue, New York, NY 10158

Routledge is an imprint of the Taylor & Francis Group, an informa business

© 2023 Anne Van Arsdall

First edition published by Routledge 2002

British Library Cataloguing-in-Publication Data
A catalogue record for this book is available from the British Library

Library of Congress Cataloging-in-Publication Data
Names: Van Arsdall, Anne, author.
Title: Medieval herbal remedies: the Old English herbarium and early-medieval medicine / Anne Van Arsdall; illustrated by Robby Poore.
Other titles: The Old English herbarium and anglo-saxon medicine
Description: Second edition. | Milton Park, Abingdon, Oxon; New York, NY: Routledge, 2023. | Includes bibliographical references and index. |
Identifiers: LCCN 2022028664 (print) | LCCN 2022028665 (ebook) |
ISBN 9780367753795 (hardback) | ISBN 9780367753771 (paperback) |
ISBN 9781003162285 (ebook)
Subjects: LCSH: Materia medica, Vegetable–Great Britain–Early works to 1800. |
Herbals–Great Britain–Early works to 1800. |
Anglo-Saxons–Medicine. | Medicine, Medieval–Great Britain. |
English language–Old English, ca. 450–1100–Texts.
Classification: LCC RS177.G7 V36 2023 (print) | LCC RS177.G7 (ebook) |
DDC 615.3/210941–dc23/eng/20220629
LC record available at https://lccn.loc.gov/2022028664
LC ebook record available at https://lccn.loc.gov/2022028665

ISBN: 978-0-367-75379-5 (hbk)
ISBN: 978-0-367-75377-1 (pbk)
ISBN: 978-1-003-16228-5 (ebk)

DOI: 10.4324/9781003162285

Typeset in Bembo
by Newgen Publishing UK

To Jay, for patiently keeping the boat on an even keel

CONTENTS

FOREWORD

It is a curious situation when a medieval text stands twice in need of rescue if it is to be understood and valued by modern readers, but that is the case for the *Old English Herbarium*. This medical and botanical treatise, written in the language of the Anglo-Saxons at the end of the first millennium, requires an accurate and lucid translation if it is to be used by those who value knowledge of the science and healing arts in an earlier era. Happily, Anne Van Arsdall has produced for this volume such a skilled and readable translation, based on the 1984 De Vriend edition.

Van Arsdall has, however, provided us with more than a useful translation from the Old English. She also has made clear why the *Herbarium* has been for more than a century neglected at best and misunderstood at worst, for the work has been available to those lacking specialized expertise in Old English only through the strange but influential 1864 translation and commentary by the Rev. T. Oswald Cockayne. Van Arsdall has rescued this text not only from the barriers presented to modern readers by Old English but also from the obfuscations and confusions of Cockayne's translation in his *Leechdoms, Wortcunning, and Starcraft of Early England*, the only modern English version available until the twenty-first century. In the process she has brought to light striking information about the sad life and death of this Victorian London schoolmaster. Cockayne's story calls to mind the sufferings of Dickens' fictional world as well as the intellectual milieu depicted in K.M. Elisabeth Murray's *Caught in the Web of Words* and Simon Winchester's *The Professor and the Madman*.

Although Van Arsdall's careful and vigorous translation of the Old English *Herbarium* and the strange story of Cockayne are reasons enough to value this book, her study makes other significant contributions. She sets this Anglo-Saxon work in an early-medieval medical context, and she clarifies its uses with recourse to contemporary practice of herbal medicine in Hispanic America that derives from medieval Europe.

The *Herbarium*, attributed wrongly to Apuleius Platonicus, was one of a number of Old English texts—occupying some thousand manuscript pages—that mark the first flowering of vernacular medical writing in medieval Europe. It is an expanded version of a late Roman treatise that survives in Old English in four manuscripts, one of them strikingly illustrated (British Library Cotton MS, Vitellius C. iii). This text is by no means a mindless translation of Mediterranean herbal remedies; rather it displays practical knowledge of plants widely available in Anglo-Saxon England through cultivation and import. Van Arsdall adds to our understanding of the uses of this text by drawing on present-day *curandera* practices in the south western United States. She makes a cogent argument that texts like the Old English *Herbarium* served as aide-mémoire for the apprenticeship system that trains traditional healers.

This volume provides insight into the origin and uses of this remedy book of some 185 plants. It also explains its vexed reception since Cockayne's mid-nineteenth-century translation, situates the *Old English Herbarium* in the context of living traditions of healing, and allows the reader to encounter it directly in a clear and graceful translation.

Linda Ehrsam Voigts, 2002

ACKNOWLEDGMENTS

My thanks to Professor Michael MacMahon of the University of Glasgow for assistance in obtaining hard-to-find information, for sharing his knowledge about the nineteenth century, and for continued encouragement with my work. I thank Professor Maria Amalia D'Aronco, University of Udine, for vital materials related to the *Old English Herbarium* and for sharing her knowledge of medieval herbals and philology over many years. I am indebted to Professor Linda Ehrsam Voigts of the University of Missouri at Kansas City for her guidance and encouragement as this work began. I am grateful to Stephanie Ball, M.D., for answering questions about medical conditions and medical practices. I thank professors at the University of New Mexico who helped shape this study when it began: in particular Drs. Helen Damico and Donald Sullivan, and Drs. David Bennahum, Patrick Gallacher, Claire Waters, and Gail Houston. Thanks to Interlibrary Loan staff at Zimmerman Library, the University of New Mexico for performing miracles. I am indebted to the College of Arts and Sciences of the university for its award of an academic fellowship supporting my study. My thanks to the staff at Harvard's Houghton and Widener libraries for their helpfulness in the fall of 1998 while I was using the Cockayne collection. I am grateful to Professor Peter Bierbaumer of the University of Graz for giving me copies of his out-of-print works on Anglo-Saxon botanical terms. At Sandia National Laboratories, for their continued support, I thank Drs. Nancy Jackson and James E. Miller, as well as my supervisors and colleagues there who often accommodated an erratic work schedule so that I could complete this work.

I thank my family for support and love through it all, and for the humor that keeps me from taking myself too seriously. Special acknowledgment to my brothers Clyde and Bob, my sisters-in-law Sybil and Inez, my sons Robby and Jonathan, and daughters-in-law Lynne and Stacy; and last but not least, Mephisto, for your long years of comfort. Finally, to Dr. Werner Paul Friederich, of the University of North Carolina, thank you for a lifetime of inspiration.

Fall 2001

For assistance in preparing the second edition, many of the above-named individuals continued their help. In addition, I am especially grateful to M.A. D'Aronco, M.K.C. MacMahon, Walton O. Schalick, M.D., and Frances Watkins. For their useful suggestions and help with various aspects of the revision, I thank M.J. Toswell and Jane Roberts; Linda E. Voigts, Vicki Pitman, Alison Denham, and Karmen Lenz. For their kindness in providing access to the University of North Carolina library system, I am grateful to Professors Mary Floyd-Wilson and Minrose Gwin, to library circulation director Joe Mitchem, and to Cheryl-Siler Jones of the English Department. And as always, my family has stood by me, enabling me to continue, most of the time with a smile.

Summer 2022

INTRODUCTION

This book began as a translation and study of the *Old English Herbarium*, an early-medieval herbal containing 185 medicinal herbs and terse instructions on their use. Almost immediately, however, the study began to morph into something larger. Naturally, I first consulted the only existing translation of the work, which was by a British minister named Oswald Cockayne. In the mid-nineteenth century, he had in fact translated and annotated all the Old English medical texts in a three-volume set he titled *Leechdoms, Wortcunning, and Starcraft of Early England*. As I unearthed more and more about this largely overlooked scholar and his voluminous undertakings, I began to see him as the epitome of an outsider in academia, the everyman in a community with unwritten but ironclad rules concerning the hierarchy of its members.

For that reason, when *Medieval Herbal Remedies* first appeared in 2002, I could not let Cockayne's life go. As much as space allows, decades of additional research are included in Chapter 1 of this new edition. His story becomes ever more poignant: his name is seldom mentioned in studies of nineteenth-century philology; his works exist on the margins of early English studies and many of his hand-written transcriptions are unpublished; many of his literary remains have long lain unnoticed, mixed with the papers of W. W. Skeat, a much more famous scholar; and he lies buried in an unmarked grave, deemed a suicide.

In addition, as I began to work on the translation intended to replace Cockayne's and to look into medieval herbals and the medicine they represent, I found that most studies said such works were impossible to follow and medically useless. It was a verdict Cockayne himself promoted. Yet everywhere around me in New Mexico, where I lived at the time, were living traditions of herbalism, both in the Latino community and as alternative practices, some of them with similarly imprecise texts. As a non-practitioner, I began to study Latino *curanderismo* and medical herbalism, and a new door to understanding the medieval texts seemed to be opening, as I mention in the first edition. In this update, I also include added insight that members of the Herbal History Research Network have given me about modern medical herbalism and its ancient roots. That insight, coupled with my experience as a science writer, led me to understand medieval medical texts as technical writings, which by necessity have both written and unwritten (explicit and tacit) components. This too is folded into Chapters 2 and 3.

This second edition, as its updated title implies, turns from a somewhat "Anglo-Saxon" focus to a broader and more inclusive understanding of these texts in the early-medieval world, a period now largely decoupled from the fall of Rome. The *Herbarium* is removed from a primarily secular Anglo-Saxon context and situated within in a medical tradition that developed throughout Western Europe from about 500–1000 CE. In almost all histories in languages other than English, this tradition has long been explained as created and spread by the Benedictine Order. It was an ill-defined system of medicine and texts, existing during a long period of political turmoil, without formal schools, using a miscellany of information taken from books carefully salvaged from libraries, whose practitioners are virtually unknown; yet one with a spirit of invention and purpose.

The contours of the book remain the same as before, beginning with a chapter about the Rev. Oswald Cockayne (1807–73), who introduced the medical works of early-medieval England to the modern world. His editions and translations of Old English medical manuscripts appeared in print between 1864 and 1866 under the fanciful title he gave them. His main interest in them was philological; he thought their contents were useless in terms of medicine. Knowing who he was and what else he studied and published helps in understanding, perhaps forgiving, Cockayne's bias toward the system of healing he was turning into literary nonsense. He was a man with the best intentions—and outsized ambitions—inside a circle of famous nineteenth-century British scholars, such as Henry Sweet and W.W. Skeat. Cockayne never achieved the fame he craved and his life's story is the stuff of a bittersweet Victorian novel. The revision adds a great deal of new information about his life and aspirations, his publications, philological interests, and it includes the final report about the circumstances of his death.

Chapter 2 discusses several modern misconceptions about medieval medicine and magic that can be linked to the *Leechdoms*, which should be considered transformations more than translations. The transformations resulted from Cockayne's arcane style of language, his biased evaluations of the medical practice of early-medieval England, and his out-of-date and often prejudicial historical viewpoints. Modern translation theory and studies of nineteenth-century philology help explain how the biases of his time slipped into many aspects of his translations and the notes to them, resulting in the healing practices of early Europe being portrayed as ludicrous. For many years, these were the only translations of medieval medical texts that were readily available. The chapter touches on recent upheavals in the field of early-medieval English studies (earlier Anglo-Saxon studies), suggesting that the changes promise to affect in a very positive manner future research on the Old English medical texts.

The third chapter focuses on why/how the *Old English Herbarium* was created and how it might have been used. Appeals to the long-lived *curandero* tradition and to modern medical herbalism shape the approach this chapter takes in weighing how these texts might have figured in the practice of healing. The study takes the *Herbarium* out of its customary "Anglo-Saxon" context and situates it in the broader pool of European texts from which it derives, notably *Rezeptliteratur*. It is a herbal with several sources; it was created in a world within or affected by Benedictine monasteries in the West. Moreover here, it is discussed as an example of technical, not literary writing. As such, it requires knowledge appropriate to its subject matter to supplement existing historical and philological studies concerning its contents. The chapter briefly touches on whether its medieval remedies actually "work."

The fourth chapter provides details about the *Old English Herbarium*, including the manuscripts in which it is found, their dates, the existing and planned modern editions, and studies of the one illustrated manuscript in which the medicinal plants are depicted. Two other vernacular medical texts from the same period are mentioned, with a discussion of their dating and relationship to each other and to the *Herbarium*. Briefly discussed is who the users might have been and how the text figured into medical treatment and knowledge transmission. The chapter underscores the need for alternatives to Oswald Cockayne's nineteenth-century translation.

The final chapter is a modern English translation of the *Old English Herbarium*. Like the Old English original and unlike Cockayne's version, it uses plain English for what could be called a first-aid manual, a reference for a practicing medieval herbalist/healer who already was familiar with medicinal plants, and how to make medications, to diagnose and treat common conditions. It contains 185 medicinal plants, many of which are still used, brief notes about the conditions each one benefits, and equally brief instructions on preparing and administering them. This is a revised and corrected version of the translation found in the first edition, the major changes outlined in a section of notes preceding it. Original drawings mimic some of the plant and snake illustrations in one early manuscript containing the *Herbarium*, emphasizing the centrality of living plants to this healing tradition. The snakes are quick markers for treating any kinds of conditions caused by poisonous bites or beverages.

About the illustrations: Through the many centuries of the late classical and medieval periods, it was traditional for manuscript illustrators to base their renditions of plant, animal, and other figures on earlier works. We continue this ancient tradition here. With the facsimile edition of the *Old English Herbarium* by D'Aronco and Cameron on a drafting table beside him, artist Robby Poore (manager at UNC Creative, University of North Carolina-Chapel Hill) took up the challenge of making original drawings of 30 plants from the *Herbarium* and a representative snake and scorpion to accompany this translation. We hope the anonymous compilers and illustrators of yore will smile on our work.

1

OSWALD COCKAYNE

The scholar whose long shadow hangs over medieval medicine

In a listing of nineteenth-century British philologists by importance, somewhere toward the end, but certainly present, would be the Rev. Oswald Cockayne (1807–73). Cockayne was the first person to transcribe and translate all the major Old English medical manuscripts, and they appeared in three volumes between 1864 and 1866 titled *Leechdoms, Wortcunning, and Starcraft of Early England*.[1] This is now virtually the only work for which he is known.

His *Leechdoms* came out in the Rolls Series, a government enterprise established to preserve the earliest writings of Great Britain. Cockayne's subtitle outlines the contents: "A Collection of Documents, for the Most Part Never Before Printed, Illustrating the History of Science in this Country Before the Norman Conquest." These three volumes are unusual in the series because of their subject matter; nearly all others are histories or literary works.

Cockayne found Old English medical works in manuscripts from the period around 1000 CE, naming them the *Old English Herbarium* (a herbal featuring medicinal plants), *Medicina de Quadrupedibus* (medicines using animal parts), *Bald's Leechbook* (a physician's manual), and *Lacnunga* (remedies, charms, etc.).[2] Thanks to him, these important early-medieval texts on healing were rediscovered and their unique vocabulary added to the Old English dictionaries being compiled in the nineteenth century.[3] Knowing the details of his life, his profession, and the scholarly milieu to which he belonged is important to understanding, perhaps forgiving, the legacy he left behind in the history of medicine and pharmacy. That legacy included slipping the negative biases of his time into the words he chose for his translations and into his notes about the native healing practices of early Europe. He was a man with the best intentions—and outsized ambitions—inside a circle of more famous British scholars. Cockayne never achieved the fame he craved and his life is the stuff of a bittersweet Victorian novel.

DOI: 10.4324/9781003162285-1

A poor curate's son makes good

On January 20, 1809, the Rev. John Cockin, curate of St. John the Baptist Anglican Church, Keynsham, baptized his first child, Thomas Oswald. By 1825, he would baptize nine more of his own offspring and bury one.[4] A small town in Somerset between Bristol and Bath, Keynsham is described as being quite poor in the first quarter of the nineteenth century when Cockin was ministering to a dwindling flock.[5] In 1824, son Oswald won a scholarship to St. John's College, Cambridge, where he had a stellar career and earned a bachelor's degree in 1828. While at university, he changed the spelling of his last name to Cockayne, the reasons rumored to be a rift with the father.[6] As an adult, he seldom if ever used his first name and always signed himself "Oswald Cockayne."

Like many university men of the time, he turned to his church for a living. Attending seminary or divinity school prior to ordination in the Church of England was not a requirement then, only a university degree. Bishops would review the records and personal information of prospective clergy and then invest them, first as deacons, then priests, or higher. Cockayne was ordained a deacon and returned to Keynsham in 1833 as curate of his baptismal church. On October 10, 1834, he became a priest and four days later married Janetta, daughter of Roger Edwards, the town's surgeon.[7] On November 6 a year later, Cockayne baptized their daughter, Florence Louisa. By now, in addition to his church duties, he was also teaching and the family was living at Tucker's Academy. (It closed soon after he left it, and the property was auctioned in May 1837.[8])

Cockayne soon managed to rescue himself from his father's path as a poor curate in a poor town. In January 1837, he beat out 43 competitors for a position as assistant schoolmaster at King's College School in London, requiring him to leave Keynsham and begin teaching that spring. Janetta, Florence Louisa, and their infant daughter Alice Eden remained behind and lived with Janetta's father; in fact, the census of 1841 shows mother and daughters still in Keynsham.

Now part of the University of London, King's College has massive stone walls that enclose a cavernous basement area, now divided into a warren of subterranean hallways and rooms. King's College School, a junior school for boys, was housed here before it moved to Wimbledon in southwest London in May 1897. The Thames is to its south, the Strand to the north, and Strand Lane to the east. From the spring of 1837 until November 1869, Cockayne taught Latin and Greek here six days a week.

Sabine Baring-Gould (1834–1924), cleric, folklorist, and prolific author who attended the school for two years (1844–46) when Cockayne was there, wrote about his alma mater:

> A more depressing set of buildings could hardly have been contrived. The College and School form the east wing of Somerset House, and were built by Smirke in 1828, fossilized ugliness. We had to descend stone stairs and pass through an iron gate in which the gas was always burning. The windows,

however, did look out onto the hard paved play yard, surrounded by high stone walls, in which not a blade of grass showed, and not a leaf quivered in the air. The place exercised a depressing effect upon the spirits, and the boys in the playground appeared destitute of buoyancy of life, crushed by the sub-terranean nature of the school and the appalling ugliness of the buildings.[9]

In their history of the school, authors Frank Miles and Graeme Cranch say that pupils regularly broke out windows of neighboring houses and went wandering into the nearby theater district, which was infamous for its loose morals. In fact, one of the school's neighbors was a bordello, and the occupants could beckon when the 400 or so boys were on the school's playground. The area around the school was dimly lit, crowded, and noisy. Dickens was describing the London to which it belonged at this very time, and in fact his eldest son, Charley, went to King's College School for one term; he left because of a serious attack of scarlet fever.

Cockayne's first 20 years in London receive scant attention in his biographies, as do the publications from that time.[10] However, these were busy years: he was a prolific writer of books for the general public and scholar of Greek philology, all the while teaching. Beginning in 1847, he is to be found living at 11 Howland Street with his wife, daughters, and three boarders.[11]

He began to write books for popular consumption as early as 1838 when, newly arrived in London, he contacted the Society for Promoting Christian Knowledge (SPCK).[12] Begun in 1698 as a missionary arm of the Church of England, the society brought Christian education to the poor in England, founding schools and training teachers for that purpose. To further its ends, the society published books that met strict suitability criteria; they were inexpensive, widely available, and on a range of topics. Handwritten SPCK ledgers at Cambridge University Library first mention "… the Rev'd Mr Cockayne as a Gentleman well qualified to afford some assistance in the preparation or examination of works" on March 3, 1838.[13]

A nearly 15-year publication relationship ensued, one more slanted toward financial gain for the society than for the author. The society paid lump sums for works it published, then kept the copyright to them.[14] Cockayne earned on average about £20 per book, a nice addition to his salary from the school (des-pite the fact that the school strictly forbade its masters taking on any outside work, according to Miles and Cranch). Early on, he negotiated a contract for four classbooks; readers filled with instructive stories and poems from various named sources.[15] All four saw several revisions and reprintings, in years afterward. He was paid to prepare the changes, generally £15; revisions were an on-going responsi-bility for years.

During the 1840s and 1850s, he proposed several more books, some of whose fate, and even authorship, is hard to determine anywhere outside the often terse SPCK committee minutes. For example, Cockayne submitted the manuscript for a book named *Margaret Trevors* to the committee on December 20, 1839, and it was approved April 3, 1840 (SPCK.MS A15/3). The minutes show the book's being sent out for printing then for reprinting, but few copies are now to be found.

Curiously, the one archived copy I located lists Jane Alice Sargant as the author; however, no name appears on the title page, just as with *Short Stories from English History*, discussed below.[16] Equally odd and nowhere to be found is *The Widow Gray* of 1846 for which he was paid £2:2; see the Council Minutes for December 4, 1846 (SPCK.MS A15/3).

Previous biographies (mine in 2002 included) have failed to identify what was certainly one of his most widely sold and long-lived SPCK books: *Short Stories Founded on English History*, 1844 ff. The small book with its winsome etchings was often reprinted with various configurations of stories, but generally without an author's name.[17] Cambridge University Library holds several copies, and its catalog attributes it to Cockayne. I found "TO Cockayne" penciled inside the cover or on several of the title pages; however, in 2004 the library could not readily explain why the name had been added. Fortunately, SPCK committee minutes prove that Cockayne is indeed the author.[18] The ledger for February 20, 1846 (Cambridge A15/3) shows: "'Short Stories from English History' (forwarded by Rev'd O Cockayne). No. 1 to VI to be set up and sent round." On May 1, it was ordered for publication and on October 16, Cockayne submitted a second series of short stories for consideration. That too was approved on November 20 and a check for £20 signed over to him for it.[19]

Even absent the ledger entries, autobiographical details tie *Short Stories* emphatically to Cockayne. In a frame story, a beloved aunt relates stories about English history to a group of well-mannered children who live in Backwell, a town in Western England a few miles from his home town of Keynsham. They are Alice, Florence, George, and Edward, the names of Cockayne's daughters and two of his recently deceased brothers.[20] The aunt's name is Louisa, surely after Cockayne's own mother. The stories are unique among Cockayne's publications because of the personal family details they reveal and their conversational style. Whether his wife and/or daughters played some role in creating this work as well as the other short-story histories, so different from his other publications, is a possibility to consider.

In addition to the SPCK books and numerous scholarly papers he wrote for the *Philological Society*, Cockayne authored a number of books for the general public that could be generally characterized as educational histories. He wrote a *Civil History of the Jews*, printed in 1841, which became a best seller for several years. In many ways it is a lively travelog to the Holy Land, with a detailed account of Jewish history, tracing the Jews in their wanderings and enslavements to creating a nation, to their near-final destruction by the Romans between 133 and 136 CE. Cockayne describes Old Testament stories and places vividly, with firm faith that they happened as described and that the miracles in them can be explained and precisely dated. He provides a list of dates at the end of the book, beginning with the Creation in 4138 BC. He often cites Roman historian Josephus and a "Mr Clinton's Fasti," which were *Fasti Hellenici* and *Fasti Romani* by Henry Fynes Clinton; popular histories that appeared during Cockayne's lifetime. In addition, he wrote a *History of France* (1848; rev. ed. 1850), *History of Ireland for Families and Schools* (1851), and a

Life of Marshal Turenne (1853; repr. 1856, 1857). Raises were extremely rare at King's College School; schoolmasters depended on per-student stipends (capitation fees), taking in boarders, and the like, so the additional income from his publications may well have been essential to Cockayne and his family.

New interests, new directions, new aspirations

Perhaps weary of producing so many books for relatively little pay, during the 1850s his contributions to the SPCK gradually dwindled, finally ceased. The 1861 UK census shows Cockayne, his wife and daughters, as many as seven boarders, and servants living in a large townhouse at 17 Montague St., near Russell Square, around the corner from the British Museum and its well-known reading room.[21] However, by that year he was no longer attending meetings of the Philological Society, which he had joined soon after its founding in the early 1840s and which he had chaired several times.[22] From the outset, the society had fostered scholarly papers on classical philology and on newer comparative studies of language. For some 15 years, Cockayne had remained with the classical, as the titles of his papers demonstrate.

Yet as detailed below, Cockayne's post-1860 publications show that he had been extremely busy for quite some time with very different kinds of studies. This personal change in focus mirrors changes within the Philological Society itself, from a preference for classical subjects to greater enthusiasm for Germanic languages, older forms of English, and exploring new concepts of what constituted philology. Members of the society fit into a large, diverse group of scholars in England who were at this time shaping "… the new philology of the 'long' nineteenth century, spanning roughly 1775 to 1925."[23] Few of them were university professors, though most of them had masters degrees from Oxford or Cambridge, many like Cockayne were ordained, and they worked in a variety of professional fields.

New linguistic studies, in particular those coming out of Germany, had been suggesting that ancient Sanskrit underlay and linked not only Latin and Greek, but even Germanic and Slavic languages. With this came the realization that a vast number of languages throughout the world—and by implication their speakers— were ultimately related, raising fundamental cultural and religious issues. Many Western Colonial nations, England certainly a major one, held biases about local populations in their colonies, and it adversely influenced how they esteemed local languages and culture. To say the Westerners looked down upon native civilizations and history would be mild. This background is important to consider, because the new philology was part of a complex story fraught with implications for understanding the thinking of the time.[24] It was not restricted to philology.

In addition, biblical literalism prevailed in the Christian West and it hindered clear-eyed language study, particularly for clerical philologists like Cockayne. One major concern was ascertaining the language Adam spoke (the date of his creation had already been precisely determined), and then ascertaining how and when the Tower of Babel account fit into the new concept of language change. Such undertakings were also affected by undercurrents of racial bias in the West.[25] These were pre-Darwin years, when fossil finds and geological strata posed enormous intellectual challenges to biblical literalism, which the new philology tended to raise as well.

First publications on Germanic philology

Cockayne's publications show that by 1861, he had clearly abandoned classical pursuits and was engaged in the new philology. In that connection, he was mastering a generally unknown language he liked to call "Saxon English," which had evolved across former Celtic Britain beginning around 450 AD out of dialects spoken by invading Saxons, Angles, and Jutes. Separate studies were developing at this time in several European countries as well concerning the evolution of the various languages of Europe. Particularly in Germany and England, the studies prompted a small number of dedicated individuals (primarily men) to seek out and transcribe manuscripts written in this early form of English. Based on these manuscripts, they wrote grammar books and dictionaries for a language they named Saxon or Gothic English, and finally and most lasting, simply Anglo Saxon.

Cockayne was among those dedicated philologists and he was not alone in veering away from the classics and toward what he called the "harsher climes." Being at Cambridge in the 1830s, his long-term position in a school closely associated with language professors at King's College, and membership in the Philological Society since the early 1840s placed him personally close to major players in language and philology, as well as to those who would soon shape early-English studies.[26]

In 1861, Cockayne published two works whose contents were based on "skin books" as he called medieval manuscripts. *Narratiunculae Anglice Conscriptae: De Pergamenis Exscribebat Notis Illustrabat Eruditis Copiam* (London: JR Smith) is a collection of short pieces he transcribed from several Old English manuscripts, one of them on a medical topic.[27] That same year his second book appeared, titled *Spoon and Sparrow, ΣΠΕΝΔΕΙΝ AND ΨAP, FUNDERE and PASSER; or, English Roots in the Greek, Latin, and Hebrew*.[28] The book was obviously intended to be a major contribution to linguistics and philology, drawn as it was from numerous languages. It consists of 1,000 paragraphs filled with dense explanations for affinities and changes among languages rather than anything resembling a method. A typical exposition follows:

> Some instinctive tests exist by which to discriminate between borrowed words and true parallels. Thus compounds can hardly be accepted [as true parallels?] ... Afformative letters added to the visible root afford a strong ground of suspicion. Yet I would say 'instinctive tests' rather than rules, for it is not reasonable to suppose but that old roots had acquired some afformative letters while still some of the kindred nations were undivided from each other.
>
> *Spoon*, 7

One or two principles may seem here sometimes to be tacitly assumed without proof; one is, that in the same syllables, or more exactly, in varied forms of equivalents, that which retains the greater number of letters is the more ancient ...

Spoon, 8

Cockayne provides no footnotes, no explanation for the reasons behind his pronouncements, and makes no appeal to any authority but his own judgment. He makes significant use of a somewhat unique approach, which is to "plot" the position of sounds in a syllable. Phonetics provides much of the underlying argument, for which he uses unfamiliar linguistic terms such as "anlaut," "auslaut," "inlaut." No specific phonetic theory is quoted as the source of Cockayne's ideas, but there are parallels with phonetic practices from the late eighteenth century onward.[29]

He often cites words and phrases heard in spoken English that are not to be found in any dictionary, very likely here echoing R.C. Trench's emphasis on the study of words, not etymology or comparative grammar.[30] And this appears to be a major reason Cockayne chose to transcribe and translate Old English medical/herbal texts; in them he was finding vocabulary used in Saxon medicine, pharmacy, and botany. Quite correctly, he thought that many ancient "Gothic" words (i.e., language of the Goths) still remained undiscovered in the manuscripts:

How many must have been the words that Ælfric never heard, how many that he refused to admit when he did hear them, how many that did not present themselves while compiling a glossary. A small examination of unpublished manuscripts will soon convince any one who can read the language, that the admirable industry of Lye and Manning had not completed the whole task: nor has any one equal to the undertaking yet appeared[31] ... Modern lexicon makers are not to be named in the same page as the old heroes of this battle.

Spoon, 10

The modern "lexicon maker" to whom Cockayne refers was Joseph Bosworth, whose well-known *Anglo-Saxon Dictionary* had appeared in 1838. Like many philologists, Cockayne included, Bosworth was a biblical literalist, at one point stating: "The minute investigation of language is not only important in examining the mental powers, but in bearing its testimony to the truth of Revelation, and in tracing the origin and affinity of nations."[32] Bosworth explained that at Babel, the Lord confused the **pronunciation** of an original language so that people could not understand one another, an explanation Cockayne seems to have at least partially accepted.

Bosworth's *The Origin of the Germanic and Scandinavian Languages* (1836) uses numbered paragraphs, and it was surely no coincidence that Cockayne chose the same format for a book in which the "lexicon makers of old" are taken to task. Obviously, Cockayne expected his book to establish him as a recognized philologist, like Bosworth. Found in his exposition of Semitic in paragraph 975 is a particularly revealing statement:

> ... convinced also that I should best win the confidence of the reader by treating of well-known words and a few of them, I set myself to examine the numerals and some proper names of common occurrence. That I am surprised at the results would be a small thing to say; though they are imperfect and partial, *I trust that they will win the assent of all scholars in Europe: and if so, they cannot fail to lead on to an application of the ordinary principles of philology* in the case of the hebrew, and to bring it more or less within the reach of illustration from other tongues [emphasis added].
>
> *Spoon, 264–5*

Only two contemporary reviews have been found for *Spoon and Sparrow*; one cursory, the other more detailed. The longer one, in *Athenaeum*, says:

> There is much less of general principle and more of detail—indeed, it is almost wholly composed of detailed matters of fact, and may be described as rather containing the raw material of a satisfactory work than a finished production ... the volume has too much the air of being a transcription of brief notes from a commonplace-book.[33]

    Spoon and Sparrow is now available free through Google Books for all to read (as are almost all of Cockayne's writings). Anyone considering reading it might consider Olender's advice: "The best way to understand them [nineteenth century philologists] is no doubt to take them seriously, to succumb to their spell ... rather than to impose a logic alien to their time."[34] The work never sold well; for years he sold it from his home address, together with other lesser known self-published works. Sales ledgers in archives of the printer, Longman's Publishing Co. at Reading University, show that five copies were sold between 1864 and 1874, when his entire remainder was auctioned off for just under £2. It included his Greek Syntax, and some of his "histories," whose titles are not given but are surely those discussed above. Those "histories" sold regularly, were reprinted several times, and obviously added at least a modest amount to his income. (The SPCK volumes and these would have been separately handled.)

    Cockayne's *Spoon and Sparrow* now remains on a stack of similar tomes, forgotten or read purely as yet another representative of experimental nineteenth-century philology.[35] He was, however, years ahead of his time in rejecting the term Anglo Saxon (anglosaxon to him), calling it an "uncouth Latinism," which he only used because it had become so established; he preferred using "Saxon English." He often asserted that the earliest Germanic inhabitants of England called themselves and their language "Englisc":

> It is now the custom to talk of Anglo-Saxon, and the term Semi-Saxon has been invented, out of a love of technicality for English between the dates

1100 and 1230. Not only, however, was the ancient language English … the whole race of people, whether Angles, Saxons, Jutes, or Friesians, were, when spoken of as one, Angel-cynn, English-kin; and the whole country, wherein they dwelt, from the Grampians to Dover was called England. While on the mainland the name of the Saxons prevailed, it gave way in this island to that of the Angles …[36]

Sadly for Cockayne, the same year these two books came out, he suffered a major personal disappointment. Perhaps bolstered by his publications, Cockayne let his ego affect how he saw his own standing at the school. On June 14, 1861, he asked the Council of King's College to grant him an honorary title, Professor of Comparative Philology. The council turned him down, "… highly as they estimated Mr Cockayne's long and faithful service as one of the Masters at the School."[37] King's College faculty and King's College School faculty were not the same, but the Council oversaw both. Granting such honorific titles would not have been unusual to university faculty. The Council's blunt refusal could be interpreted both as putting Cockayne in his place as a schoolmaster and indirectly censuring him for breaking the school's strict rules prohibiting activities outside teaching.[38]

Attack on Bosworth, lion of Old English scholarship

Despite being turned down for a title he believed he deserved, and perhaps angry as well, in 1863, Cockayne sent a letter to Oxford demanding he be named joint or chief editor of a new *Anglo-Saxon Dictionary* Bosworth was then heading up. Cockayne wanted his name on its title page and expected to be well paid for his services. If Oxford did not meet his demands, he threatened to publish a pamphlet outlining its current editor's deficiencies in Old English. (Bosworth had been the Rawlinson Professor of Anglo-Saxon there since 1858.)[39] He even sent Bosworth a draft of the pamphlet. Cockayne received no reply and as a consequence, in 1864 "Dr. Bosworth and His Saxon Dictionary" appeared. It was in a series Cockayne self-published titled *The Shrine, A Collection of Papers on Dry Subjects.*[40] Eleven pages of bitter indictments unfolded, among them the bet that the new dictionary might include philology;

> … it is not comparative philology (filology) nor Bopp nor Pott nor an army of German fanatics in languages, that we want in a Saxon Dictionary.[41] We look for a work that shall reassure young students, that shall shew them their way in old English sentences, that shall convince them that our old tongue was grammatical and that its periods will bear the ordinary tests.
>
> *Shrine, 2*

C.B. Thurston, an Oxford associate, replied in a pamphlet titled "A Few Remarks in Defense of Dr. Bosworth."[42] In it, he said Bosworth heard a Mr. Cockayne was writing a pamphlet against the dictionary and they finally ascertained he was an under-master at King's College School, London, establishing Cockayne's lowly status vis-à-vis the Oxford Professor. Thurston said he used Bosworth's own notes to reply to each accusation, concluding "It is clear that … his [Cockayne's] Anglo-Saxon studies have not been close, nor minute, nor of long duration, not having commenced before 1855, and perhaps some years later." Thurston claimed the prevailing feature of Cockayne's attack was a depreciation of others and praise of himself.

Cockayne replied in *The Shrine*: "Postscript on Bosworth's Dictionary." "To some private representations, I reply, that in Dr. Bosworth's dictionary I see just the small merit that I admitted; it is no more trustworthy of footing than a Welsh bog." (*Shrine*, 1864, 27). Nothing further happened. Cockayne had taken on a lion of the establishment and did not even merit a personal reply.[43]

His famous pupils, W.W. Skeat and Henry Sweet

As teenagers in high school, well-known philologists Walter William Skeat (1835–1912) and Henry Sweet (1845–1912) were in Cockayne's classics classes at King's College School, separated in time by about ten years. Remarkably coincidental to their being in his classes was Cockayne's interest in early English manuscripts. Yet how much the schoolmaster influenced his pupils' future paths is not easy to establish.

Skeat was in Cockayne's fourth form in the early 1850s; later, in a book of reminiscences, he wrote:

> During part of the time when I was at King's College School, in the Strand, it was my singular fate to have for my class-master the Rev. Oswald Cockayne, well known to students as a careful and excellent Anglo-Saxon scholar, perhaps one of the best of his own date. He was an excellent and painstaking teacher, and it was, I believe, from him that I imbibed the notion of what is known as scholarship. In after life, it was my good fortune to know him personally, and I always experienced from him the greatest kindness and readiness to help. After his death, I acquired some of his books, including his well-known and useful work intitled *Anglo-Saxon Leechdoms*, and some of his carefully executed transcripts. His transcript of Ælfric's *Lives of the Saints*, in particular, has often proved useful.[44]

We know too from Skeat that Cockayne had been working on an Anglo-Saxon dictionary:

> At the time of his death, he had actually completed, on clearly written slips, the letters A to E [for a new Anglo-Saxon Dictionary,[45] because he was dissatisfied with Bosworth's]; and these came into my hands with the other papers.

Pastime, viii–ix

Here Skeat mentions that he passed along Cockayne's dictionary notes to Professor T. Northcote Toller to use in a supplement to Bosworth, which Skeat called "only a translation of Lye and Manning."

Most biographical sources list Harvard University as the major repository for Cockayne's literary remains.[46] Yet in 1999, while searching there for Cockayne's transcriptions of Old English medical manuscripts, I ascertained that the papers Skeat said had come into his hands were not included in the Harvard collection, nor was material for the *Leechdoms* to be found there. Much later I learned that in 2018, Professor M.J. Toswell had discovered several folders of what she suspected was Cockayne material while looking through boxes of Skeat's papers in the archives of King's College London (KCL). Toswell discusses the discovery in her paper "The Lost Women of Old English Studies."[47] After being Cockayne's student, Skeat remained a friend and colleague. It seems reasonable to think he approached Janetta Cockayne after her husband's death about acquiring some of his papers, and that is how they came into Skeat's hands. (Skeat's family donated a portrait of Cockayne to the UK National Portrait Gallery, where it can be viewed on-line.)

Toswell was investigating women in what she calls "Skeat's atelier," women who transcribed and in several instances translated early works for the famous scholar without receiving any pay or much credit. Recent work by Toswell and other feminist scholars is revealing that such unacknowledged women's help was quite common at the time.[48]

In her paper, Toswell notes that in addition to what were believed to be Cockayne's transcriptions, she found "a very neat hand … small, neat, and pointed—not Cockayne nor Skeat" (note 33). On reading this, I immediately suspected that the hand Toswell had spotted in those transcriptions belonged to Cockayne's wife and/or his daughters. The reason was that in 2004 I had found a ledger in the archives of the British Museum titled "Signature of Readers" showing Cockayne there on November 26 and 27, 1858.[49] His signature did not appear again until 1861, and that on November 20, but a librarian at the museum said that if a person were known to the library, it would not be unusual for them not to sign in. Among the reader's cards for that year was the name Alice Eden Cockayne on October 23, her father as sponsor. She renewed the card for several years more, joined in 1862 by sister Florence, and in 1864 by mother Janetta. In 1865, only Alice and her father had reader's cards and the name Cockayne does not reappear thereafter, but they could have continued to use the library. Cockayne's flurry of publications on Old and early Middle English coincides with the period when Alice, Florence, and Jannetta all had cards. If they helped him, he never openly acknowledged it.

Spurred by Toswell's findings, and with the long COVID epidemic subsiding, in April 2022 I verified in the archives of KCL that many of Cockayne's distinctive notebooks and other papers are indeed mixed in with Skeat's. Identical notebooks are in the collection at Harvard; 8×9 ½-in. ruled paper pages sewn in signatures, the covers made of cardboard covered in thin leather. Many of the notebooks are complete but missing covers; however, a number of the signatures exist as separate entities, unrelated to the materials with which they are stored. It is clear that transcriptions of Aelfric's *Lives of Saints* are prominent in Cockayne's notebooks, as Toswell points out.

Boxes at KCL marked Skeat 4 and 6, which Toswell specifically names in connection with the *Lives of Saints*, suggest in their style of notebook, hands, transcription style, and apparent numbering system in some notebooks that more Cockayne material may in fact be scattered throughout the entire Skeat archives. Transcriptions of manuscripts related to the *Leechdoms* were not found in the boxes I saw, save for one small piece of paper folded in four in box KCL Skeat 4/2/1, though other transcriptions of herbal material are present. Much of what I examined in boxes KCL Skeat 4 and 6 that can be securely identified as being Cockayne's are transcriptions of variety of works in Old and Middle English, in several hands but always in the distinctive notebooks, even more strongly bolstering the theory that Cockayne's womenfolk helped with his work.[50] Of particular interest is a transcript of the botanical folios (13–57) from British Library MS Sloane 5, an important Middle English herbal.[51]

The initials "OC" in his hand appear beside many transcriptions, as though they had been checked off for some reason, and several instructional asides can be found here and there; e.g., "Latin and Saxon letters are mixed, so take care." The Cockayne collection inside the Skeat collection awaits a careful sorting out and evaluation, with the potential to add important information to studies of both men, notably the remarkable number of as yet unacknowledged manuscripts that Cockayne chose to transcribe or have transcribed.

Skeat's acknowledgment that he found Cockayne's transcriptions of Aelfric's saints lives "useful" was tucked away in his 1896 memoir. Cockayne's notebooks in Skeat's archives are filled with transcriptions of Aelfric's lives of the saints, homilies, and notes about them as well, as Toswell points out. Yet only scant acknowledgement of using such notebooks appears in Skeat's 1881 two-volume edition of the work for the Early English Text Society (EETS).[52] Evidence points to Cockayne's having been at work on the saints' lives for quite some time; as early as 1864 he vigorously proposed several times and was repeatedly turned down to edit them for the Rolls Series.[53]

A decade younger than Skeat, Henry Sweet was in Cockayne's classes in 1862–63, having entered in 1860 and leaving in 1863 to study philology in Heidelberg.[54] It is interesting that both Cockayne and Sweet often voiced strong disagreement with philologists in Germany. Sweet's work on the *Student's Dictionary of Anglo-Saxon* is said to have begun during his teenage years (MacMahon, 167) and he was 18 years old when he left King's College School for Heidelberg.

Upon his return to England in 1868, Sweet enrolled at Oxford, where Bosworth was revising the Old English Dictionary. We know from Skeat that Cockayne was compiling his own entries for a new dictionary at that very time, obviously undeterred by Bosworth's earlier snub, or perhaps spurred on by it. Might Cockayne have heard that young Sweet was asked to work with Bosworth, as Momma suggests?[55]

In discussing Cockayne, historians Miles and Cranch said (without giving a source): "Sweet, who was an eccentric in many ways, always boasted that he was self-educated, but he clearly kept in touch with Cockayne in later years, and the two reviewed each other's philological books."[56] Whether they actually kept in touch is uncertain, but they did review a few of each other's works—unfavorably and over minutiae for the most part. Cockayne's less than stellar professional and scholarly reputation late in life may have played a role in Sweet's rejection of any notion that his old schoolmaster sparked his interest or helped him in any way with Old English.[57]

Much like Cockayne, Sweet argued against such theories as Grimm's laws of language change, saying:

> Grimm's law has been compared to a rolling wheel; it has been described as a primary and mysterious principle, like heat or electricity; but I am unable to see in it anything but an aggregation of purely physiological changes, not necessarily connected together.[58]

Sweet scholar MacMahon finds the strongest link between Cockayne and Sweet to be an interest in phonology. In *Spoon and Sparrow*, Cockayne "plots" the position of sounds in a syllable, and phonetics provides much of the underlying argument. Although no specific phonetic theory is quoted as the source of Cockayne's ideas, there are parallels to his in phonetic practices from the late eighteenth century onward.

In 1871, Sweet paid Cockayne at least one small compliment. In the Preface to his translation of the Old English *Pastoral Care* by King Alfred, Sweet wrote in a footnote that Cockayne was the only editor in England or abroad who "did not ignore the genuine West-Saxon manuscripts" in studying King Alfred's language, others preferring "garbled reflections."[59]

In 1872, Sweet wrote an unflattering review of Cockayne and Edmund Brock's *Liflade of St. Juliana*, saying,

> The translations are on the whole very accurate but some of the renderings require criticism … This style of translation not only makes the old language ridiculous, but also exercises an injurious influence on English scholarship, by deadening the modern reader's perception of the changes (often very delicate) of meaning which many old words preserved in the present English have undergone.[60]

Cockayne preferred a style in translating older works that he must have believed connected the reader more closely to the past. It involved using antiquated words and phrasing, and, to make it read even more oddly, Cockayne used what became customary for him, a preference for the Old English letters Þ and ð for "th" not only in his translations but also in modern English prose. A brief example follows from his translation of *Juliana*:

Juliana þe blessed, Jesus Christs leman, out of his blissful love, made herself bold and sent to him all openly by a messenger to say: þis word she sends þee; for nought hast þou toiled, be as wrað as þou may, do as þou wilt. [61]

Medicine and pharmacy, saints' lives, and herbs

Behind the scenes during this period, Cockayne was working on a massive project for the newly created Rolls Series. In 1858, Her Majesty's Stationary office had begun this series with the goal of publishing historical records from the earliest days of the country (understood as post-Roman England forward, beginning with the Germanic invasions). The entire project was lavishly funded at £3000 a year for ten years, the sum exclusively for editors' compensation; printing was covered separately. Editors were to be well paid for their efforts; eight guineas per sheet of 16 pages, the average volume to be about 500 pages. [62]

Cockayne's *Leechdoms, Wortcunning, and Starcraft of Early England: Being a collection of documents, for the most part never before printed, illustrating the history of science in this country before the Norman Conquest* (1864–66) are in three volumes that together make up volume 35. They contain transcriptions of a number of Old English manuscripts in a font mirroring the original script, his translations of them, numerous notes, and highly abbreviated citations of references he had consulted. In addition, he provided a long preface for each volume, each one his musings on a wide variety of topics.

The UK National Archives hold the ledgers of the Rolls Series and correspondence connected with it. They also have some of Cockayne's correspondence from 1862 to about 1869 with the Master of the Rolls and his Deputy Keeper, who were responsible for selecting works to be included in the series and paying the editors to ready them for publication. [63] Cockayne's original proposal to them for the *Leechdoms* suggests that he already had suitable material in hand by 1862 and was at work on it when he sent the proposal off. It was handwritten on three sheets of letter paper, sent from King's College London dated only February 1862, and began:

A proposal to Master of Rolls to publish some works in Saxon and half-Saxon English as follows:

1. The herbarium a collection of receipts for various ailments taken from Apuleius, the author of the Golden Ass. It has half more matter than the Latin "De virtutibus Herbarum" and is the foundation of the leechcraft of our cullers of simples and herbalists … it will be a valuable contribution towards a better knowledge of the genders of Saxon English substantives, many of which are scarce known, and an enlargement of the vocabulary of the dictionaries …
2. Medicine de Quadrupedibus … a continuation of the Herbarium, also in Saxon.
3. Liber Medicinalis also in Saxon in the King's Library, British Museum

PRO 37/25:8/28, page 123

Cockayne ended the proposal with a suggestion to include additional material if space allowed "to complete the view of Saxon science by adding some short treatises once printed in detached portions, usually known as 'de termporibus', 'de caelo' etc. In that case the volume might be entitled 'Illustrations of Saxon English science.'" An acceptance letter came quickly from Sir John Romilly, Master of the Rolls, dated February 14 that same year (PRO 31/13, pp. 123–5).

The major justification Cockayne gave for publishing the Saxon English works, which he would repeat in future proposals, was their value as witnesses to gradual language change (grammatical and phonetic) and their ability to add many words to the lexicon of early English. Such reasons help explain why Cockayne spent years working with texts he considered only the relics of leeches and cullers of simples. However, the generous anticipated payment may well have been another. Another hardbound Rolls Series ledger book (PRO 37/18) contains a handwritten summary of the payments made to him for each volume of the *Leechdoms*: £262.10 for volume one; £239.8 for volume two; £256.5 for volume 3, all of it paid out between 1863 and 1866.

Cockayne penned a preface that is 105 pages long for the first volume containing the *Old English Herbarium*. Including his translations and notes, it runs an additional 400 pages. In that preface, Cockayne warns readers about the Teutonic superstition and folly they will find: "It will be difficult for the kindliest temper to give a friendly welcome to the medical philosophy of Saxon days" (Cockayne 1965, 1:ix). He notes that Germanic tribes (he sometimes calls them Goths) were in awe of Rome, which might be true, but then he claims they were incapable of mastering much of what the superior civilization offered. He extends such prejudice to the corpus of early-medieval medical texts:

> Not only the Engle and Seaxe, the warrior inhabitants of our own island, but all the races of Gothic invaders, were too rude to learn much of Gallenos, or of Alexander of Tralles, though they would fain do so. The writings of Marcellus, called Empericus, the Herbarium of Apuleius, the stuff current under the name of Sextus Placitus, the copious volumes of Constantinus Africanus, the writings of St. Hildegard of Bingen, the collections out of Dioskorides, the smaller Saxon pieces, are all of one character, substituting for the case of instruments and Indian drugs, indigenous herbs, the worts of the fatherland, smearings, and wizard chants. Over the whole face of Europe … the next to hand remedy became the established remedy, and the searching incision of the practiced anatomist was replaced by a droning song.
>
> *Cockayne 1965, 1:xxvii*

The excerpt captures the spirit of the prefaces and translations that followed in the next two volumes, and the following chapters discuss his *Leechdoms* in detail, particularly the *Old English Herbarium*. Suffice it to say at this point that Cockayne's translations helped introduce a widespread negativity toward early-medieval healing practices that continued for many decades, even to the present. However, his work did add significant vocabulary to the Old English dictionaries being compiled then and provided many examples of philological changes in the old language. They did introduce the early English medical texts to the world, the earliest of their kind in any European vernacular.

As the final volume of *Leechdoms* neared publication, Cockayne sent a letter to the Rolls dated November 6, 1866 indicating that he clearly anticipated continuing what he believed to be a long-term commitment on both sides to publish Saxon remains. He began the letter:

> The last sheets of the third Saxon volume that I had the honour to edit under your Lordships [sic] direction are now passing through the press. I have now to submit to your Lordship an account of the materials that wait for continuing the publications of Saxon.

Cockayne outlined an impressive and nearly endless list; i.e., works issued by King Alfred, many still unedited; Handbook of Brihtferð, a work

> cognate to the volumes already edited by me; some lives, which would be of saints, from Ælfrics unedited Homilies and the Martyrology; Ælfric's abridgement of the Historical Books of the Old Testament; and some charters similar to those J.M. Kemble had edited.

Cockayne concluded the letter, "Awaiting your Lordships commands I have the honour to remain" and signed it (PRO 23/25).

Only the final "command" sent to Cockayne remains in the archives, and that a copy. Cockayne obviously had sent a series of proposals, justifications, and reductions in scope of works to be prepared, but they are missing. However, certain of his responses to the answers he received do remain. It appears that the Rolls had at first been polite, then firm, then emphatic that his association with them was over. At one point, Cockayne must have questioned the right of the Master of the Rolls to have the final say on what was to be included in the series, demanding to know his rationale for making choices. The reply, in an unsigned copy from Romilly reads in part:

> I should think there could be no doubt as to the meaning of my previous communication, to which I have nothing further to add. I must, therefore, with all courtesy, decline entering into any further explanation of my motives for not accepting the proposal you submitted to me for publishing Aelfric's Lives of Saints.
>
> *PRO 37/13, p. 353*

Cockayne would soon turn elsewhere to publish.

From the long list of titles in the complete Rolls Series, it is clear that the majority are accounts of various parts of English history written in Latin during periods that qualify as early; for a complete list see https://the-orb.arlima.net/rolls. html. Only two are in Saxon English; Cockayne's and the *Anglo-Saxon Chronicle*, edited by Benjamin Thorpe in 1861. And too, Scotland, Ireland, and Wales were not part of the original scope, but written summaries of their individual histories were reluctantly included because of political pressure, as a long document in the same section of the archives shows (PRO 37/73). Neither Old English literature in the original nor its language seems to have captivated the popular nor scholarly mid-nineteenth century world early on, when Cockayne and others became so enraptured by all things "anglosaxon." Classicism still had firm grip on most of education and taste.

Given that situation, to make Old and Middle English writings more widely known and available, a subscription series was begun in 1864, thus approximately at the same time as the Rolls, sponsored by the EETS: see https://users.ox.ac. uk/~eets/. But unlike the well-funded government sponsored Rolls, the EETS struggled even to meet printing costs, and editors worked because of their own fervor and for a modicum of recognition within their own small circle.

After repeated refusals from the Rolls after 1866 to accept three quite similar early English works, Cockayne turned to the EETS to publish *Seinte Marherete: The Meiden Ant Martyr* (1866), *Hali Meidenhad: An Alliterative Homily of the Thirteenth Century* (1866),[64] and *The Liflade of St. Juliana* (1872). All of them extol virginity and chastity as the highest forms of Christian life and were written by male clerics for cloistered nuns. They date to a period slightly later than the Old English medical texts. We know from the 1862 proposal to the Rolls that Cockayne was already interested in and working on two of them. In the 1866 EETS edition, he provides three chronologically different versions of the Margaret story, saying that "Having before us specimens of our language at different times, we shall do well to turn our attention to some of its changes" (74). At least for his interest in the Saint Margaret poem, it is possible to conclude it was primarily linguistic; Cockayne's remarks there on changes in Old English over several decades are interesting to read.

However, *Juliana* and *Maidenhood* are more than language studies, though Cockayne's stated reasons for studying them were such. They contain vivid depictions of delicate bodies being tortured, martyrdoms endured by the virgins while they remained steadfast in faith—they are torn apart and bloodied, beaten, boiled in cauldrons. "Holy Maidenhood" tells of another kind of torture, describing childbirth as being painful and filled with terror; sexual intercourse fares no better, nor the travail of enduring a husband's dominance. Cockayne explains: "þis treatise on þe high state of virginity contains so many coarse and repulsive passages, þat it was [initially] laid out for printing wiþout a modernized version." Anywhere a modernized version was deemed necessary, he tells readers that "the most objectionable portions have been Latinized" (v). (In translating Old English medical texts as well, Cockayne often substitutes Latin and does not translate the Old English original when women's bodies are involved.)

A not-too-comfortable juggling act unfolds as Cockayne translates the subject matter, which at times condones sexual intercourse in marriage but at the same time damns the act itself and praises virginity. In fact he feels it necessary to explain that it was written for nuns, not married couples,

> Hence it is plain þat to speak evil of þe marriage estate is no tenet of any large body of Christians, or of þe early church, and it editing þis work it was filling to declare a distance from such teaching.
>
> *Meidenhad, vi*

Certainly, Victorian prudery would not allow a frank treatment of sex or medical matters dealing with intimate topics. With a story similar to that in St. Margaret, *Juliana* was the last book Cockayne published.[65]

Yet at the time he died in Cornwall, he was almost certainly working on a book that has never before been attributed to him. In 1872, "*Jon the Gardener, &c, An Early-English Herb-Book*, ed. Rev. T.O. Cockayne" appears in a list of four books planned by the EETS for 1875.[66] It never appeared again in their lists and they never published it. Planned EETS publications listed in 1866 show "*Mayster Jon Gardener and other early pieces on Herbs, etc.* To be edited from the MSS by W. Aldis Wright, M.A."[67]

A clue that Wright's work on gardener Jon languished and Cockayne was asked to take it on turned up in 2022 among Cockayne's jumbled papers in Skeat's archives at KCL. It was in a small stack of miscellaneous letters and receipts on the backs of which Cockayne had scribbled notes, and was a letter dated September 26, 1871 from F.J. Furnivall, the editor of the EETS concerning a "treatise on the virtues of herbs which you have in hand for us," (KCL Skeat archive, box 4/3). Furnivall concludes the letter saying, "I hope we shall be able to make room for the herbal volume in 1873." Cockayne's death may have intervened, and Skeat may have passed on Cockayne's work to the person who finally published it.[68]

Twilight then darkness

Unfortunately, Cockayne's scholarly publications and his requests for recognition in the 1860s coincided with a difficult period at King's College School.[69] Though its reputation was always stellar, enrollment dropped in the 1860s, a new headmaster was hired, and what could be seen as legacy staff came under scrutiny. Cockayne was one.

Within ten years of embarking on early English studies, Cockayne was fired from the position he had held for decades. Although Miles and Cranch describe him as "a most distinguished scholar … and the leading philologist of his day," they also say he was "a highly idiosyncratic teacher," complaints having been lodged about him in 1864 and 1866. In November 1869, Cockayne was formally accused of talking to his class "unnecessarily of subjects which could only tend to corrupt them."[70] By then he had been an assistant master at the school for 27 years.

A Committee of Five, including the Headmaster, investigated. Notes in school archives reveal that several boys claimed Cockayne had made inappropriate remarks in class, and several parents had threatened to withdraw their sons if he remained their teacher. Cockayne was summoned before a sub-committee on November 15 and did not deny he had said much of what was alleged. In his defense, he said it was better to speak openly of such things so the boys would "have the evil effects of vice clearly set before them." Cockayne's frank reply to several accusations are revealing:

> That I had spoken of diseases coming upon fornicators, and had alleged that no exemption attaches to bad women riding in carriages. Reply: that we had Horatius before us, a free liver, a pig of the herd of Epicurus, with his Chloes and Lydias and Barines, a fresh name at every ode, giving an autobiography of his amours, it was desirable, speaking to lads mostly of fifteen, sixteen, and seventeen, to warn them that his sin is visibly punished by God. Especially that by a direct providential interference about the year 1500 A.D., God seeing men vicious in this respect, notwithstanding the teachings of religion, had sent a heavy plague to deter them.[71]

In their book about the school, Miles and Cranch describe the area around it as abounding in theaters and bordellos. It is not at all surprising that his teenage students had such topics on their minds, but convention demanded silence. Subsequently, a few of the accusations against Cockayne were withdrawn, but most were left standing. A final report was sent to the full committee; it voted to terminate Cockayne immediately, and he was summoned to appear before them in the deserted school late on Saturday, November 20 to hear the decision. The room where the committee usually met around a large wooden table is directly across the hall from the school's stately maroon and white chapel, and the scene that quiet afternoon can be imagined even today. Six mornings a week for most of his life, Cockayne had entered the chapel to worship with his students and colleagues. However, on this day, he walked down a deserted hallway into the committee room to be dismissed.

Cockayne may have earlier seen the handwriting on the wall because by November 20, his address had already changed to a London suburb at some distance from the school. In the self-published *Narrative*, which was already printed before the actual firing, he claims that one person ("a Delator") made the accusations against him, that he was never given a copy of the evidence against him, and that the boys mentioned had been in his class as much as five years earlier. He said that the Committee was embarrassed by the flimsiness of its own evidence, adding, "The chairman of the committee, with sarcastic generosity, offered me, not the evidence, but the report seasoned to his own taste, and said I might publish it in the 'Times'." He appended ten letters of sympathy and support from parents and former pupils. Obviously, Cockayne had sent them the "Narrative" to elicit support, but it was to no avail.

On the Monday after his dismissal, he sent two letters to school secretary J.W. Cunningham, both from 13 Manor Park, Lee. One suggests he must have been asked to leave immediately after being fired, without even collecting his personal belongings. He wrote, "The keys are in the school drawer and I will send up the key of the drawer tomorrow. Some articles of private property are in the drawer and cupboards and them I suppose I can have through the porter." The other reads, "The parents of my boarders shall have the news from me anon. The boys themselves would of course let them know if I failed to do so."[72] School records show that Cunningham's son had been straightaway promoted to Cockayne's now vacant position. Ironically, Richard Morris, the early-English scholar and philologist, was hired as First Form Master that same year.[73]

To make his life even sadder during these stressful months, Cockayne's elder daughter Florence was suffering from the effects of advanced breast cancer. Operations were unthinkable ordeals at the time since anesthesia was not always an option, moreover rampant sepsis was a constant danger in hospitals. Her condition must have been such that there was no alternative. On January 8, 1870, Florence had an operation in a large hospital on Harley Street and died of infection on the 10th. She was buried on the 24th in London's Norwood Cemetery.[74]

The home to which the Cockayne family had moved in Lee is large and it still stands on a rise inside a neat yard. The census of 1871 shows boarders living with them, suggesting a school of some kind. But few records can be found about their life now, outside his publications. What income Cockayne, wife Janetta, and daughter Alice lived on after November 1869 is unknown. He may have sold part of his personal library, and earnings from the Rolls Series may have been a factor. Glued into his copy of Benjamin Thorpe's 1842 *Codex Exoniensis: A Collection of Anglo-Saxon Poetry*, now at Harvard, at page 355 is a scrap of paper with note from Trübner and Co: American Continental and Oriental Literary Agency: 60 Paternoster Row, London dated May 10, 1872. It reads, "Mr Trübner presents his compliments to Mr Cockayne and will have much pleasure in looking at Mr Cockayne's collection any day next week. Mr Trübner will be in every day between 12 and 2 o'clock."

Another bit of evidence for Cockayne's strained circumstances is in a handwritten notebook at Harvard. On the back of hand-numbered page 330 is a torn sheet of printed blue paper from the North Western Railway of Montevideo Company, Limited, advertising that the company was putting in miles of railway in Uruguay and claiming that a decree of the government from December 12, 1870 "guarantees to the Company a certain amount of revenue for 40 years from the date of opening of each section of the Line."[75] At page 331 of the notebook is more blue paper, dated June 14, 1872 with an offer to invest, rewards guaranteed based on the success of a similar railway in Brazil. Whether Cockayne actually made an investment in the company is not known, but points to his at least having looked into it, perhaps as a way to try to find money on which to live.

Other than these few clues, for this time in Cockayne's life, MacMahon found

absolutely no reference to Cockayne in the philological literature of the 1870s. For whatever reason or reasons, he simply slid from view. Even Furnivall, that gregarious character of the Philological Society--and many others--seems to have overlooked him.[76]

If Cockayne's publications earned him little attention in his lifetime, sadly, his death was publicized in newspapers throughout England, Scotland, and Ireland.[77] His own family may well have learned of it through headlines. This is what happened.

Sometime in late May 1873, Cockayne left his wife and daughter either in Lee or more possibly while on a visit to Keynsham, saying he needed a short trip to Hastings for his health.[78] On June 18, an inquest began into the death of an unidentified man whose body had been found June 15 at Carrack Dew, a boulder-strewn area beside the ocean in the Parish of St. Ives in southwest Cornwall. The cause of death was determined then to be: "Killed by a pistol bullet through his head, but no evidence by whom such pistol was fired." On June 18, a headline in the *Cornish Telegraph* read, "Discovery of the Body of a Traveller who had Committed Suicide a Fortnight Since" followed by this story, which is quoted nearly in full:

> The greatest possible excitement was created in the town on Sunday afternoon by a report that the dead body of a man had been discovered by some children near the edge of cliffs, a little to the westward of Cardew, and which proved to be true ... A pistol was found in his breast-coat pocket, with which he had shot himself. The body was rapidly becoming decomposed by the fortnight's exposure, and appeared to be that of a man between 50 and 60 years of age ... on turning over the body, it was found that the man had been shot through the eye, from which worms were now crawling. The ball had passed out at the back of the head, and the body was quite black from being so long dead. The only articles found in the pockets of the deceased were a map of Cornwall, a lock of hair (of a light colour), a pistol in his coat pocket, and a powder and shot flask. The pistol had been fired off, the cap being split.
>
> There were also 6s 10 1/2d in money, and the wearing apparel consisted of an overcoat, a black coat, vest, striped trowsers, boots with cloth tops, drawers, and stockings. Deceased is supposed to be a man about 60 years of age. He had grey whiskers, and was about 6 feet high, but it is not yet known who he was. He arrived at the "Western" hotel, on Sunday fortnight, and left the hotel on the Monday afternoon, between 3 and 4 o'clock. After paying his bill he had 6s 10 1/2d in change. He said he was only going on the hills to see the sea. Deceased left a carpet-bag at the hotel, locked.

That same day, the Rev. John Balmer Jones of St. Andrew Church recorded he had buried "a male person found shot" in an unconsecrated portion of the St. Ives cemetery.[79]

The inquest continued through June 23. At some point before it concluded, a male relative came to St. Ives to look at the dead man's effects and, from them, conclusively identified the person as Cockayne. The *West Briton* of June 23 (see addendum) published the full inquest results, giving a wealth of detail about the deceased, such as his being tall, upright, and intelligent and wearing boots of a very peculiar make. The inquest reported he had asked a person he encountered about various herbs growing in the area and had oddly replied "from the moon" to being asked where he had come from. The account states, "*The jury, after deliberating, returned a verdict of 'Found dead, the cause of death being a pistol shot, but by whom fired unknown.'*" [italics added]

On Wednesday, June 25, 1873, the *Cornish Telegraph* elaborated on how Cockayne's identity had been established:

> On Friday the police officer at St. Ives received a telegram from a gentleman asking for information relative to the deceased's description. The reply induced the gentleman to visit St. Ives on Saturday, when he was enabled, without hesitation, to identify the deceased, from the description given and from his clothes – his body having been previously buried.
>
> … About a week before the fatal occurrence his relatives were shocked to receive a letter from him, bearing a Western postmark; and that stating that he should never return home again. Their suspicions and fears were at once aroused, and they instituted a searching but fruitless inquiry after him. Newspaper paragraphs, announcing the sad occurrence, arrested their attention, and induced them to extend their inquiries to St. Ives, which ultimately led to the discovery of deceased. … Deceased appears to have been of an eccentric disposition, and latterly shewed unmistakable signs of melancholy. Many years ago he was one of the masters of King's College School, London, and singularly enough the Rev. J.B. Jones, vicar of St. Ives, on whom devolved the duty of paying the last sad rites to deceased, was one of his pupils at King's College at that time. . . .

Cockayne had many reasons to be depressed in 1873, and suicide could have easily been the result. However, the official inquest ruled the death was from … *a pistol shot, by whom fired unknown*. Questions about Cockayne's alleged suicide linger, among them, why he went to St. Ives, a town he obviously did not know, why there with a map and travel schedules, and how he was able to shoot himself in the eye and return the gun to an inside pocket. It was the newspaper article that pronounced a verdict of suicide, not the official inquest, and the article set in concrete a verdict that has been passed on unquestioned ever since.

In the summer and fall of 1873 as the newspaper announcements of his demise appeared, silence was the reaction to them. No eulogies or public tributes to Cockayne have yet been found. Likewise, his grave in St. Ives cemetery cannot be easily located. With other nameless dead who lie in unmarked plots on a grassy slope, Cockayne shares a beautiful if somber eternal resting place. The coroner's office in Penzance does maintain an official map of cemetery plots that identifies those in them. And so, on a summer's day well over a century after his death, I laid flowers on his grass-covered plot to remember him at least for a moment in time.[80]

Eventually, Cockayne's wife and daughter Alice moved out of the large home in Lee and always remained living together. In 1881 the UK census lists them as teachers in Dovercourt, near Harwich. By 1891 they were living at Bromley College, a home for poor relatives of clergy in Bromley, Kent. Alice moved back to Keynsham after her mother died in 1894 and rented a room in the High Street home of a baker/confectioner named Wilkins. On March 27, 1897 she was found near death inside her locked, smoke-filled room. A physician who was called had to climb a ladder and force his way in through her window. He reported she had suffered a fit of some kind, fallen onto her fire grate, caught on fire, and was badly burned. She died about 15 minutes after he arrived. On March 29 a coroner ruled the death accidental, and Alice Cockayne was buried March 30 in the town where her father had baptized her 60 years earlier.[81]

Addenda

West Briton, June 23, 1873.

ST. IVES. SUICIDE AT ST IVES. The inquest relative to the death of a man found at Carhew Point, near St Ives, on Sunday last had been concluded after repeated adjournments. It will be remembered that deceased was discovered lying on the ground in an unfrequented spot, and on examination it was found that he had been shot through the head. A discharged pistol was also found in his left breast coat pocket. The evidence on the inquest went to shew that deceased arrived at Hodge's Western Hotel, St Ives, on Sunday, the 1st inst. He slept at the hotel that night, and the boots of the hotel, who gave evidence, was called to identify deceased by his boots, which were of a very peculiar make. Deceased was last seen alive on Monday evening, the 2nd inst, by Mr William Bennets. Deceased asked Mr Bennets several unimportant questions, such as the names of the various kinds of herbs growing in the locality; and Mr Bennetts described him as a tall, upright, intelligent gentleman. They parted near the village of Aya, deceased going down toward the cliffs. Mr Bennets saw deceased about half an hour afterwards in a field close to the place where he was discovered. It appears that deceased was observed by some boys on Sunday the 8th inst, but the boys, thinking he was asleep threw stones at him and ran away. In the deceased's carpet bag at the hotel were found a night shirt, night cap, pocket handkerchief, scissors, brushes and combs, a lock of hair, and a pair of black kid gloves. He appears to have taken great pains to prevent identification, for the handkerchief and his carpet-bag had each a piece cut out of it (probably where the name was), and the name was also cut out of the high hat he wore.

Having stated at the hotel that his luggage was at St Ives road station, the inquest was adjourned to ascertain if it was correct, and if so, to examine the luggage. The adjourned inquest was held on Friday afternoon. A young man named Monk stated that he had a long conversation with deceased on the

2nd instant. Deceased appeared to talk very rationally for some time, and enquired about the nature of the different kinds of herbs growing in the locality. Witness asked him where he came from, and he replied, with a laugh, "From the moon." Mrs. Hodge, the landlady of the hotel, also spoke as to the deceased's manner, and described him as being gentlemanly and showing no signs of insanity. The jury, after deliberating, returned a verdict of "Found dead, the cause of death being a pistol shot, but by whom fired unknown." Since the inquest the deceased has been identified as a clergyman--the Rev. Thomas Oswald Cockayne, formerly curate of Keynsham, and subsequently head master of King's College, London. He was the author of several learned treatises. He left his home, near Bristol, a few days before his suicide, with the intention of going to Hastings for the benefit of his health.

Shepton Mallet Journal. April 2, 1897, Friday

KEYNSHAM An elderly maiden lady, Miss Alice Cockayne, who had been lodging at Mr. Wilkins's, confectioner, was burnt to death on Saturday. Just before seven the servant thought she heard moans as she was passing Miss Cockayne's door. A ladder was procured and Dr. Harrison, who happened to be passing the time, went up and looked through the window, and saw the room was full of smoke. Upon smashing the window and getting into the room, he found the lady with her head on the fire grate, where she had fallen, supposedly, in fit. The police were once sent for, and the coroner has been communicated with. The deceased lady is daughter of the Rev. Mr. Cockayne, former curate of Keynsham.—On Monday evening the coroner for North Somerset (Mr. S. Craddock) held inquest at Keynsham on the body Alice Eden Cockayne, aged 60 years, who died Saturday. Allen Sanger, servant, said that on Saturday morning, about nine o'clock, she took some breakfast up to the deceased, who was lying in bed, and in her usual condition, and about quarter of hour afterwards witness went again, and noticed nothing unusual. But about eleven o'clock, hearing some groans, she called Mrs. Wilkin's attention. They found deceased's bedroom door locked, and they called to Dr. Harrison, who was passing at the time, and he procured a ladder, smashed a window, and got into the room. Charles Harrison, surgeon, of Keynsham, said that on entering the bedroom, be found the deceased lying on the floor, with her head in the fire. She was burnt very badly, and she died about a quarter of hour afterwards. It appeared that the woman had had fit, and had fallen into the fire.

N.B. Wilkins was a baker and confectioner on Keynsham High Street.

Inquest March 29, Monday, rules accidental death. She is buried the following day.

Notes

1 Rev. Oswald Cockayne, ed., *Leechdoms, Wortcunning, and Starcraft of Early England: Being a Collection of Documents for the Most Part Never Before Printed, Illustrating the History of Science in this Country Before the Norman Conquest*, Rolls Series, 3 vols, Vol. 35 (London: Her

Majesty's Stationery Office, 1864–66). Reprint (London: Kraus Reprint Ltd., 1965), cited as Cockayne 1965. British historian of medicine and science, Dr. Charles Singer (1876–1960) removed Cockayne's prefaces, substituted his own and reprinted the volumes under the same title and author as the original (London: The Holland Press, reprint 1961); cited in text as Cockayne 1961. Cockayne never used his given name, Thomas, preferring only Oswald, his middle name, often abbreviated simply as O.

2 The major medical works in Cockayne's Rolls Series volumes have recently been re-edited and re-translated as *The Old English Herbal, Lacnunga, and Other Texts*, ed. and transl. by John D. Niles and Maria A. D'Aronco, as volume one for Harvard University's Dumbarton Oaks Medieval Library (Anglo-Saxon Medicine). Planned for the future is the *Leechbook of Bald*, ed. and transl. by Debby Banham and Christine Voth as volume 2.

3 Because of recent developments in the field of Anglo-Saxon studies, in this revised edition, wherever possible the term "Anglo-Saxon" has been replaced by an alternative, such as early-medieval English, pre-Norman, Old English. The issue is discussed at the very beginning of chapter two.

4 Keynsham Historical Society Website (keysalthistory.org.uk); his birth may have been late 1808; only his early 1809 baptismal record survives. This revised chapter adds substantial new information about Cockayne aided by Professor Mike MacMahon, whose collaboration is gratefully acknowledged. It augments the 2004 *Oxford Dictionary of National Biography* T.O. Cockayne entry by Daniel Kenneally, which is based on his unpublished 1999 MA thesis titled "Thomas Oswald Cockayne," King's College London; and it uses information in Daniel Kenneally and Jane Roberts, "Oswald Cockayne," *Poetica*, Vol. 86 (2016): 107–37. The article contains new research by Roberts as well as her insightful evaluation of Cockayne's publications and skills as a philologist. Kenneally's thesis can be consulted at the London archives of King's College.

5 Elizabeth White, ed., *Keynsham and Saltford: Life and Work in Times Past 1539-1945* (Keynsham and Saltford Local Historical Society, 1990). John Cockin was curate from 1809 to about 1825, when he and the family moved away. I am grateful to Mrs. White for her unflagging help with research on Cockayne, his family, and Keynsham generally.

6 Mrs. White provided this detail. See Kenneally and Roberts pages 1–2 for his many honors. Cockayne earned his MA in 1835 also from Cambridge, gained by applying for it soon after graduating and providing letters of recommendation. Records at St. John's College Cambridge show he studied Greek, Latin, and Hebrew, all of which figured into his later writings on philology. Old English was not yet part of any customary university program in England at that time.

7 Roger Edwards (d. 1855) was probably a general practitioner/apothecary-surgeon, not a university-trained surgeon; no records are found of him from a university or medical school. For "surgeons" of the period, especially in the provinces, see J.F. Kett, "Provincial Medical Practice in England 1730-1815," *Journal of the History of Medicine and Allied Sciences*, Vol. 19, No 1 (January 1964): 17–29.

8 *Bath Chronicle and Weekly Gazette*, May 4, 1837.

> To be sold (in fee) by auction on May 18 ... Large dwelling house together with orchards, garden, and excellent close of pasture land adjoining ... lately occupied by the Rev TO Cockayne. The house large and commodious, comprising dining, drawing, and breakfast rooms; a room lately used as a school room, seven bed rooms ... besides dressing rooms and attics; kitchen, back kitchen, wash house etc.; coach house and stable and a cottage detached.

9 Quoted in Frank Miles and Graeme Cranch, *King's College School: The First 150 Years* (London: King's College School, 1979): 19–20. Cockayne's starting salary was £150 a year, much later £242, with no pension, according to Frank Miles in a letter to MacMahon, April 15, 1977. The description of the school is Van Arsdall's based on a visit in 2010.

10 Kenneally's unpublished MA thesis and the Kenneally-Roberts paper outline Cockayne's several publications on classical Greek language and literature, in particular the many papers he delivered and wrote for the Philological Society between 1843, when he joined it, and the late 1850s, when he left it.

11 UK census for 1851. On May 13, 1847, Cockayne wrote to King's College Council: "In compliance with what I understand to be your regulations, I have the honour of requesting your sanction to my opening a house for the reception of boarders." King's College London (KCL) archives KA/1C/C 31.

12 The SPCK gave its archives and library to Cambridge University Library (CUL) in 1998, marking the society's 300th anniversary. CUL Manuscripts Department holds the largely hand-written archives; the older books are in Rare Books. For more information about this collection, see (www.lib.cam.ac.uk/collections/departments/rare-books/collections/society-promoting-christian-knowledge-spck).

13 Minutes of the Committee of General Literature and Education, Cambridge, CUL, SPCK/MS A15/2. Committee records are under SPCK.MS.A15, beginning A15/1 continuing /2 onward in chronological order in ten-year segments.

14 Committee report of June 10, 1835, "… it is not the plan of the Committee to allow to authors any reserved copyright in the publications which they undertake" (CUL, SPCK/MS A15/2).

15 His first contract was finalized June 24, 1838: "First Book by the Rev'd O Cockayne … that £10 be paid to the author for the copyright and that it be laid into type by Mr J.W. Parker. The price to be fixed afterwards." (Parker was the SPCK's usual printer for many years.) The second was approved on October 6. He received the same for each of the four books, worth about a month's salary at the school (CUL, SPCK/MS A15/2).

16 The minutes read: May 28, 1840. Margaret Trevors. Agreed, that £5:5 be sent to the Rev O Cockayne for the author of this work. June 5, 1840. Read a letter from the Rev O Cockayne thanking the Committee for the sum of £5:5:0 for the MS of Margaret Trevors. The connection between Cockayne and Sargant, the author of several SPCK books, is as yet unknown. *Margaret Trevors* is listed in the catalog of London's Hackney Archives (https://hackney.gov.uk/archives-collections) with Sargant as the author. I am grateful to its staff for information about the book and for making and sending electronic images of some of its contents.

17 In fact, I have yet to find a copy with his name printed in it as the author; the same situation as with *Margaret Trevors*.

18 I am grateful to the US National Endowment for the Humanities for a fellowship in 2004 to attend its summer seminar on Anglo-Saxon England which enabled research at Cambridge University, the British Museum, Oxford libraries, and, indirectly, for a visit to Keynsham and Cornwall. It was a summer of Cockayne. Professor M.K.C. MacMahon contributed research help from Glasgow, particularly dealing with Henry Sweet, from then to the present. I acknowledge and am grateful for his assistance, but take responsibility for any errors once the information provided was put in final form.

19 The Committee minutes show that Cockayne was paid anywhere from £15 to £20 per book; he negotiated several iterations of the Short Stories series in the late 1840s and early 1850s, one for France and possibly one for Spain. Other of his SPCK volumes also sold well; *Outlines of the History of France* (1846), *Outlines of the History of Ireland* (1851).

For Longman's Travellers' Library, he wrote *The Life of Marshal Turenne* (1853), which sold well, but no records have been located to find what he earned for his efforts.

20 George Alfred Cockayne (b. 1819–40); Edward Cockayne (1813–35); on-line baptismal records of St. John the Baptist Anglican church in Keynsham; on-line records of burials of St. Bartholomew's church in Sydenham.

21 The house number is listed at times as 16, then, 17; several of the stately townhomes with these numbers in 2022 were part of a fashionable hotel named The Montague on the Gardens. Indeed, a large garden still exists behind what were townhomes.

22 A complete set of the prestigious society's minutes is at Cambridge University Library; titled "Proceedings of the Philological Society" to 1854, "Transactions of the …" thereafter. I searched vols. 1–21, from its founding in 1842 to 1874. Cockayne presented a paper in 1842 and was elected to membership June 9, 1843 (vol 1); was chair from 1851 to 1854 (vols 3–7); is listed as a member up to 1861 (vol 13). No list of members is in the society's "Transactions" for 1862–63 (vol 14) and in the following volume Cockayne is not there. In fact, he never again appears as a member.

23 Haruko Momma, *From Philology to English Studies: Language and Culture in the Nineteenth Century* (Cambridge: Cambridge University Press, 2012): xiii–xiv.

24 Momma addresses these cultural issues thoroughly. Hans Aarsleff, *The Study of Language in England, 1780-1860* (Princeton: Princeton University Press, 1967) covers the period directly preceding as well as the period when new philology was being created, focusing in detail on philology rather than the larger issues.

25 For a thought-provoking overview, see Maurice Olender, *The Languages of Paradise: Race, Religion, and Philology in the Nineteenth Century* (Cambridge: Harvard University Press, 2008).

26 Influential and popular Richard Chenevix Trench (1807–86) was one of them; see Aarlseff and Momma for detail on the controversies and on Trench himself. Roberts suggests it was Trench's lectures on language given to the students at King's College School in 1854 that kindled Cockayne's interest in English philology; see Kenneally-Roberts, 10. The Philological Society too was at the center of the new philology, and Cockayne was by no means alone in catching the Old English fever.

27 The preface and notes are in Latin as are the titles Cockayne gives them, but the transcriptions are in Old and early Middle English. They are *Epistola Alexandri ad Aristotelem, De Rebus in Oriente Mirabilis, Passio Sanctae Margaretae Virginis, De Generatione Hominem Excerptum, Mambres Magicus*. For the rest of his life, he was known for his careful and accurate transcriptions.

28 O. Cockayne, *Spoon and Sparrow, ΣΠΕΝΔΕΙΝ AND ΨAP, FUNDERE AND PASSER; or, English Roots in the Greek, Latin, and Hebrew: Being a Consideration of the Affinities of the Old English, Anglo-Saxon, or Teutonic Portion of Our Tongue to the Latin and Greek; with a Few Pages on the Relation of the Hebrew to the European Languages* (London: Parker, Son, and Bourn, 1861).

29 MacMahon provided insight into Cockayne's aims and methods in philology.

30 See Aarsleff, 241–59. Cockayne is not mentioned in any of the nineteenth-century studies cited in this section.

31 Ælfric was an English abbot around the year 1000 and a prolific writer in both Latin and Old English. Edward Lye (1694–1767) did not live to see the publication of his *Dictionarium saxonico et gothico-latinum*, which was edited and published with his memoirs in 1772 by Owing Manning (1721–1801). It was a standard authority in the nineteenth-century, often referred to simply as Lye and Manning. Note the use of "Gothic" for Germanic.

32 The Rev. J. Bosworth, *The Origin of the Germanic and Scandinavian Languages and Nations: With a Sketch of Their Literature, and Short Chronological Specimens of the Anglo-Saxon, Friesic, Flemish, Dutch, the German from the Meso-Goths to the Present Time, the Icelandic, Danish, Norwegian, and Swedish: Tracing the Progress of These Languages and Their Connection with the Anglo-Saxon and the Present English* (London: Longman, Rees, Orme, Brown, and Green, 1836): 2.

33 Anonymous review in *The Athenaeum*, No 1782 (December 21, 1861): 840–1. Page 599 of *The Westminster and Foreign Quarterly Review* of April 1, 1862 has more a notice than a review of the book, omitting the lengthy subtitle after *Spoon and Sparrow*.

34 Olender, 16.

35 Kenneally and Roberts, 10–12 present an alternative understanding/evaluation of *Spoon and Sparrow* and of Cockayne as a philologist.

36 Oswald Cockayne, *Seinte Marherete the Meiden Ant Martyr*, EETS (London: Trübner, 1866): 75. The author's dislike of the term Anglo-Saxon grows as time passes and can be traced in the introductions and notes to several works. He uses "anglosaxon" in *Spoon and Sparrow* without comment, then turns against it very soon.

37 KCL Archives, KA/C5/M2. Council Minutes, May 1861–November 1865, June 14, 1861, Friday, Letter from the Rev T.O. Cockayne, and the council's response. Also, Kenneally thesis, 10–11; Van Arsdall, 2002, 6. Because of space concerns in the second edition, some details about Cockayne had to be cut to make way for newer information; see the first edition for more material. A future biography could present everything.

38 Undeterred it seems, in a letter to the Council on June 23, 1865, Cockayne asked permission to accept the Professorship of Saxon at University College "should such an appointment be offered to him." Again, the Council refused. Such professorships were largely honorary; language study outside the classics came late to universities in England.

39 For Bosworth, see Dabney A. Bankert, *Joseph Bosworth and the Making of His Old English Dictionary, 1820-1921*. University of Toronto: Pontifical Institute of Medieval Studies, Publications of the Dictionary of Old English, 2022.

40 *The Shrine: A Collection of Occasional Papers on Dry Subjects*, a series of 13 pamphlets Cockayne wrote, published, and sold by subscription or appeared individually sporadically between 1864 and 1871. For the most part it contains his transcriptions of miscellaneous Old English manuscripts. See Kenneally and Roberts, 17–18 for more detail about this publication.

41 The "German fanatics" to whom Cockayne refers were Franz Bopp (1791–1867) and August Friedrich Pott (1802–87). See Aarsleff for a complete account of the controversies at this time in the field of philology and discussion of the major personalities. It should be noted that Cockayne is not mentioned in either Aarsleff or Momma.

42 C.B. Thurston, *A Few Remarks in Defense of Dr. Bosworth and His Anglo-Saxon Dictionaries* (London: Macmillan and Co., 1864). The pamphlet is nearly 20 pages long. J.J.R. Tolkien quoted from Cockayne's attack on Bosworth to begin his landmark 1936 lecture on "*Beowulf: The Monsters and the Critics*," calling the attack unfair. See *The Monsters and the Critics and Other Essays*, ed. C. Tolkien (London: George Allen & Unwin, 1983): 5.

43 While in the silent gloom of the stacks at Oxford University in 2004, I came across a newspaper clipping with Cockayne's 1873 obituary glued without comment into the front cover of Bosworth's copy of the *Leechdoms*.

44 Rev. Walter W. Skeat, *A Student's Pastime: Being a Select Series of Articles Reprinted from "Notes and Queries"* (Oxford: Clarendon Press, 1896): viii.

45 Cockayne advertised his dictionary as well as an Anglo-Saxon Grammar, both as forthcoming, on the last page of the final issue of *The Shrine* in 1871.

46 In 1878, only a few years after Cockayne's death, the American book collector William Medlicott already owned most of Cockayne's personal library and some of his hand-written notebooks. When Medlicott offered his extensive library for sale that year, Harvard purchased most of the Cockayne material, and it remains in the Houghton and Widener libraries. See J.R. Hall, "William G. Medlicott (1816–83): An American Book Collector and His Collection," *Harvard Library Bulletin*, Vol. 1, No. 1 (Spring 1990): 13–46.

47 Paper presented at the Oxford Medieval Seminar October 21, 2020. I am extremely grateful to Professor Jane Roberts for putting Professor Toswell in touch with me after she heard the paper, and to its author for sharing a copy with me, giving me permission to quote from it.

48 See Jane Chance, ed., *Women Medievalists and the Academy* (Madison: University of Wisconsin Press, 2005).

49 I found the ledger at the British Museum in 2004, two years after the first edition of this book was published. Alice renewed her card May 7, 1862; January 9, and September 22, 1863; May 5 and November 23, 1864; May 26, 1865. Florence Louisa obtained a card January 23, renewed October 7, 1862; renewed November 12, 1863; renewed July 25, 1864. Mrs. Janetta Cockayne obtained a card January 22, 1864, renewed September 27 of that year.

50 A thorough search through the Skeat collection at King's College London and Cockayne collection at Harvard could produce a detailed list of all the manuscripts Cockayne transcribed or had transcribed; his little known work, the *Shrine* gives a clue as to the large number involved. However, the focus of my study has been on manuscripts relevant to the *Leechdoms*. Obviously, along the way, the life of Cockayne began to exert a spellbinding curiosity over me.

51 Facing a publication deadline, I am able only to note at this point that this herbal does not appear to have been much studied to date, the exception being a first critical edition by David Moreno Olalla, *Lelamour Herbal (MS Sloane 5, ff 13r-57r): An Annotated Critical Edition* (Pieterlen: Peter Lang Verlag, 2018). In an e-mail to me in May 2022, Olalla said he was unaware of Cockayne's transcription when preparing his edition. It was indeed well hidden, and other of Cockayne's transcriptions might well be hiding with it in the Skeat folders at King's College London.

52 Preface to volume 2 of W.W. Skeat, *Aelfric's Lives of Saints*, Early English Text Society, Original Series (London: Trübner, 1881). There, Skeat does give Cockayne credit for being one of the first to correctly identify the author of the saints' lives as Aelfric **of Eynsham.** The identification had appeared in Cockayne's preface to volume three of his *Leechdoms*, an unlikely place to look for information on the Old English churchman and author. (A matter of debate at one time was the correct identification of the author of these saints' lives, as there were several Old English contenders named Aelfric.)

53 Letters in The National Archives records, Public Records Office (PRO) PRO 523 and 525. I am extremely grateful to Frances Watkins, PhD, member of the Herbal History Research Network, for visiting these archives for me several times early in 2022 during COVID restrictions. She examined the handwritten ledgers and letters pertaining to Cockayne, and provided the information in them to me; I vouch for their completeness and take responsibility for any errors.

54 M.K.C. MacMahon, biography of Henry Sweet in Helen Damico, ed., *Medieval Scholarship: Biographical Studies on the Formation of a Discipline* (New York: Garland Press, 1998).

55 Haruko Momma, "Old English as a Living Language: Henry Sweet and an English School of Philology," Paper presented at the International Society of Anglo-Saxonists, Palermo, Italy, 1997, 2.

56 Miles and Cranch, 28.

57 Remarks on Cockayne's relationship with Sweet are based on communications with MacMahon that span several years. We often speculated about the personal interactions Cockayne and Sweet may have had while Sweet was a student in his class and in later years, but have never come to any conclusions.

58 Henry Sweet, "The History of the TH in English" (1869) in H.C. Wyld, *Collected Papers of Henry Sweet* (Oxford: Clarendon Press, 1913): 176. (First printed in the *Transactions of the Philological Society* 1868–69: 272–88.)

59 Henry Sweet, *King Alfred's West Saxon Version of Gregory's Pastoral Care* (1871; London: Kegan Paul, Trench, Trübner & Co., Ltd., reprinted 1930): v.

60 Henry Sweet, review of *Liflade of St Juliana*, *Academy* III, 52 (July 15, 1872): 278. In 1871, in the Preface to the *Pastoral Care* (x), Sweet was careful to point out that in his own translation he "carefully avoided that heterogeneous mixture of Chaucer, Dickens, and Broad Scotch, which is affected by so many translators from the Northern languages."

61 Rev. O. Cockayne and Edmund Brock. *Þe Liflade of St Juliana, from Two Old English Manuscripts of 1230 AD with Renderings into Modern English* (London: EETS by Trübner & Co., 1872): 9.

62 See "The Rolls Series" in David Knowles, *Great Historical Enterprises* (New York: Nelson, 1962) for an extensive account of the entire series. One guinea equals one pound one shilling, or 21 shillings ($£1.05$). All the records of the series are at The National Archives (UK) formerly named the Public Records Office.

63 They can be found in The National Archives records, Public Records Office (PRO) 37/25 (proposal for *Leechdoms*); 37/17–18 (payments for *Leechdoms*); 37/13.

64 Oswald Cockayne, M.A., *Seinte Marherete: The Meiden ant Martyr* (London: EETS, Trübner & Co., 1866); *Hali Meidenhad, An Alliterative Homily of the Thirteenth Century* (London: EETS, Trübner & Co., 1866). They are known as the Katherine Group of works in early Middle English. See Bella Millett, "The Saints' Lives of the Katherine Group and the Alliterative Tradition," *Journal of English and Germanic Philology*, Vol. 87, No 1 (January 1988): 16–34.

65 His final publication was a short article in *Notes and Queries* No. 281 (May 17, 1873): 397–8 about where King Oswald of Northumbria died (a matter of some discussion in that area). It is available on-line in *Transactions of the Shropshire Archaeological and Natural History Society* (Shrewsbury 1897).

66 It appears in the volume with his *Juliana* in 1872. Lists of current and planned publications, costs, and news about the EETS were generally printed at the end of every book and often ran to several pages. Some modern libraries have bound their copies without these lists; an omission borrowers may discover to their dismay.

67 Wright (1831–1914), also a Cambridge man, published many early English literary texts, in particular Shakespeare, for use at universities in a Clarendon Press series and was a regular contributor to the EETS. Wright worked for several years on a very long romance named *Generydes* (ca. 1440), which appeared in three volumes during in late 1860s–70s, possibly the reason he left off work on the gardening tract.

68 Jon's practical handbook from ca. 1440 was finally published in 1894 in *Archaeologia* as "A Fifteenth Century Treatise on Gardening. By 'Mayster Ion Gardener,'" with remarks by the Honorable Alicia M. Tyssen Amherst. Baroness Amherst there acknowledges Skeat's help (159–60). Among the papers from Cockayne that Skeat acquired may well have been his work on this handbook for the EETS, and Skeat may well have given them to the baroness. The short work is fully covered in a more recent "The First English Garden Book: Mayster Jon Gardener's Treatise and its Background" by John. H. Harvey

in *Garden History*, Vol. 13, No. 2. (1985): 83–101). Whether Sloane 5 and the Lelamour herbal figures into this story too is also a possibility (see note 51 above).

69 See Miles and Cranch for full details about the school's history while he taught there. Salaries were adjusted, many changes were made, and several older staff left or were let go. Also see Van Arsdall 2002, chapter one, and Kenneally and Roberts.

70 Miles and Cranch, 66.

71 Quotation is on page 3 of a slender pamphlet Cockayne seems to have produced as the hearing was taking place. It is titled "Mr. Cockayne's Narrative" and quotes are from a photocopy made in KCL archives, ref. IC/68. For more on the firing, see Miles and Cranch, 65–7; Van Arsdall 2002, 18–20; Kenneally, 18–26; Kenneally and Roberts, 5–9.

72 Letters are in KCL archives KA/1C/C69.

73 Charlotte Brewer, in her chapter on Walter William Skeat in Damico, *Scholarship*, 139–50, says that Skeat acknowledged Morris' considerable influence on his work in Middle English.

74 She was 34 years old. Number 33060 in the Bishop's Transcript, Church of England Deaths and Burials. Comments: Reused graves at Norwood, London Metropolitan Archives, Ref DW/T/0931. Found through Ancestry.com.

75 Both items found at Houghton Library, Harvard University, MS 641.1, Vol. 2.

76 MacMahon, e-mail of February 1998. Frederick James Furnivall (1825–1910) directed the Early English Text Society publications for many years and was outspoken and opinionated.

77 Verified by a search in the British Library's *British Newspaper Archives*, available on-line: www.britishnewspaperarchive.co.uk/. The initial inquest, No. 120, was written up on June 18, 1873 by CP Grenfell, Deputy Coroner for Cornwall, Penzance, sub-district of, St. Ives, No. 120.

78 In addition to the famous town by the same name, a small, rural Hastings exists in Somerset not too far from Keynsham, and might have been Cockayne's stated destination, had he had been in Keynsham.

79 A later entry to this record reads, "Subsequently identified as Rev Thomas Oswald Cockayne of London." Ironically, Jones had been in Cockayne's class at King's College School, but probably never saw the body he buried. It was in terrible shape and most likely in a shroud or coffin.

80 Details are from a personal visit to the cemetery in 2004. I am grateful to St. Ives Visitor Information Centre on Gabriel St. for obtaining directions to Cockayne's unmarked grave, and for cheerfully providing a wealth of other information and assistance.

81 *Shepton Mallet Journal*, April 2, 1897.

2

COCKAYNE'S *HERBARIUM*

Transformations

Many modern misconceptions about medieval medicine and magic can be linked to Cockayne's nineteenth-century *Leechdoms, Wortcunning, and Starcraft of Early England*, where the *Old English Herbarium* is found. This chapter discusses how the translations and notes he wrote for them transformed straightforward medical texts into literary curiosities. As curiosities, they have long adversely affected the way in which early-medieval medicine is generally regarded. Cockayne's archaizing translation style, prejudicial notes about the medical practice of early-medieval England, and his biased historical viewpoints were all contributors to the effect.[1] In addition, his work is usually classified under the broader field of "Anglo-Saxon studies," which has recently experienced its own significant transformations. The changes deserve mention here because going forward, they will most certainly affect how the entire Old English corpus is studied.

"Anglo-Saxon" has been used to describe an era, a place, a people, and a field of study since at least Cockayne's time. However, in 2019 because of cultural sensitivities connected with the term, the International Society of Anglo-Saxonists (founded 1983) voted to change its name to the International Society for the Study of Early-Medieval England (ISSEME) and suggested but did not mandate avoiding the term Anglo-Saxon from then on. The move has been both welcomed and criticized. The history and rationale for the change are explained at its website: isseme.org. There, dates for early-medieval England now are listed as c. 450–1100 CE, including Norman England, no longer ending with the Norman Conquest in 1066. These changes signify that studies of early-medieval England should consider the mixed parentage out of which the nation grew, open to Celts, Scandinavians, Normans, as well as Angles, Saxons, and Jutes.

DOI: 10.4324/9781003162285-2

The effects of these changes will undoubtedly be evidenced in many disciplines affected by or rooted in the concept of an Anglo-Saxon England. One of them will be medicine. The Old English medical texts have often been considered to be Anglo-Saxon products, and studies based on that premise seek out their most distinctive traits. Yet the traits sought are not medical as we understand the term, but involve for the most part searches for magic, superstition, and vestiges of pagan beliefs. These studies tend to downplay or simply omit mention of the role of monasteries in the healing practices of this period. Instead, they privilege seeking out secular reasons behind extra-medical components in the medical texts. This revised chapter incorporates several sources not yet available when the first edition was written.

Cockayne's "odd volumes"

In an 1898 review of the *Leechdoms* titled "Odd Volumes" by the Right Hon. Sir Herbert Maxwell, the author turns to "a collection of Anglo-Saxon treatises on medicine," which he says were admirably edited by Cockayne.[2] It begins:

> … one turns indolently to it [Cockayne's work] to see what mad or blind pranks our forefathers played with their constitutions, and to thank God that we are not such blockheads as they. In truth, many of the remedies prescribed seem worse than the diseases they professed to cure: unspeakably nasty, some of them …
>
> *Maxwell, 660*

Maxwell then discusses in some detail the dreadful nature of the contents under review, echoing widespread opinions of his time concerning early medicine. They include a certainty that even the medieval physicians and wise men of the day did not believe in the remedies they prescribed, simply passing on written remedies blindly without knowing why. Maxwell mentions magic in Anglo-Saxon medicine, as well as superstition, prayers, and pagan charms. The essay very much reflects the mindset of Cockayne's own time: looking at the childhood of the English nation from the vantage point of a superior age.

Cockayne's *Leechdoms* contain translations of the vernacular medical texts of early-medieval England (ca. 1000 CE), which are now known to be the earliest medical texts in a European vernacular. However, they are not simply translations with comments. A number of Victorian writers used the same translation style as Cockayne to reflect a bygone age; however, many ridiculed it. The result was that his style in the translations transformed medical texts written in simple prose into preposterous-sounding material. In all fairness, perhaps he did not intend them to have this effect. However, he also supplied prefaces to each volume suggesting that such healing practice could not have worked much, if at all, coming as he did from a background shaped by the classics. They reflect Cockayne's scathing evaluation of medicine during the childhood of the English nation. Such views on early medicine are echoed in the small number of studies on the topic that began soon after his volumes appeared, spread into general histories and histories of medicine, and have now become more or less received wisdom.

From Cockayne's prefaces emerges an image of Saxon leeches, as he liked to call the healers of the time, vainly seeking to comprehend classical remedies that were beyond their intellectual reach while chanting gibberish and saying nonsensical words reflecting native magic.[3] This image encouraged later scholars, beginning notably with historian Charles Singer, to seek out native medico-magic content and to study primarily such extra-medical material in the medieval works. The texts indeed have such material, mingled with translations from classical Latin and possibly Greek medical works and they belong to a tradition that very early combined magic/religion in healing practices.

Cockayne's prefaces reflect a smug assumption that he comes from an age of advanced medicine; yet ironically, we would consider the medicine and pharmacology during Cockayne's lifetime to be closer to the medieval than the twenty-first century. In the few places where Cockayne addresses the medical practice of Saxon leeches, not early-medieval-English culture in general, it was to express horror or dismay. Yet from a modern vantage point, those are our reactions to the much of the nineteenth-century medicine Cockayne knew. To be able to understand Cockayne's background somewhat better, a brief overview of the state of medicine he knew and the translation strategies popular when he was writing follow.

Medicine in early-nineteenth-century England

Cockayne had more than passing familiarity with medical practice in his lifetime. His father-in-law, Roger Edwards, was a surgeon in his hometown of Keynsham, a medical title that meant something different then than it does now. "Barber-surgeon" is what we now use. No university education was required to become a surgeon; instead, several years of apprenticeship to a licensed practitioner were required. A surgeon's practice then resembled that of a modern general practitioner, treating myriad medical conditions, including performing minor surgery, setting bones, treating skin conditions, lancing boils, pulling teeth, treating wounds … the list is endless. At this time, male surgeons (male midwives) were beginning successfully to oust female midwives from their customary role in attending childbirth, citing superior qualifications to gain clientele. Theirs was the kind of hands-on work no physician of the time would stoop to do; the surgeon's work was considered merely a craft. Physicians knew theory and stood apart and above surgeons and also apothecaries, the men who supplied medicines the physicians prescribed.

Only men from Oxford or Cambridge could become physicians in England at that time, and most of them had lucrative practices in London. At university, they first obtained Bachelor of Arts degrees in the classics followed by a medical curriculum based on Hippocrates and Galen. This theoretical basis was then supplemented by in-person training (observation, not hands-on practice) at teaching hospitals. Historian Irvine Loudon fills in the details:

> The position of physicians as the highest of the three orders or estates demanded that they undertook no form of manual operation and that they prescribed but did not dispense medicines. Indeed, they scarcely touched their patients, keeping their distance both literally and metaphorically. But their superior education was, nevertheless, supposed to embrace the whole of surgery and pharmacy conferring on the physicians the right to oversee the work of the surgeons and apothecaries.[4]

At least some of Cockayne's classmates pursing the same degree as he at Cambridge would have been aspiring physicians. That Cockayne shared a common educational foundation with the physicians of his time may explain why he felt qualified to expound on and judge "Saxon" medicine as well as medicine in general.

Apothecaries were legally bound to physicians, who had a monopoly on the "practice of physic," and their only role was supposed to be the filling of prescriptions physicians wrote, which were generally made of extremely caustic ingredients and cost a great deal. Apothecaries were governed by a Society of Apothecaries, and despite governmental regulations, many of them sold medicines over the counter without a physician's prescription. Apothecaries commonly dispensed medications and medical advice. Theirs was a lucrative practice; like the barber-surgeons, they too acted as quasi-general practitioners. Some apothecaries even made house calls (see Loudon, 20–3). In spite of vehement protests from physicians, in 1815, Parliament passed the Apothecary Act, giving the society power to license and oversee a kind of health provider we now call a general practitioner. Of course, this changed the dynamic between surgeon and apothecary and encroached even more on the physicians' realms.

Social historian M. Jeanne Peterson describes an increasingly chaotic situation in English health care at this time.[5] It happened because of the competition between these three estates, as she calls the three kinds of providers, and they reflect widespread social changes of that time. Unquestioned privileges of the upper class, which included physicians, were being questioned and challenged on many fronts and there was widespread popular dissatisfaction with the hierarchical medical system. Physicians controlled the system, but were vastly outnumbered by surgeons and apothecaries, the people who did the bulk of hands-on practice.

In the mix of health-care providers, but increasingly separate from these three estates, were numerous herbalists, who had practiced in England since 1542 under a Herbalists Charter granted by King Henry VIII. Histories of medicine do not generally include this profession in their discussions, because medicine and pharmacy as they have evolved tended to exclude this ancient field. In the mid-1800s, physicians, apothecaries, and surgeons were altering their training requirements and methods of practice in vying with each other for legitimacy and licensing. Herbalists too had to fight for their position in general health care, and in 1864 "a National Association of Medical Herbalists was founded to promote professional practice and to set education standards."[6] Years of debate over licensing, qualifications, specialties, and the like resulted in a power struggle to control laws and licensing in all areas of health care, and herbalists were adversely affected by it.[7]

Histories of medicine in the nineteenth century detail great changes that were gestating then, changes that emerged at different times in different countries as the century progressed, each one in some way or another leading to increased specialization. Wellcome Institute historian W.F. Bynum evaluates the situation this way:

> In terms of concepts, institutions, and professional structures, the medicine of 1900 was closer to us almost a century later than it was to the medicine of 1790 ... modern medicine was the product of nineteenth century society.[8]

Cockayne's lifetime spans these widespread changes; however, he was formed by the age of surgeons and apothecaries being controlled by physicians, and herbalists freely practicing and dispensing as well. This world of medicine was fast changing while he worked on medical texts belonging to a much earlier tradition.

Louis Pasteur (1822–95) began to publish his pioneering discoveries in bacteriology in the 1860s, explaining how epidemics spread. Because of his writings, use of vaccinations and "pasteurization" became more widespread, and disinfectants were increasingly used to prevent contamination and infection. At the same time Cockayne was writing about the surgical skills of the Greeks and Romans, many surgeons were just beginning to use anesthesia, and it took until the turn of the century for anesthetics to win acceptance. (The first successful demonstration of ether was in 1846 at Massachusetts General Hospital and the use of anesthesia spread rapidly; even so, it was not universally used.) Needless to say, for much of Cockayne's life, surgery was a last resort for many, the patient preferring death to submission to the knife.[9] Life expectancy throughout Europe during Cockayne's lifetime was 40 years, by 1900 it was 50, and in 1950 it was 70, a fact that is generally attributed to improvements in preventive medicine in the late nineteenth century and to continued improved nutrition, which began even earlier.[10]

Many medical historians attribute swift advances in medicine in the later nineteenth century to the Industrial Revolution with its rapidly increasing urban population and the attendant woes related to health under crowded and unsanitary conditions. Yet this sad phenomenon also enabled clinical observation to be made on large numbers of people and statistics to be kept on diseases, treatments, and success with cures.[11]

Public interest in health issues was on the increase at the time, as evidenced by the number of periodicals devoted to the topic: "For various reasons, the nineteenth century saw huge growth in the number of medical journals including from 1823, weeklies which dispensed a varied diet of news, opinion, scholarly articles and so forth."[12] Chemical and medicinal preparations made up the majority of the advertisements, and the medical literature showed that physicians were divided as to their opinion toward them. The situation sounds much the same as it is today, with hundreds of remedies readily promising myriad cures.

On a more personal level, Sabine Baring-Gould, who was a student at King's College School soon after Cockayne began teaching there (1844–45), vividly remembered details of his own medical treatment as a child in the mid-nineteenth century as he penned his memoirs in 1922. Having received great relief from pleurisy when his mother applied mustard poultices to his chest, Gould's opinion toward them soon changed:

> I had them [mustard poultices] not only applied to my chest and to my back, but also on one occasion behind and below my ears. There the poultice was kept on so long that when removed it carried off my skin with it, and the fresh growth was brown as the hide of a West Indian. ... Not only did the windows of apothecaries display in those days outspread yellow wax-bedaubed chamois leathers, but also, what was more interesting, globes full of water, containing leeches. I have on my chest to this day the triangular scars produced by the bites of those blood-suckers. ...
>
> My constitution must have been robust, in spite of the opinion of the physicians, or I could not have survived the draughts of castor-oil, the blue pills followed by drenches of senna and salts, the powders barely disguising themselves in raspberry jam, the ipecacuanha doses, the gargles, the plasters, the blisters, the cotton-wool paddings before and behind the ribs, the leeches, the cuppings and the bleedings.[13]

In brief, this was the world of health care in England at the time Cockayne was reading and evaluating early-medieval medical manuscripts. It was medicine that many today would not consider modern but "medieval," as often used today to mean primitive.

Transformational translations

Cockayne was the first person to write about early-medieval English medicine and the first to reveal its texts to the world. However, he brought certain attitudes toward the England of 500–1066 CE that affected how he read these texts, believing the barbaric newcomers were cultural children, lacking the refinements and skill of the classical world. As a result, he thought of their medical texts as being the product of such a culture. His translations and comments reflected his thoughts, and for the work under consideration here, resulted in what might be called "Cockayne's *Herbarium.*" Its legacy proved to be long lived.

In all fairness to Cockayne, and to every translator, the jury is still out on whether translation is by its very nature a form of transformation. It appears to be likely, no matter how careful or accurate any translation may be, if only because of nuances inherent to different languages. Cockayne's *Leechdoms* are his personal legacy and also a legacy shaped by values of his time. In this, he shares a bond with all translators past and present.

Lawrence Venuti, both a translator and historian, studies translations from many angles, cultural as well as linguistic. In *The Scandals of Translation*, he shows how translations can influence the way one culture receives another, arguing that translations reflect a translator's perception not only of the work itself, but of the culture from which it comes.[14] (Here, Venuti's primary interest is literary translations and the problems in translating—or failing to translate—the literature of marginalized cultures. In many ways, Cockayne saw early-medieval English culture as marginal—in our words, as of a third-world country.) Venuti argues that choice of words, omissions, paraphrases, and adaptations involved in translating any text from one language to another constitutes a reworking of the original text, no matter how "literal" the translation is intended to be:

> Translation wields enormous power in constructing representations of foreign cultures. Foreign literatures tend to be dehistoricized by the selection of texts for translation, removed from the foreign literary traditions where they draw their significance. ... Translation patterns that come to be fairly established fix stereotypes for foreign cultures, excluding values, debates, and conflicts that don't appear to serve domestic agendas.
>
> *Venuti, Scandals, 67*

Although Venuti is primarily concerned with modern literature and the power translations wield over how foreign texts are received in dominant cultures, his ideas are very much applicable to Cockayne's treatment of the Old English medical texts, which belonged to an essentially foreign culture considered primitive in many ways at the time. They are creations of a nineteenth-century antiquarian whose historical prejudices and stereotypes are obvious. In the following chapter, I discuss the original milieu in which the Old English medical texts were created and the reasons for their creation. I suggest viewing them as technical writings created with a defined audience and intended use in mind. Yet that is not the way they are generally studied, nor is translation theory of any kind applied to them.[15]

In fact, few translation studies have ever dealt with technical texts, a type to which medical writings certainly belong. Yet because of a few scholars, medieval translations of medical texts into the vernaculars of Europe was the focus of several conference sessions in 1997 (to which there has unfortunately been little follow-up). A paper by historian William Crossgrove summarizes some of the topics addressed there stressing the unique aspects of technical texts.[16] A primary concern is the audience for which the work is intended, and that has always been true. Crossgrove writes:

> In the case of technology, there are texts for experts, written down as technologists begin participating in vernacular written culture, that are virtually unreadable by lay persons who are not familiar with the practice being

described. Meanwhile, other technology texts apparently aim to provide general information about a particular technology for literate readers and would be of little interest to practitioners. … Medical texts cover a broader spectrum because some medical practitioners are academically trained and others have received only a practical training. Texts run the gamut from remedy books, to more general advice for lay persons for use in treating themselves or their families, to translations of academic texts for practitioners.

Crossgrove, 49

Yet theory concerning the translation of literary texts can in many instances be applied to translations of technical subjects, because of changes that can occur when any type of writing (or speech) is translated from one language to another. A translator's background and prejudices will affect word choices, phrasing, and so forth, as they affected Cockayne. Josephine Helm Bloomfield, for example, suggests that Frederick Klaeber's venerated edition of *Beowulf* (1922) strongly reflects values in Prussian Germany at the turn of the twentieth century, a situation analogous to what Cockayne did with the medieval medical texts. Klaeber favored "kind" and "kindness" in notes, articles, and glosses when the words used referred to Queen Wealhtheow, Bloomfield argues, but elsewhere, in masculine contexts, those same words were given such meanings as "lordly," "glorious," and "fitting." Klaeber did not alter the character of Wealhtheow by conscious intent, Bloomfield suggests, but explains that Klaeber (like Cockayne) was shaped by his own culture and it necessarily affected his scholarship:

> Even a scholar so great as he [Klaeber] might not have been able to escape or override the influences of his own culture in such areas as gender and gender roles (or indeed in such areas as family relationships and political authority).[17]

Although outrageously convoluted at times, the style Cockayne chose for his translations was in tune with literary trends in England at the time, trends toward escapism into earlier eras, especially the Middle Ages, as seen in the works of, for example, Sir Walter Scott, John Keats, Samuel Taylor Coleridge, Robert Browning, Dante Gabriel Rossetti, William Morris, and Alfred Lord Tennyson. Cockayne consciously chose one particular style that was controversial and quickly went out of vogue. Its intent was to recall a by-gone era by using antiquated words and turns of phrase. The following is an excerpt from chapter 18 of the *Old English Herbarium*, on the medicinal uses for the tuberous plant cyclamen (sowbread):

3. For stirring of the inwards, take this same wort, work it to a salve; lay it to the sore of the inwards. It also is well beneficial for heartache.
4. For sore of the milt *(spleen)*, take juice of this same wort one cup, and five spoonsful of vinegar; give (this) to drink for nine days; thou wilt wonder at the benefit. Take also the root of the same wort, and hang it about the mans swere *(neck)*, so that it may hang in front against the milt *(spleen)*;

> soon he will be healed. And whatsoever man swallows the juice of this wort, with wondrous quickness he will perceive relief of the inwards. This wort a man may collect at any period.
>
> *Cockayne 1965, 1: 113; entry XVIII for cyclamen*

In discussing translation strategies of the past, Venuti explains the background of the style Cockayne chose. It mirrors F.W. Newman's in his 1856 translation of the *Iliad*:

> Newman adopted a discourse that signified historical remoteness—archaism. He argues against a modern style for ancient works in translation. He even argues for using 'Saxo-Norman' for Homer, because his [Homer's] style is nearer the old English ballad [style] than the polished verse of Pope.
>
> *Venuti, Scandals, 122–3*

In fact, Newman published a glossary with his translation to define the archaic terms he used.

Matthew Arnold (1822–88), Oxford professor of poetry and literary critic, thought Newman's was a very bad translation—so bad that he roundly criticized it in a lecture series published as *On Translating Homer* in 1861. The pejorative term "to Newmanize" originated in this lecture; Arnold "coined a satiric neologism for Newman's translation discourse—to 'Newmanize'—and for the next 25 years this word was part of the lexicon of critical terms in the literary periodicals" (Venuti, 140). Leading literary magazines kept the subject alive, and it is reasonable to assume that Cockayne was aware of the controversy.

Only one contemporary review of the *Leechdoms* praised its style. In what amounts to a 14-page essay on ancient and medieval medicine and magic, much of the information gleaned from Cockayne's prefaces but unacknowledged, an unnamed reviewer in the *Dublin University Magazine* for May 1867 wrote:

> The translation fully possesses the compactness and rough strength of the original. Any reader of philological taste will scarcely arise from the perusal of the volumes without a deeper liking for unadulterated English than he entertained before, so well does it combine clearness, compactness, and vigour, and fitness.[18]

Part of Cockayne's intent in rescuing the medical manuscripts from museum storage was to document healing practices during the infancy of Britain. His prefaces were intended to outline how the texts should be understood, and one notion he introduced while doing so became particularly influential. It was a suggestion that the works he had named *Leechbook of Bald* and *Lacnunga* clearly reflected the practice of their time because barbaric charms and magic abounded in them. On the other hand, he said that the *Old English Herbarium* belonged to another tradition entirely, i.e., a classical tradition. Many later scholars in a field until recently known as "Anglo-Saxon studies" were interested in those magical and folkloric aspects and made much of them, to the exclusion of the *Herbarium*. The latter was often deemed merely a translation of a classical text and as such, more or less useless to the practice of its time. Countless studies perpetuate this perceived difference between the Old English medical texts, differences unsuited to their original complex and variegated nature, as discussed in more detail in the following chapter.

Even though the Celtic tradition was and is strong in large parts of Great Britain, Cockayne and most of his contemporaries did not look into or talk about the Celts (Britons) at any length; after all, they had been conquered and moved elsewhere or were living as slaves in the kingdoms the Germanic tribes created.[19] Naturally, no Celtic medical tradition that might have made any contribution was discussed; the goal for most scholars of "Anglo-Saxon" England was to find the roots of what they considered to be true English culture.[20] In fact, quite a bias against the Celts, whom they considered inferior, is evident in their many publications.

Popular nineteenth-century historian Sharon Turner even asserted that the Celts lost the moral virtue they needed to survive, in contrast to the superior Saxons who completed their destiny in laying the foundation for Great Britain.[21] Cockayne too claimed the Saxons were given "the Keltic careless tribes for a prey" (Cockayne 1965, 1: x). Moreover, few modern works attempt to deal with ancient Celtic medicine itself, scholars preferring to study Celtic divination and magic (reflecting the preferences in studying the Old English medical works as well). However in *Magie, médecine et divination chez les Celtes*, Christian-J. Guyonvarc'h looks closely at Celtic medicine and finds that healing was part of the duties of the druids, that medicine and spiritual practices were intertwined.[22] Because the druids learned everything orally in a secret 12-year apprenticeship, nothing was written down. Thus, only remnants of the druids' healing practices may have survived the years of their being outlawed under the Roman Empire and being suppressed by Christianity. Therefore, precious little—if any—of the Celtic (druidic) healing tradition survives. Recent work by Diana Luft and a ground-breaking article by Deborah Haden in *Speculum* on the relationship between Irish and Old English charms may signal increased interest in studying Celtic medicine and the monastic medicine of early-medieval England during its formative years. [23]

The *Leechdoms'* legacy

An evaluation of healing practices during the so-called Dark Ages as summarized by S.G.B. Stubbs and E.W. Bligh in *Sixty Centuries of Health and Physick* is fairly typical for general medical histories even into the twenty-first century. In a chapter titled "A Thousand Years of Darkness," they write:

> We have chosen to attempt a brief note on the medieval background rather than to present strings of names of tedious writers and lengthy specimens of the futilities of medieval recipe books. It is obvious that if this attempt be a fair representation nothing in the way of medical science as we understand it could exist. In fact it did not—in Europe.[24]

Theirs is certainly not an isolated evaluation, and although Cockayne himself did not cause all the negativity, his translations and prefaces contributed to it.

Forty years after the publication of Cockayne's *Leechdoms*, in a stated effort to spark interest in the history of English medicine, Joseph Frank Payne, M.D. gave two lectures before the Royal College of Physicians in June of 1903, citing "lamentable apathy and but little industry" on the part of British medical historians toward studying the history of their profession in England from the earliest time.[25] Central to his topic were the Old English medical texts Cockayne had translated, texts Payne said he regretted had still not received the attention they deserved. He told his audience that Cockayne's works presented all that was left of the medical library of early-medieval England, yet in a prefatory note to the published lectures, he acknowledged having received help from Henry Bradley, who he said "corrected a large number of inaccuracies in Mr. Cockayne's translation of the Anglo-Saxon texts" (Payne, v). Bradley was an editor of the *Oxford English Dictionary*. Nothing more was said in the lectures or in notes in the book about Bradley's alleged corrections to Cockayne's work, and the content and extent of these corrections are not known.

Payne portrays Old English medicine in a much more sympathetic light than Cockayne, praising the intelligence and ingenuity of speakers of Old English:

> In no other European country was there, at that time or for centuries after, any scientific literature written in the vernacular. ... This is proof that the Anglo-Saxons possessed high intelligence and activity of mind; though not necessarily that they possessed deep learning. ... The other quality which we find in the medical as in the pure literature, and which seems characteristic of the Anglo-Saxon mind, is that readiness to learn from all sources, that hospitality to ideas, of which I have already spoken.
>
> *Payne, 33*

However, Payne said that notwithstanding the merits of the texts, they could not transcend the time in which they were written. Echoing Cockayne, Payne described the early medieval period as "the time when European medicine stood at its very lowest level; and if any period deserved the name of the dark ages it was this" (Payne, 57).

Yet he displayed a remarkably tolerant attitude toward the allegedly superstitious elements of early medicine, saying that what we call superstition has been part of every known medical system to the present. Like Cockayne, Payne touched on the possibility of being able to trace charms and superstitions to a locale or a tribe, responding to a keen interest in this topic at the time. He took the position that they came out of a tradition spanning a great deal of time and a huge geographic area (including countries surrounding and affecting the West), at a time and place when superstition and healing were inextricably intertwined.

Many of the topics Payne discussed in 1903 were repeated almost verbatim in the 1920s by physician/historian Charles Singer, whose works do not acknowledge or cite Payne. Singer's writings are numerous and ubiquitous and have long been part of the essential reading on medieval medicine.[26] Like Payne, Singer saw in the Old English (indeed in all medieval) medical texts a conglomeration of traditions, one of which was the end of Greek rational medicine, in his words "… the last stage of a process that has left no legitimate successor, a final pathological disintegration of the great system of Greek medical thought." Throughout his many works, this message resounds: medieval medicine is monstrous and preposterous.

As mentioned earlier, Singer reissued the three-volume *Leechdoms* in facsimile in 1961 and substituted his own prefaces for Cockayne's, saying: "Each of the three [original] volumes had a long preface. These we omit because they are misleading in the present state of knowledge" (Cockayne 1961, 1: xx). And so in this edition of the *Leechdoms*, the bias in Singer's 1952 *Magic and Medicine* was even more closely linked to the Old English works, much of it gleaned from what Cockayne and Payne had said without crediting them with the ideas. The following was typical for Singer in talking about early-medieval English medicine:

> The Anglo-Saxon leech had no originality. That quality, for him, would have a negative value. He had no understanding of even the rudiments of the science of classical antiquity. His sources were very various and the demonstration of them provides the chief interest of these volumes of Cockayne. The general level of this medicine will be found far lower, far more barbarous, than the common accounts of Anglo-Saxon culture suggest. The sources of this debased material, if accurately and completely displayed, would reveal much of the social circumstances of England for several centuries before and for a century after the Conquest.
>
> … thus Cockayne's *Leechdoms* should be regarded as an end not a beginning. They provide good examples of the darkest and deliquescent stage of a [sic] outdated culture.
>
> *Cockayne 1961, 1: xix–xx, and xlvii*

About ten years later, Wilfrid Bonser, one of Singer's pupils, continued Singer's ideas in detail in a book whose title, *The Medical Background of Anglo-Saxon England*, is misleading, and whose subtitle actually tells the truth: "A Study in History, Psychology, and Folklore." The preconceived notions about medicine and what motivated its healers that are seen in Cockayne and Singer are repeated and amplified here. Though the following statement is not attributed to Singer, it perpetuates the ideas he promoted about early-medieval medicine generally:

> Western medicine stagnated for more than five hundred years from the later Imperial Roman times until it began to revive in the hands of the Arabs. The chief reason for this stagnation was the lack of that inquiring spirit to which one is accustomed today. … Most leeches were content to copy dead material without questioning this authority.[27]

In what proved to be a ground-breaking work, historian Loren MacKinney disagreed with Singer, his contemporary, on the question of exactly what medieval medicine represented:

> Dr. Singer, the eminent English scholar, has defended medieval medical history on the ground that it is a study in the pathology of civilization. But it is more than this; it is the birth and growth of a new civilization. Early medieval civilization consisted of two healthy elements, and one that was old and pathological. In the West, although classical civilization was sick unto death, much of it was preserved through its union with a vigorous young religion (Christianity) and a sturdy new race of rulers (the Germans). These two furnished the active elements by which a practically new civilization was created. *The early middle age is a period in which the clergy, originally dedicated to supernatural healing, and the Germanic people, addicted to primitive folk medicine, slowly progressed to the point where they could appreciate classical medical science and apply more intelligently the results of their own practical experience* [emphasis added].[28]

MacKinney cited several scholars who display bias such as Singer's toward the "Dark Ages," writing pointedly, "Many an educated man's conception of the early middle ages is merely an amplified image of the term dark age, the sole remnant of youthful acquisitions in a history class." (MacKinney, 21)

Stanley Rubin, writing a bit later on the subject, shares MacKinney's objectivity toward medieval remedies in thinking they might have helped patients. However, *Medieval English Medicine* also demonstrates a personal bias similar to that in Cockayne, Singer, and Bonser against the whole tradition of medicine in early-medieval England. Rubin does cite interesting archaeological evidence that few other works use. However, instead of being grounded in the concrete, the work is replete with assumptions prefaced by words like "undoubtedly" and "no doubt" and postulations of what might have been.

Rubin repeatedly underscores terrible living conditions that he thought must have prevailed at the time, but not from an objective archaeologist's point of view. For example, citing no sources, he describes the dwellings of the early Germanic invaders as being miserable, semi-sunken and says: "Refuse would quickly accumulate and general squalor prevailed. ... Domestic hygiene was impossible under these conditions and infectious diseases and others caused by squalor and dirt would have been common and widespread."[29] The evidence now available for living conditions and medical treatment at that time certainly does not put them on a level high enough to satisfy the sanitary concerns of the modern Western world, but "squalor" is not a term to be used lightly. If Rubin had cited as much archaeological data for descriptions of life in early-medieval England as he did for diseases shown in skeletal remains, his picture would have much more validity. Even more recently in dissertations on the Old English medical writings, Barbara Olds and Frieda Hankins adopted Rubin's technique of reaching a number of "doubtless" conclusions, and they both cite Rubin's work.[30] A newer way of looking at medieval medical practices at variance with this long-established tradition is discussed in the next chapter.

"Native" vs. "classical" elements in the Old English medical texts

Cockayne made a clear distinction between native and classical medical traditions in the works he was translating; the points he made have subsequently become received wisdom. In his and Singer's wake, other scholars seeking early-medieval pagan folklore and folk medicine began to deem the *Old English Herbarium* useless to early England. They believed *Bald's Leechbook* and *Lacnunga* were goldmines of hidden information about native culture because of original material in each. Such evaluations come easily when discussing a culture defined as "Anglo-Saxon." Regarded instead as part of a complex European tradition, to which it clearly belongs, that culture begins to look different.

For the same reasons, because it is a fairly straightforward translation of Latin works, the *Old English Herbarium* has often been said to have had comparatively less value to native healers. Such a point of view is stated as fact in the two dissertations just mentioned. Hankins lists the main sources for Old English medicine and magic as MSS Harley 585 and Royal 12. D. xviii: here is where *Lacnunga* and *Bald's Leechbook* are found. Hankins characterizes the *Herbarium* as "… an Anglo-Saxon translation from the Greek Apuleius, … a description of herbs and plants" (Hankins, 2). Likewise, in speaking about Cockayne's translations, Olds claims that "Of all these writings, the most studied and the most useful for an understanding of Anglo-Saxon medicine are the *Lacnunga* and *Leechbook*" (Olds, 2). Olds characterizes the *Herbarium* as a compilation based on Pliny written in North Africa at the end of the fifth century. Numerous publications have continued this line of thought. For example, work by Karen Jolly contrasts the "rational" or "classical" medicine in the *Herbarium* unfavorably with what is considered useful "native" material in the *Lacnunga* and *Bald's Leechbook*.[31] (Such studies nowhere mention the numbers of medical texts in Latin known to be in monastic and cathedral libraries at this same time, nor, for example, the large amount of Latin in *Lacnunga*, much of it used in prayers. Many Latin works were not translated into the vernacular and yet show evidence of having been used.)

Both Olds and Hankins cite Charles Talbot's *Medicine in Medieval England*, which touts the importance of *Bald's Leechbook* and *Lacnunga* because they alone reflect actual practice.[32] Talbot characterizes the *Herbarium* as classical and mentions it only as an aside to the two other works. At the same time, however, he acknowledges the known and suspected classical sources that can be found everywhere in *Bald's Leechbook* and also in *Lacnunga*.

Talbot is unusual in devoting considerable space to Latin medical texts that would have been available in monasteries in England.[33] There, Latin (and perhaps Greek) medical texts are known to have been kept and shared, and some kind of medicine was practiced. He lists some of the classical authors and compliments the contents in *Bald's Leechbook* that came from them. For example:

> The Leech-Book embodies the teaching of Greek writers as transmitted by Latin translations. … In short, far from the Leech-Book being a tissue of folk remedies and irrational ideas, it embodies some of the best medical literature available to the West at that time. … Indeed even the irrational remedies which appear from time to time in the Leech-book are the same as those used by Galen and Celsus.
>
> *Talbot, 18–19*

Talbot cites only two sources for his chapter on early-medieval English medicine: the 1904 work by J.F. Payne, *English Medicine in Anglo-Saxon Times*, and Grattan and Singer's *Anglo-Saxon Magic and Medicine*.

Not everyone has made a great distinction between classical medicine and magical native Germanic practices in the old texts. A study by Faye Getz, though concentrating on late medieval medicine in England, stresses the interrelationship of Latin and vernacular medical texts already in the earlier period and traces what she termed an encyclopedic medical tradition from the ruins of Rome through the early Middle Ages, one that very early encompassed magic. Getz describes it as combining medicinal herbs, simple remedies, and charms, and she links it to the medical tradition of the Benedictine monasteries and the texts associated with it (including all the Old English texts).[34]

Two conferences also pointed up the union of magic and medicine in the medieval period. Donald G. Scragg, one of the organizers of the 1987 and 1988 conferences at Manchester, England, wrote in an introduction to some of the papers published after the conference:

> No one in Anglo-Saxon England would have distinguished magic and medicine in the way that we do today, and it was logical therefore that, after the successful conference in Manchester in 1987 on Anglo-Saxon medicine, there should be a follow-up conference to look at magic and at those credited with supernatural healing powers.[35]

The eight papers in the two publications cover a wide range of medical subjects, and treatments using herbs are mentioned in many. The conferences are mentioned here to underscore their focus on medicine and magic together.[36]

As seen in the studies cited, a trend since Cockayne's time has been to approach past traditions by breaking them into defined parts: with medieval medicine broken into Greek, Roman, Germanic, magic, folkloric traditions, and so forth. This has contributed to magic and superstition being taken out of the original texts in which they were embedded and studied in isolation. As a consequence, that small part of early medicine has received a disproportionate amount of attention.

Cockayne often talks about magic and superstition. For example, in the Preface to Vol. 1 of the *Leechdoms*, he describes the medicine of the northern leeches during the "rudest ages" as being a combination of medicinal plants, charms, and incantations (xxvii). He then likens the superstition of the Germanic tribes to superstitious practices of the Roman Church in the "earlier ages of our modern period" (xxviii), practices such as "medicine masses, and blessing of worts out in the field." He quotes Germanic and Scandinavian sources to show the widespread belief in the power of witches, dwarfs, wizards, even by such famous men of the day as Bede and Theodore of Tarsus, Archbishop of Canterbury from 668 to 690. Not only in his prefaces, but also in his copious notes to translations of medical texts, he points out superstition, magic, pagan worship in the same breath as "popish" practices. The comments were intended to guide a reader's understanding, and they have guided many. Others read the same texts differently and find his asides to be misleading if not downright biased, and not just toward barbaric beliefs.

The reasons behind such a slant in studies of Old English medical texts are probed in E.G. Stanley's *The Search for Anglo-Saxon Paganism*.[37] There, Stanley discusses how the quest to find pagan Germanic elements began with Jacob Grimm's philological work and was taken up by nineteenth-century Old English philologists, becoming a standard feature of Anglo-Saxon scholarship. This quest for native paganism penetrated into and used Cockayne's translations.

Like Stanley, Allen J. Frantzen in *Desire for Origins: New Language, Old English, and Teaching the Tradition* examines the fundamental role of nineteenth-century scholarship in Anglo-Saxon studies. Frantzen showed how repercussions from those seminal years can be found in many subsequent studies. Though he does not directly treat the Old English medical texts, the search he describes for paganism and other "Anglo-Saxon" (especially non-Christian) elements in Old English texts can be seen as responsible for splitting the *Herbarium* apart from the other two medical works. Frantzen's underlying thesis is that nineteenth-century scholars created the origins they sought, and that it then formed the basis for many subsequent studies.

Godfrid Storms, however, was a scholar who challenged the idea that magic or even more specifically pagan magic could be easily identified as such in medieval medical texts (in this he echoes Payne). In *Anglo Saxon Magic*, Storms discusses magic, its origins, and how magic was used to heal; hence, the two Old English works thought to contain the most magic, *Bald's Leechbook* and *Lacnunga*, are the center of his study.[38] (The *Herbarium* is not excluded, and a number of its remedies are said to have a magic element.) Storms did not limit his study to an Anglo-Saxon England, but tied the three Old English medical texts to a pan-European tradition. Yet, his goal was to find the *Ur*germanic and the *Ur*Indo-European in them, a quest like Sir James George Frazer's in the *Golden Bough*, which he cited. In addition, Storms clearly states how difficult it is to separate native from classical sources in any of this material.

Storms determined that the Germanic tribes in England and on the continent had no general denomination for magic, nor did the Romans. He explains that the Old English referred to the way magic actions were performed, rather than to magic in general, and that it used abstract terms made with *craeft* to describe magical practices. He cites four elements on the cause of disease as unique to pagan Teutonic ideas: (1) flying venoms, (2) the evil nines, (3) worm as the cause of disease, and (4) the doctrine of elf-shot. Yet he concludes that with the exception of the last, elf-shot, "… we can hardly speak of distinguishing characteristics because the same elements occur in classical magic as well, as was admitted by Singer," (Storms, 118).

Segregating the "classical" *Old English Herbarium* from other Old English medical texts has tended to diminish its importance to its time and its medical tradition. Apropos such imposed contextualization, medievalist A.J. Minnis, though speaking about studies of medieval literary texts, wrote:

> Cultural change is one thing: cultural imperialism is something else. One can only hope that the greater awareness of medieval literary theory and criticism will help us go back to the texts and their contexts with the desire to listen and learn, not to shout down and dominate.[39]

My study has Minnis's admonition in mind in studying how Cockayne's legacy lived on in the *Leechdoms*, and how that affected the status of the *Old English Herbarium* in the pantheon of Old English medical texts. Regarding it as a rational, classical work has tended to isolate it and make it considered less valuable to the medical practice of the time than *Lacnunga* and *Bald's Leechbook* in a field that has privileged "anglo-saxonism."

In the following chapter, both the medical texts in Latin and those based upon them in Old English are considered to be part of an early-medieval monastic system in Europe. There, the *Herbarium* is placed back on the shelf beside *Lacnunga* and the *Leechbook*, all three representing texts that were valuable for their time. (In all fairness, the Latin medical manuscripts from the same period should be included and studied as well.) All belong to the same basic tradition, just with a different mix of sources. The same medical texts as in early-medieval England were found throughout the monastery libraries of Europe, with the same evidence for their having been used.

Old English scholar J.D.A Ogilvy characterized the *Herbarium* as "Apparently the standard medical text of the later Anglo-Saxons. … It is really a complex of Dioscorides, Pseudo-Apuleius, Pseudo-Musa (*De Herba Bettonica, De Taxone*) and Sectus Placitus Papyriensis *De Med. ex Animalibus.*"[40] By the time it was translated into Old English, the *Herbarium* complex in England also included the additions and revisions of those who had copied, translated, and used it. In reality, the main reason the Old English medical texts are important, other than for their value to philology, is that they are the earliest translations of Latin medical texts into a Western European vernacular. The actual medical practice these Latin and Old English writings represent is another topic entirely, one that awaits serious study. Studies of the magical aspects of the medical texts and philological studies have been the most numerous to date.[41]

Positive transformations

The importance of these Old English medical texts to philology cannot overshadow a much more negative view outside language studies toward this early-medieval period generally. Most histories of medicine written in English place early-medieval medicine into a historical Dark Age that was defined to a great extent by the nineteenth-century studies covered here.[42,43] Another way to view these early texts is as part of a unique period of significant change.

What might be called infirmary medicine spread throughout Europe thanks to Benedictine monks and nuns. Their medical practice is ill-defined, many of the Latin and possibly Greek texts they owned and shared are scattered in numerous libraries or have been lost. Theirs was medical practice during a fraught and unsettled time in European history, and the Old English medical texts are one window into it. The following chapter discusses that tradition with a focus on the *Herbarium* and, to the extent possible, the medical practice that went with it.

Notes

1 A good general history of the medieval period is John M. Riddle, *History of the Middle Ages 300–1500* (Lanham, MD: Rowman & Littlefield, 2008); rev. with Winston Black, 2015.

2 Herbert Maxwell, "Odd Volumes – I," *Blackwood's Edinburgh Magazine*, Vol. 163 (May 1898): 652–70.

3 The Old English *lacnan/laecan* with their many variants and compounds connote healer, physician, as well as the aquatic worms used medicinally. The Oxford English Dictionary lists both uses in 900 CE. Like starcraft and wortcunning, in 1864, the word leechdom would have had an odd connotation for anything connected with medicine. At that time, it was in general use only for the worms used medicinally that were often sold at pharmacies.

4 Irvine Loudon, *Medical Care and the General Practitioner 1750–1850* (Oxford: Clarendon Press, 1986), 3, and 85–99 for discussion of these practices. Also W.F. Bynum, *Science and the Practice of Medicine in the Nineteenth Century* (Cambridge: Cambridge University Press, 1994) for details of medical training and changes in medicine during the nineteenth century.

5 M. Jeanne Peterson, *The Medical Profession of Mid-Victorian London* (Berkeley, CA: University of California Press, 1978), 11–53 for background on the material here.

6 Graeme Tobyn, Alison Denham, Margaret Whitelegg, *The Western Herbal Tradition: 2000 Years of Medical Plant Knowledge* (Edinburgh: Elsevier, 2011), 16–19, 29–35. Also the related Hananja Brice-Yisma and Frances Watkins, eds., *Herbal Exchanges: In Celebration of the National Institute of Medical Herbalists 1864–2014* (London: Strathmore Publishing, 2014), 1–39.

7 For more detail on the general history of herbalism, refer to the books cited in note 6 and Susan Francia and Anne Stobart, eds., *Critical Approaches to the History of Herbal Medicine: From Classical Antiquity to the Early Modern Period* (London: Bloomsbury, 2014), and Barbara Griggs, *Green Pharmacy: The History and Evolution of Western Herbal Medicine* (Rochester, VT: Healing Arts Press, 1997).

8 W.F. Bynum, *Science and the Practice of Medicine in the Nineteenth Century* (Cambridge: Cambridge University Press, 1994), xi. The eighteenth and especially the

nineteenth centuries were seminal for all. The United States only came into its own in medicine about 1900.

9 For a riveting account of the history of anesthesia in the West, including a first-hand account of a patient who underwent surgery without it, see E.M. Papper, *Romance, Poetry, and Surgical Sleep: Literature Influences Medicine* (Westport, CT: Greenwood Press, 1995); also Victor Robinson, *Victory Over Pain: A History of Anesthesia* (New York: Henry Schuman, 1946), which includes classical and medieval attempts at anesthesia and Thomas E. Keys, *The History of Surgical Anesthesia* (1945; New York: Dover Publications, 1963).

10 Consult William H. McNeill, *Plagues and Peoples* (New York: Doubleday, 1976), especially chapter 6, "The Ecological Impact of Medical Science and Organization since 1700," and Alfred W. Crosby, Jr., *The Columbian Exchange: Biological and Cultural Consequences of 1492* (Westport, CT: Greenwood Publishing Co., 1972) for a discussion of nutrition.

11 Earlier assessments of medicine in the later nineteenth century are found in Brian Inglis, "The Doctor and the Quack" in his *A History of Medicine* (Cleveland, OH: The World Publishing Company, 1965) and Erwin H. Ackerknecht, "Public Health and Professional Development in the Nineteenth Century" in his *A Short History of Medicine* (New York: The Ronald Press, 1955).

12 Peter Bartrip, "Secret Remedies, Medical Ethics, and the Finances of the British Medical Journal," in Robert Baker, ed., *The Codification of Medical Morality: Historical and Philosophical Studies of the Formalization of Western Medical Morality in the Eighteenth and Nineteenth Centuries*, Vol. 2 (Dordrecht: Kluwer Academic Publishers, 1995), 196.

13 Sabine Baring-Gould, *Early Reminiscences: 1834–1864* (New York: E.P. Dutton & Co., n.d. [1922]), 112–13, a goldmine of information on details of life in mid-nineteenth-century England and France. In addition, W.M. Thackeray's novel *Pendennis* of 1850 describes the life of a contemporary apothecary by that name.

14 Lawrence Venuti, *The Scandals of Translation: Towards an Ethics of Difference* (London: Routledge, 1998). Translations and their widespread cultural effects have become an increasingly important field of study in this global age, and Venuti's remains an important voice. Particularly relevant is his *Translation Changes Everything: Theory and Practice* (London: Routledge, 2013), one of his numerous publications. Another important aspect of the field is ascertaining why certain works are *not* translated; discussed in Eugene A. Nida and William D. Reyburn, *Meaning Across Cultures* (Maryknoll, NY: Orbis Books, 1981) who argue that translators evaluate what they are translating in terms of the biases of their own culture, and this bias is necessarily reflected in the translation.

15 Additional insight into issues of translation is found in Rita Copeland, *Rhetoric, Hermeneutics, and Translation in the Middle Ages: Academic Traditions and Vernacular Texts* (Cambridge: Cambridge University Press, 1991).

16 William Crossgrove, "The Vernacularization of Science, Medicine, and Technology in Late Medieval Europe: Broadening our Perspective" in *Early Science and Medicine*, Vol. 5, No. 1 (2000): 47–63. Organized by Crossgrove and Linda Voigts, several sessions were part of the 32nd International Congress on Medieval Studies in 1997 at Western Michigan University, Kalamazoo MI. Technical writing is now recognized as a stand-alone field of rhetoric.

17 Josephine Helm Bloomfield, "Diminished by Kindness: Frederick Klaeber's Rewriting of Wealhtheow," *Journal of English and Germanic Philology*, Vol. 93 (April 1994): 186.

18 "Anglo-Saxon Leechdoms: Medicine and Astronomy in the Dark Ages," *Dublin University Magazine*, Vol. 69 (May 1867): 533. What the reviewer may have meant in praising the "compactness" of the language is not entirely clear.

19 David A.E. Pelteret, *Slavery in Early Medieval England: From the Reign of Alfred until the Twelfth Century* (Woolbridge: The Boydell Press, 1995). It begins "The existence of

slavery as an integral part of early English society comes as a considerable surprise to most people."

20 For an interesting interpretation of cultural biases associated very early with the term/concept "Anglo-Saxon," read Oxford historian Bryan Ward-Perkins, "Why did the Anglo-Saxons not become more British?" *The English Historical Review*, Vol. 115, No. 462 (June 2000): 513–33.

21 Sharon Turner, *The History of the Anglo-Saxons: Comprising the History of England from the Earliest Period to the Norman Conquest*, 4th ed., Vol. 3, 1799–1805. (Reprint. London: Longman, Hurst, Rees, Orme, and Brown, 1823): 1: 196–242.

22 Christian-J. Guyonvarc'h, *Magie, médecine et divination chez les Celtes* (Paris: Payot, 1997), 224.

23 Diana Luft, *Medieval Welsh Medical Texts: Vol. 1, the Recipes* (Cardiff: University of Wales Press, 2020); Deborah Hayden, "Old English in the Irish Charms," *Speculum*, Vol. 97, No. 2 (April 2022): 349–76.

24 S.G.B. Stubbs and E.W. Bligh, *Sixty Centuries of Health and Physick*, in a chapter on the early Middle Ages titled "A Thousand Years of Darkness" (London: Sampson Low, Marsten and Co., 1931), 86 .

25 Joseph Frank Payne, *The Fitz-Patrick Lectures for 1903: English Medicine in the Anglo-Saxon Times* (London: Clarendon Press, 1904), 4.

26 For example, Charles Singer, *From Magic to Science: Essays on the Scientific Twilight* (1928; New York: Dover Publications, 1958), and his "The Herbal in Antiquity," *The Journal of Hellenic Studies*, Vol. 47 (1927): 1–52.

27 Wilfrid Bonser, *The Medical Background of Anglo-Saxon England: A Study in History, Psychology, and Folklore* (London: The Wellcome Historical Medical Library, 1963), 6.

28 Loren MacKinney, *Early Medieval Medicine* (Baltimore, MD: The Johns Hopkins Press, 1937), 57–8.

29 Stanley Rubin, *Medieval English Medicine* (New York: Barnes and Noble, 1974), 14.

30 Barbara M. Olds, "The Anglo-Saxon Leechbook III: A Critical Edition and Translation," Ph.D. dissertation, University of Denver, 1984; Freda Richards Hankins, "Bald's *Leechbook* Reconsidered," Ph.D. dissertation, University of North Carolina at Chapel Hill, 1991.

31 Karen Louise Jolly, *Popular Religion in Late Saxon England: Elf Charms in Context* (Chapel Hill, NC: University of North Carolina Press, 1996). Although Jolly talks here about a composite and partly unwritten medical tradition, she excludes the *Herbarium* and works like it entirely from the realm of medicine as it was practiced in early-medieval England.

32 Charles H. Talbot, *Medicine in Medieval England* (London: Oldbourne, 1967).

33 A recent and very complete study is to be found in Conan Doyle, "Anglo-Saxon Medicine and Disease: A Semantic Approach," Ph.D. dissertation, Corpus Christi College, Cambridge, 2011, with its comprehensive bibliography including foundational philological studies. An earlier discussion of the texts that were available to early-medieval healers in England is in M.L. Cameron, "The Sources of Medical Knowledge in Anglo-Saxon England," *Anglo-Saxon England*, Vol. 11 (1983): 135–55.

34 Faye Getz, *Medicine in the English Middle Ages* (Princeton, NJ: Princeton University Press, 1998). Of particular relevance is chapter 3, "Medieval English Medical Texts." What Getz calls the encyclopedic tradition appears to be the same that Jerry Stannard and others called *Rezeptliteratur*, a genre discussed in detail in chapter 3. Getz does not reference Stannard or the standard writers on *Rezeptliteratur*, although she does cite Bonser, who mentions the genre in several places.

35 Donald G. Scragg, *Superstition and Popular Medicine in Anglo-Saxon England* (Manchester: University of Manchester, 1989), 7. A companion volume is Marilyn Deegan

and Donald G. Scragg, eds., *Medicine in Early Medieval England* (Manchester: University of Manchester, 1989).

36 Other views on this subject are found in, for example, Audrey L. Meaney, "Extra-Medical Elements in Anglo-Saxon Medicine," *Social History of Medicine*, Vol. 24, No. 1 (2011): 41–56; and for later medieval England Lea Olsan, "Charms and Prayers in Medieval Theory and Practice," *Social History of Medicine*, Vol. 16, No.3 (Dec. 2003): 343–66; Catherine Rider, "Medical Magic and the Church in Thirteenth Century England," *Social History of Medicine*, Vol. 24, No. 1 (2011): 92–107.

37 E.G. Stanley, *The Search for Anglo-Saxon Paganism* (Cambridge: D.S. Brewer, 1975), viii. The book was originally published as articles in *Notes and Queries* 1964–65.

38 Godfrid Storms, *Anglo-Saxon Magic* (1948; The Hague: Martinus Nijhoff, 1974).

39 Alastair J. Minnis, *Medieval Theory of Authorship*, 2nd ed., (Philadelphia, PA: University of Pennsylvania Press, 1984), xvii–xviii.

40 J.D.A. Ogilvy, *Books Known to the English, 597–1066* (Cambridge, MA: Medieval Academy of America, 1967), 75. For more information on availability of books in these early years (as well as later times), consult *The Book in Britain: A Historical Introduction*, ed. Zachary Lesser (Hoboken, NJ: John Wiley & Sons, 2019), 9–47. Its scope is wider than "Anglo-Saxon" England and includes all of the British Isles and Ireland.

41 For example the 2011 Doyle dissertation, which is "a semantic approach."

42 For example, Roy Porter, *The Greatest Benefit to Mankind: A Medical History of Humanity* (New York: W.W. Norton & Co., 1997). Lizabeth Hardman, *The History of Medicine* (Detroit, MI: Lucent Books, 2011), aimed at impressionable high school students. Both stress the darkness and horrors of early-medieval medicine, with illustrations to drive the point home. In 2022, at Jordan High School in Durham, NC, USA students were still being taught about the Middle Ages as the "Dark Ages" in high-school history classes (personally verified by the author).

43 For a push back against such prejudice in science history, one that began long ago with MacKinney, see "Unity and Disunity in Academia," and "The Dark Age That Wasn't" in *Viewpoint*, the on-line magazine of the British Society for the History of Science at www.bshs.org.uk/wp-content/uploads/Viewpoint116_ONLINE.pdf. Also see historian James T. Palmer's related blog on technical topics connected with the early-medieval world of northern Europe at merovingianworld.com.

3

NEW CONTEXTS FOR THE *OLD ENGLISH HERBARIUM*

An observation made by physician–historian Jacalyn Duffin is relevant to ever-changing ideas about the Old English medical texts; "Historical ideas, like disease ideas, can be both hereditary and communicable."[1] Setting herself apart from the customary "ages in the history of medicine" approach, Duffin elaborates:

> Medical history, like all history, and like medical practice and medical science, is about questions and answers, evidence and interpretation. Some questions are better than others; some sources are more to be trusted than others; and some interpretations are stronger than others. Good historians are aware of the danger in projecting their own desires and values into historical scenarios and texts. History invites students to ponder why things came to be as they are and how they change. It challenges them to explain how something that is so wrong now could once have seemed right. And it reminds them of the future probability of having to relinquish the very ideas and "facts" that they are about to study. As a result, history is a brilliant instructor in the ideals of lifelong learning.
>
> *Duffin, 6*

Following Duffin's suggestions about studying medical history, the questions posed in this chapter are why/how the *Old English Herbarium* was created and how it might have been used. I suggest that the answers require first taking this text out of a primarily "Anglo-Saxon" context and putting it into the broader realm of European texts from which it derives. It is a herbal with several sources; its genre is technical writing. To unravel its mysteries properly, physicians, medical herbalists, language scholars, historians, archaeologists, and specialists in related disciplines would ideally collaborate. This study does not claim to address all approaches, but hopes to provide useful suggestions.

DOI: 10.4324/9781003162285-3

The *Old English Herbarium,* related vernacular texts, and early-medieval medicine

The *Old English Herbarium* is a translation of what had originally been several Latin works on medicinal plants and herbs, generally classified as herbals.[2] Its Latin sources are of interest because they shed light on related texts circulating in Europe and on those that managed to reach England.[3] More detailed studies and translations of the entire pool of available Latin works out of which the *Old English Herbarium* was created (including those omitted) could greatly add to understanding medical practice and treatment at the time the compilation was made.[4]

However, important to remember here is that many Latin writings on topics related to medicine and pharmacy circulated throughout early-medieval Europe and some reached England well before the year 1000, though actual dates of arrival and use are still debated.[5] The longest, the *Herbarium Apulei Platonici traditum a Chirone Centauro, magistro Achilles,* is believed to have been written or compiled in about the fourth century CE. Attribution to "Apuleius" might have been added to suggest that the work originated with the God of Medicine, Aesculapius.[6] Its immense popularity in early-medieval Europe is evidenced by the large number of surviving manuscripts, many of them illustrated, and this popularity continued into the age of the printed book; it was the earliest herbal printed, and that was in Italy (1481).[7]

Almost always appended to the Latin *Herbarium* was *Medicina ex Animalibus* (or *de Quadrupedibus*), remedies using animal parts/fluids, attributed to Sextus Placitus but itself a composite text. This type of medieval pharmacy draws censure in modern times; however, its ingredients are commonly found in remedies from antiquity forward. German has a particularly descriptive term for it: *Dreckapotheke,* a pharmacy of filth.

Classical authors echoed in these Latin works include Dioscorides (d. A.D. 80), whose *De materia medica (The Materials of Medicine)* became a model for later herbals; he began the tradition of listing uses for each plant, how it grows, and how it can be identified.[8] Important also in the background of the *Herbarium* is the encyclopedic *Natural History* by Pliny the Elder. This comprehensive first-century Latin work served as an uncited source for numerous early-medieval compilations.[9]

Echoed as well are some of the humoral theories of Galen (d. A.D. 200), the undisputed authority on medical and pharmaceutical matters throughout the Middle Ages and most of the Renaissance. Much of his treatment was based on a theory of humors in the body (blood, black bile, yellow bile, and phlegm) whose imbalance explained disease, and whose balance assured a healthy life. This system became more important in later medieval medicine; in this early period, some of his drug preparations were known, including simple medicines and mixtures using exotic ingredients, such as clays and earths from many locations around the world.[10] His writings were incorporated without attribution into many collections of medical texts, but usually only in part.

Medical historian Jerry Stannard found bits and pieces of Galenic theory persisting in many medieval remedies (often called *Rezepten*, lacking a suitable English equivalent) without their authors necessarily being linked directly to a knowledge or study of Galen. As he explains it,

> ... acceptance of the doctrine of humors and its corollaries is seldom explicitly defended in the [medicinal] recipes themselves. Its defense or promulgation is usually reserved for separate, introductory chapters in leechbooks and assumed thereafter in recipes. But, as the principal explanatory basis for medical, botanical, and pharmacological theory, some form of humoralist doctrine is frequently found in recipes.[11]

Examples are references in texts to hot plants, cold plants, and hot and cold conditions. In addition, many remedies are based on the concept that opposites effect cures.

However, after Dioscorides, Pliny, and Galen, no clear path made by any medical authority leads through late antiquity and the early-Middle Ages (often disparaged as the Dark Ages). The period as a whole is acknowledged to be hard to define, in constant flux, with peoples and boundaries changing regularly.[12] To increase the complexity, the decades-old custom of using the fall of Rome (476 CE) as its primary reference point is giving way to newer perspectives allowing greater nuance. During these unsettled centuries (ca. 350–700), medical texts were copied whole or in part, most of the time without any attribution, and their transmission and dissemination present enormous challenges to later scholars who want to trace any given work to its source(s). If instead these writings are studied as salvaging selections of medical knowledge to use in infirmary-like settings, sources become understood as being irrelevant to their users even though of great importance to historians, and at that moment, content takes center stage.[13]

Pointing out the dearth of named sources in the Old English texts is, however, common. In a 2011 volume of the journal *Social History of Medicine* devoted to early-medieval medicine, for example, Debby Banham writes about medicine in England as follows:

> Although English vernacular medicine of the late ninth to twelfth centuries draws heavily upon the classical and sub-classical tradition, classical authorities are almost never cited. In fact, citations of any kind are very rare, and the majority of authorities cited in texts before the Norman Conquest are themselves English. This suggests a rather self-sufficient medical community in England, with limited historical awareness or contact with wider developments, at least until new Latin medical texts came in from the continent in the eleventh century.[14]

Whether the authorities mentioned were pure "English," uncontaminated by information from elsewhere remains to be seen.

In the same volume, Audrey L. Meany writes a comprehensive article on the "extra-medical elements" in the Old English medical works, "… elements which are not strictly medicinal … amulets, incantations, rituals and special exotic ingredients."[15] Especially pertinent to the present study is another article in that same volume, one that gets to the issues Banham and Meaney discuss, as well as to those raised here. In writing about "what is wrong with early medieval medicine," historian Peregrine Horden addresses problems in interpreting this elusive era in medical history:

> The contrast between the concentrated vigor of work on medicine surviving in the Old English vernacular and the inevitably diffused efforts of those dealing with continental European Latin medicine is instructive. Stray remedies and glosses apart, Anglo-Saxonists have to work with a substantial corpus of around 500 folios but embodying only five major works, three of which survive in unique manuscripts. I certainly do not mean to suggest that interpretive difficulties are much reduced, but the focus is at least clear.[16]

Medical writings in Old English in the area called "Anglo-Saxon England" (ending precisely at 1066 CE) have long been a focus of study. Now, with the scope of the period extending to ca. 1100 and including every culture in early-medieval England, even Norman, views about those same medical writings may well change. This study embraces the latter focus and includes, to the limited extent possible, consideration of how both Latin and Old English texts figured into medical practice and training. The drawback is that many of the Latin texts have never been studied.

Long ago, historian Loren MacKinney was one of the first to discuss this medical tradition without inherited "Dark Age" prejudices. He begins it in Southern France, coming out of a Roman world, and by the early Middle Ages, it is already mixed with other elements (including magic and charms) from many sources:

> The second phase of supernatural healing was a combination of pagan and Christian superstition. [The first was the early Christian emphasis on Divine healing.] In Roman folk-medicine, incantations, charms, and magic played an important part. The pages of Pliny's *Natural History*, and Marcellus Empericus' handbook of medicine bear ample evidence of the fact … [In spite of Christian prohibitions against things pagan] medieval folk-healers continued to use magical lore, under cover of Christian prayers and often with the sign of the cross. In similar fashion Germanic and Celtic superstitions persisted in the Christian world of medicine.[17]

The number of medical writings increases during the early Middle Ages, largely in France and Italy, but their contents do not change appreciably, additions being wisdom supplied by practitioners as the compilations evolve over time. Apropos these texts MacKinney writes,

Apparently those medical men who delved into the manuscripts that were available read much the same sort of material as had circulated in the West since the fifth and sixth centuries. And until the eleventh century, medical literature was to continue thus.

MacKinney, 99

It must be kept in mind that in this kind of healing the recipes and the ingredients vary widely, and substitutions are common.

In comparing the botanical content of classical and medieval medical texts, historian Stannard found that medieval *materia medica* takes on a distinctive bent, tending more toward prescriptions and charms, to practical uses, than to Dioscorides' almost text-book approach to medical botany. Stannard notes that

> Generally speaking, much of the content of Graeco-Roman materia medica was retained but it was modified over many centuries by values, needs, and institutions of an incipient culture. One stage of the transition from ancient to medieval materia medica is represented by Marcellus of Bordeaux.[18]

Stannard remarks here that Marcellus, a physician living in southern Gaul and writing ca. 395–410 CE, is generally ignored by historians of pharmacy, but studied by folklorists, notably Jacob Grimm. It is a great shame that no English translation of Marcellus's important work exists; the only one in a modern European language is in German, dating to 1968. Marcellus's writings are a forerunner to a characteristic type of medieval medical literature, in which the names of plants are often given in two or three languages (as they are in the *Old English Herbarium*) and other elements included, such as comments about the efficacy of the recipes, charms, and other information. About the genre, Stannard says:

> The change from describing medicinal plants to discussing their names is intimately connected with the development of medieval materia medica. The northward and westward expansion of European civilization away from its earlier Mediterranean homeland to the south, meant an encounter, not always quickly recognized, with a new and different flora. As a consequence, many of the locally abundant plants were unrecognized or unknown except insofar as they could be identified with the plants of the *flora classica*. Because of the uncertainty regarding the identity, hence the properties, of these plants, names and synonyms assumed the role formerly played by descriptions.

Stannard, "Marcellus," 49

Concerning the Old English version of the *Herbarium* and its handling of plant names, its facsimile editors, M.A. D'Aronco and Cameron explain:

> The Anglo-Saxon translation observes the tradition of adding the name to a list of synonyms in other languages. It should however be emphasized that

the translator chose as the key name first on the list not the name in his own language, but the Latin, or sometimes Greek, term for each plant. The Anglo-Saxon plant name was always inserted in last place, evidently because it was considered a kind of synonym. … This occurs not only in cases where the plants are native to the warmer zones of the Mediterranean basin, and therefore not necessarily common in Britain, but also for plants like equisetum or horsetail, found in all parts of Europe including the British Isles, whose English name the translator appears to be unaware of.[19]

Marcellus, who used the Latin *Herbarium*, is often said to anticipate medieval practices by including pagan and semipagan charms, incantations, and magical formulas as intrinsic parts of the therapy, and it appears that with this kind of medical writing, we are no longer dealing with "rational" medicine in the sense of the classical Greek tradition, though much of it can be ultimately traced to that source. Roman medicine, in contrast to Greek, always included a certain amount of what we term superstition, though Cockayne and Singer did not distinguish Greek from Roman in their concept of "classical." Important to this argument is the fact that Greek rational medicine very early became part of a fluid mass of medical knowledge that was passed on in texts and in practice, and this included charms, prayers, and rituals that were pan-European. The *Herbarium* belonged to this tradition, not only to the purely classical Greek one.

In an article on medieval medical practice, historian John M. Riddle also describes a composite tradition in the early Middle Ages, out of which works like the *Herbarium of Pseudo-Apuleius* arose. Here, he probes the relationship between theory and practice as seen in drug therapy ("the way most medicine was practiced") during the entire Middle Ages. Both Roman and medieval medicine consisted of noninstitutionalized, informal practice based on essentially the same medical education, he finds. Its medical practice was not totally dependent on written texts but was based on a pharmacy that preserved older knowledge and also recognized and used new drugs.[20]

Riddle also argues that the rise of universities and expansion of the scope of medical texts beginning in the eleventh century promoted the importance of theory in medical practice. He sees a growing gap between theory and practice because some of the theories were unworkable in practice. Based on a complex theoretical system involving—among other things—the use of opposites to effect healing, the new remedies included more and more exotic ingredients that were in theory supposed to work because their philosophical *raisons d'être* proved they must work.

Absent many alternatives and by necessity classifying certain early-medieval writings simply as "medical" may put them into a category into which they do not comfortably fit because of modern conceptions of what constitutes medicine. Because they are abbreviated written (explicit) instructions, in order to be able to follow them, a user must possess a certain amount of tacit (unwritten practical) knowledge.[21] Early-medieval medical texts will always suffer by comparison to modern writings that are considered truly medical and/or scientific because of the difference in how they are written. Perhaps it would make sense to adopt the German term *Rezeptliteratur* (remedy texts) for them until an English alternative is adopted.

Medieval remedy texts as technical writings

Latin texts on science, technology, and medicine that were translated into the several vernaculars during the later Middle Ages, together called *Fachliteratur* (specialist texts), were the focus of the series of papers delivered at the International Congress on Medieval Studies in May 1997 mentioned in the preceding chapter.[22] As the issues with Cockayne's translations/transformations demonstrate, understanding medieval technical texts presents challenges quite different from those in other genres.

At the time of the conference, a suitable name for the genre was an issue: the already established German terms *Fachliteratur* or *Sachliteratur* became customary. Today the field of technical writing is flourishing and it could certainly be used as the general category for such writings from the past. (Apropos this topic, an unusual website, the Merovingian World, covers a host of early-medieval technical subjects, including medicine: https://merovingianworld.com/). In the paper cited earlier, Crossgrove admits that histories of modern science and rational medicine will not find much in the vernacular technical texts of the Middle Ages with direct bearing on their fields in comparison with learned Latin writings. However, he asserts that the vernacular texts do contain extremely valuable information:

> The history of technology, on the other hand, relies heavily on vernacular texts, if there are any texts at all, because technologists did not routinely participate in written culture and the Latin technical treatises preferred by learned authors seldom had much relevance for contemporary practice. The history of medicine has a lot to learn from vernacular texts about medical practice, but it does not necessarily learn much from such texts for the history of academic medicine. There are evidently important distinctions that are easily glossed over when we refer to *Sachliteratur*, but the partial similarities also illustrate why it remains useful to discuss the vernacularization of medieval science, medicine, and technology as part of a single larger purpose.[23]

With reference to the need for alternative terms, it may also be misleading to mention "physicians" using the early-medieval remedy books because today the word implies practitioners with formal training in written theory and hands-on practice probably at the university level. Yet, it is common to do so because references to physicians occur in the early texts. However, there is no evidence for schools of medicine anywhere in the post-Roman West before 1100. If instead we call those medieval practitioners "medics" or simply the less formal "doctors," their role is clearer in a modern context. On-the-job learning coupled with practical writings was their training; such healers have ministered for centuries, for example, the nineteenth-century barber-surgeons discussed in the previous chapter.

Earlier, historian Riddle anticipated Crossgrove's words:

> To Roman and early medieval people, medicine was an art, not a *scientia*; so Hippocrates had said and so the early Middle Ages believed. It could no more be formally studied than woodcarving, plowing, or butchering. Medicine was neither a science nor chance but a skill, a trade. Isidore said medicine was not a "subject" because it deals in all areas, not singular themes. Early medicine was practical. The distinction was dropped between medicine as a practice (art) and medicine as a theory (science), a distinction made by Aristotle and noted by Pliny who railed against illiterate practitioners knowing no theory. … As Christianity divided into eastern and western halves, the western monastic orders stressed the basic practical values as compared with the more ascetic an theoretical attitudes of eastern Christianity.[24]

In his article, Crossgrove also outlines the distinctive requirements technical disciplines have in terms of how their literature is written and, by the same token, how their literature should be read. These requirements of course cannot be met when medical, scientific, or technical documents are read as literary works and discussed as such, as they have been in the past. Skill, specialized knowledge, familiarity with terms having specific connotations in the technical field, and the tacit knowledge to fill in what is not explained in words; all are needed to read, follow, or interpret such texts. Yet technical writings from the past continue to lack a place on the shelf of their own. As recently as 2018 in writing about the Middle English Lelamour Herbal, David Morena Olalla lamented the "historical neglect of Fachprosa," saying that it "remains a textual Cinderella."[25]

Of the known Old English technical writings on healing and health care, one is a herbal with remedies, botanical lore, and, in only one of the manuscripts, plant illustrations; one is a healer's manual with techniques and remedies; one gives advice, remedies, and prayers/charms/incantations. Centuries after their creation, who can understand them as their authors intended? The answer really depends on who is reading or translating them and the use for which they are intended. Most of the time, it is assuredly not the one their medieval authors had in mind. An extensive body of literature on remedy books exists in German under the name *Rezeptliteraur* [remedy literature]. These studies are instructive on how the *Herbarium* and the other related Old English writings might be evaluated and interpreted when freed from the confines of belonging exclusively to "Anglo-Saxon medicine."[26]

Need for an English name for *Rezeptliteratur*

Medical historian Henry E. Sigerist sought out and studied *Rezeptliteratur* because he was seeking traces of classical medicine. He credited monasteries with transmitting both medical texts and practice, the latter similar to a master-apprentice system of learning a craft. Although Sigerist believed that *Rezeptliteratur* formed the basis of medical knowledge at the first medieval medical school at Salerno, he discovered that no two of the collections were alike: "The common foundation that they [the Salernitan texts] have is nothing other than the medicinal recipe material from the sixth and seventh centuries, to which over time new remedies came or old ones in new forms."[27] The texts within this genre changed continually, as unusable information was thrown out, additional material incorporated, and new compilations were made. About the genre, Sigerist concluded, "Thus I believe that in most cases we have original compilations before us, collections that the scribe assembled for the needs of his monastic/medical uses" (Sigerist, 186).[28]

These writings have been studied extensively, investigators even splitting the remedies into types. Ulrich Stoll, for example, wrote of a fundamental difference between what he termed short and long remedies, tracing the long ones to Dioscorides and Galen and their tradition, the shorter versions to the Latin world.[29] Stoll put the *Herbarium of Pseudo-Apuleius* into the short-remedy type, i.e., an early-medieval, Latin type. Gundolf Keil envisioned short remedies being addressed to patients or to their caregivers, and he believed that the monastery door was where medical prescriptions were passed on orally, even being translated there. He thought this oral transmission of information was crucially important in early-medieval medicine. In fact, both Keil and Stoll found that short prescriptions, or medical bits of advice, made up most of the literature and general medical lore circulating in Europe—and in England, it is fair to assume (see U. Stoll and Keil and Schnitzer, "Einleitung," 7).

The genre is rich, varied, and defies modern characterization that does it justice within our accepted norm for what constitutes medicine. It is medical, herbal, religious, imprecise by modern standards, superstitious, and tailored to individual patients in its diagnoses and prescriptions. Its practitioners were trained healers. And below I show that many of its practices and remedies are withstanding modern trials.

Role of the monasteries

Evolution of the medical tradition in early-medieval Europe is a thread that runs throughout the seminal articles a book about the Lorsch monastery remedy book and early-medieval medicine, *Das Lorscher Arzneibuch und die frühmittelalterliche Medizin*, which brings together papers from a 1991 medical-history symposium in Lorsch, Germany. The symposium centered around a Latin medical manuscript called *Das Lorscher Arzneibuch* (also known as the *Bamberger Codex*), the first medical compilation made in German lands and similar in nature to the Latin *Herbarium of Pseudo-Apuleius*. It dates to about 790 CE and was likely associated with Carolingian reforms, particularly Charlemagne's ordinances known as *Capitulare* that dealt with the social good.[30]

The Lorsch contributors portray Benedictine monasteries as major sources of medical knowledge in Europe in the early Middle Ages, including England. Not only were medical texts like the *Herbarium of Pseudo-Apuleius* copied, excerpted, and used as references by monks who treated sick people, but the monks and their infirmaries/hospitals were also a source for medical information on healing, medicines, and growing and collecting medicinal herbs.[31] This knowledge was passed orally and in written form from monks and nuns to others within their orders, to patients, and to lay persons who also served as healers outside the monastery walls. According to Gundolf Keil, "Monasteries established themselves as central locations for medical care in populated areas, and finally, monasteries determined to act as arbiters in transmitting the breadth and variety of the medical tradition."[32]

An admittedly small sample of general histories of medicine in German and French suggests that the role of monasteries is simply accepted as an integral part of early-medieval medicine everywhere. For example, in the early twentieth century at about the time Payne gave the lecture mentioned above, Max Neuburger, professor of medicine at Vienna, wrote a detailed history of Western medicine during the medieval period. Unlike similar studies in English that tend to focus on "Anglo-Saxon" medicine in isolation, this German study included Anglo-Saxon England as a matter of course in relating what was going on throughout Europe. Though not downplaying the long hiatus in medical progress and the extremely hard times during centuries of invasion and recovery everywhere, Neuburger does describe in some detail what was happening in caregiving, the texts that were being written, the role of the Benedictines in keeping learning alive, their establishing hospitals, and so forth.[33] Rather than seeing *Klostermedizin* (monastic medicine) as an abomination, he portrays it as a bastion of safety.

More recently, Karl-Heinz Leven echoes this assessment in describing how early-medieval medicine developed while invasions and tribal migrations were raging, affecting the entire West. In a slender handbook aimed at general audiences, the German physician/historian speaks of a system of monasteries and infirmaries being founded by Benedictine monks. It was based on the early Christian church's embracing what he calls an entirely new concept of charity formulated in the New Testament.[34] As far as how Dark Age medicine fares against classical, Leven says that it is difficult, looking backward, to try to break medicine into periods; he finds that medieval medicine was for the most part grounded in the classical tradition, so that no meaningful separation can be made between the two. In fact, he finds many aspects of early modern medicine before about 1800 could be called "medieval," so even this differentiation is not clear.[35]

In a more detailed recent study, French physician and historian Roger Dachez devotes chapter six to the "shadows and highlights of medicine during the Middle Ages" ("Ombres et Lumières de la Médecine au Moyen Age"). It is essentially the same story as found in the two German works, with a similar detailed account of monastic medicine as in Neuberger. He relates that about AD 530, Benedict founded the first monastery in the West at Monte Cassino in Italy, and created an order of monks and a written rule for them to follow:

> From that foundation, numerous other monasteries spread throughout most of Europe, first in Italy near Pavia, then into Germanic countries, such as at

St. Gall or Cologne, finally into England at Oxford, York, or Canterbury. Later other orders of monks were founded, notably in France at Cluny, Clairvaux and Cîteaux.

author's paraphrase of the French original[36]

Monastic medicine continues to be studied, for example, at the University of Würzburg, Germany in the Forschergruppe Klostermedizin, founded in 1999, but with roots going back to the 1980s in several departments. Here, an interdisciplinary group of researchers studies several aspects of the tradition and its time, including texts, medicinal plants used, and their efficacy (information at www.klo stermedizin.de). Its website explains the scope of its studies:

> Monastic medicine is seen first of all as a period in the history of medicine, not a type of medical treatment. For this reason, no information about the so-called medicine of Hildegard von Bingen will be found here, but instead historical information about her and her works. The research group understands its mission to be fundamental research into the history of pharmacy and medicine in cooperation with clinical pharmaceutical studies.
>
> *author's paraphrase of German original*[37]

It has long been acknowledged that learning and books began arriving in early-medieval England as early as the seventh century with Benedictine monks.[38] Philologist and historian M.A. D'Aronco notes in several publications that in early Western Europe, monastic duties included care of the sick, monasteries had infirmaries, and monastic gardens in which medicinal plants were grown became famous.[39] These infirmaries are an important part of the history of hospitals, and they are often called hospitals in the literature. However their supposed size and level of available care might mark them more as infirmaries, as the term is understood today.[40]

Yet mention of monks, monasteries, and faith, and their role in the medical tradition of early-medieval Western Europe seems to be sparse in the English-speaking countries whose background has been staunchly Protestant for centuries. This neglect, possibly unconscious, may have begun as it did in other areas with the biases of nineteenth-century scholars. Many of them, like Cockayne, were ordained Church of England clergy. Their biases have cast long shadows, apparently one of them over the role of Christianity in medicine during this period. At that time in the West, Christianity was of course the very early Roman Catholic Church with its expanding network of monasteries. Given the rigorously secular modern mindset in parts of the world, and given certainly deplorable twists and turns within that church over the thousand years since the Old English *Herbarium* was created, the exclusion of such topics as monasticism and medicine from any field is understandable, but shortsighted.[41]

The role of faith in healing was publicly asserted in the 1879 founding of the Christian Science Church (First Church of Christ, Scientist) and is echoed in the writings of at least one modern physician, Victoria Sweet, who studied the philosophy and medicine of medieval abbess Hildegard von Bingen.[42] However, such voices have remained far in the background. A slight but palpable nod to the role some form spirituality has always played in medicine is in no small part due to increased public interest in and resurgence of what are often called complementary healing methods. They include herbalism in its several forms and systems outside mainstream evidence-based medicine; for example, Eastern healing systems, acupuncture, energy work, meditation, and yoga.[43] Yet bringing any hint of mainstream religion into a discussion of medicine or healing appears to have its own perplexing aspects, while superstition and charms in systems considered primitive are sought after. (What is called the "placebo effect" in medicine is another topic entirely.)

A collection of papers by several noted medieval scholars titled *Religion and Medicine in the Middle Ages* is an example of such exclusion. The book focuses on medicine after 1100 and does not consider monastic medicine at all, which three reviewers note.[44] Linda Voigts, one of them, although praising the papers, concludes, "Its lacunae, particularly 'monastic medicine', also proclaim how far we still have to go."[45] Two decades later, the lacunae have not yet been filled. In a discussion of translation in the previous chapter, I note that exclusion plays an important role in which books are chosen to be translated, and which are not. Silence, acting as exclusionary concerning monastic medicine in early-medieval England, is deafening in many studies.

On the other hand, a recent inclusive study by Ciaran Arthur ties the *Old English Herbarium*, the *Leechbooks*, and *Lacnunga* together both through the dates of the manuscripts in which they are found and spiritually. Breaking with earlier studies that see charms, incantations, and other supposed non-medical material as primarily local and heathen, Arthur ties them to the liturgy of the Roman Catholic Church, and to its prayers and practices.[46] Presenting similar ideas with equally convincing evidence—particularly concerning the vast number of overlooked texts in Latin—is Claire Burridge's "Healing Body and Soul in early-Medieval Europe."[47] Admittedly the *Herbarium* has the least "extra-medical" material of the three major Old English medical texts; however, any study of healing practices and the texts known to have been available and used anywhere in Europe cannot be complete if it excludes the interlinked system of monasteries. It is crucial to understanding the medical texts and medicine as practiced nearly everywhere.

Demonstrable evidence of how Christianity spread is the basis for *The Introduction of Christianity into the Early-Medieval Insular World* by a group of researchers using archaeology, artifacts, and related tangible evidence.[48] Excavations of small and large monasteries and the settlements they were in, including England, are part of it, showing evidence of infirmaries and gardens, or the lack of any such places, and providing many more details about the interactions of the monasteries and the communities in which they were located. Archaeology, ethnobotany, herbalism, art and art history, literature, hagiography: any field that might shed light on the period are used or suggested as sources to consider. The same approach specifically to medicine in early-medieval England would help to understand the practice and transmission of medical knowledge at that time. Many studies assume the transmission was primarily in written form and use it to explain why translations of the material were made into Old English.

For example, with regard to early-medieval medical texts, the editors of a volume titled *Agents of Transmission, Translation and Transformation* sum up nicely an ideal, primarily textual approach to a manuscript complex such as medical texts that were copied, translated, excerpted, and appropriated in widespread locations over many centuries:

> What was transmitted, translated and transformed was the legacy of the civilizations that emerged around the Mediterranean in the last two millennia BCE, particularly in Greece, Rome and the near East. More specifically, our project stressed the importance of the interchange of ancient legacies for understanding medieval textual cultures (transmission and translation), by recognizing that reception is a creative cultural act (transformation).[49]

However, missing—outside the scope of almost all such studies—is attention to the medical text itself and how it was used. The real study of such texts should very much involve the moment when a medical writing is in the hands—or more often in the head and memory—of a user. This was a healing practice that was disseminated both orally and in writing, and we tend to look at only one part of it.[50]

In the first chapter of *The Book in Britain: A Historical Introduction*, Siân Echard considers such details as who read books, who did not read books but heard them, who copied books, and why, in the earliest decades of Anglo-Saxon England (Echard points out that the Celts in Roman Britain and afterward were literate to some extent, unlike the Teutonic invaders). The chapter examines a place and time where oral transmission was the way in which stories and knowledge were customarily spread, and it assesses how the written word and a belief system based on texts impacted it.

Supremely foreign to modern thinking is a world that functions well largely without the written word (note that Roman aqueducts and Christian cathedrals were built without it). Echard explains that

> Throughout the Middle Ages, "textual communities" could organize themselves around the centrality of a book like the Bible, and even though the vast majority of people in those communities could not read, whether in Latin or in the vernacular, their lives could be profoundly influenced by books.[51]

It would be interesting to consider whether medical texts were assembled and translated and some actually written in Old English primarily to be able to read them aloud in the vernacular to others. In this way, the information could be used to transmit information or to train infirmary workers and practicing medics. Perhaps the translations were **not** intended to be transmitted primarily in written form. And yet that is how they continue to be analyzed, primarily as writings, with language and textual tradition, etc. as the focus. Witness the title of a recent study, *Medical Texts in Anglo-Saxon Literary Culture*.[52] Emily Kesling's work is comprehensive, insightful, and the most recent a long line of Anglo-Saxon studies; the author does address medical practice of the time, but in a theoretical manner for the most part.

The *Old English Herbarium* belongs to a medical tradition nurtured and to a great extent spread by monasteries in both its textual and practical aspects, just like the kindred *Leechbook of Bald* and *Lacnunga*. Some details especially in the two latter works could be unique to early-medieval England where they were created, but they become fully comprehensible only when considered as parts of a larger medical continuum in which Benedictine monasteries played an important role.

Using living traditions of healing to comprehend early-medieval medical practice

This study began some time ago simply as a translation and scholarly study of a medieval herbal. However as the work progressed, and in contrast to what was being said in existing studies about it, I began to have a hunch that the *Old English Herbarium* could actually have been used by healers of the time (and by extension so could similar writings).

The medicinal herbs in it made me wonder whether herbalism as practiced in New Mexico, where I lived, might help me understand the text. I began to explore the local *curanderismo* tradition in workshops and lectures, then to take classes in modern herbal medicine, both as a non-practitioner.[53] Undertaking such practical study was suggested, if indirectly, by many of the approaches to medieval medicine cited here, especially by the ground-breaking work of Voigts, Riddle, D'Aronco, Cameron, and Bart Holland. Using what I was learning from practicing healers, I realized that the *Old English Herbarium* was clearly a text with meaningful—if cryptic—content. To understand it was no mystery, but essential to understanding it was familiarity with how herbal medicine is practiced and how its remedies are made, much like understanding terse recipes by learning how to cook.

Some years later, I was part of a conference in London at which the Herbal History Research Network (HHRN) was launched.[54] There I became acquainted with modern herbal practitioners in the United Kingdom and their related but much more learned practice of medical herbalism. It became obvious to me that theirs was a different system from the one in New Mexico, though both are closely related. Medical herbalism involved rigorous training, standardized diagnoses, and treatment based on theory using both texts and experience—in other words, a tradition closer to medicine/pharmacy as it developed when the early-medieval system became one that was increasingly text based.

Understanding the value and methods of a healing system using medicinal plants as the primary therapeutics requires a shift in expectations and a need to open up to a different practice than is customary in the West. Becoming familiar with such systems while studying medieval medical texts can allow textual scholars to get closer to the mindset of medieval healers and helps in interpreting their texts. Consulting with medical herbalists who share an interest in older texts while engaged in the study is even more ideal.[55]

To understand how a partially unwritten body of knowledge about plants and healing survived fairly intact over many centuries and in many geographical locales, the living, ancient *curandero* (folk-healer) tradition of the Southwestern United States not only serves as a model, but its roots can be traced to part of the medical tradition discussed here. *Curanderismo*, a folk practice stemming from medieval European medicine and its texts, persisted for centuries largely by means other than through texts, similar to what happened in the early-medieval world. (Modern medical herbalism has the same roots as well, but can trace its lineage unbroken to the texts and practice of Western Europe.[56])

Curandera/os—healers using herbs and ritual—came to the New World from medieval Spain with remedies from Europe and even Morocco. Through the years, the tradition picked up information and ingredients from indigenous populations in the New World, and added even more to the stock of information as settlers moved into the Southwestern regions of the United States beginning in about 1700. The European medical tradition from which it stemmed included university-trained physicians, herbalists, apothecaries, and folk healers who practiced at the same time, but in different social strata. The colonizers of New Mexico were not the upper class for the most part. The medicinal ingredients for all healers were essentially the same no matter the social class, yet university-trained physicians tended to use expensive imports along with the common herbs.

No small part of the common medical culture was the body of knowledge, written and unwritten, about medicinal plants, which made its inexact way through the hands and words of many during the course of two millennia—and which continues. For example, there is evidence that Phillip II of Spain provided funds to Francisco Hernandez, one of his physicians, to go to New Spain in 1570 to record the plants and animals—the *materia medica*—of the New World. Hernandez based his information on a written Aztec codex and on exhaustive interviews with local inhabitants and one personal experience with the drugs. The outcome was his *Rerum Medicarum Novae Hispaniae Thesaurus*, which had an unhappy subsequent history. But the point here is that, along with a search for gold, the old world was looking at the new for a new pharmacopoeia, presumably largely in plant form.[57]

An appeal to the living and changing *curandero* tradition in the Southwestern United States lends credibility to the argument that by considering the presence of a common, largely unwritten, and constantly evolving tradition of healing during late antique and early-medieval periods in Europe, the medical tradition of those times can be better understood. The *curandero* tradition is similar to the medieval one, because of its roots in medieval Europe, and because the situation under which it began in the United States (then a Spanish territory) shows remarkable similarities to the situation in early-medieval England, or for that matter to most of Europe then.

It was a world where peoples were conquered, sometimes repeatedly, or over time merged with the conquerors or migrated into unfamiliar locales and adapted, taking much with them in their memories and adding new information to it. The knowledge any healer had, Saxon leech, monastic healer, or Spanish *curandero*, was for the most part passed down from person to person and it was based on knowledge of the use of plants—this kind of treatment can be traced in the texts. Ritual was part of healing from the earliest days. When familiar plants were not available, new ones with a similar appearance or smell were tried. In New Mexico, local Pueblo Indians shared their medical lore and plants with the Spanish/Mexican settlers.[58]

As mentioned above, Clemens Stoll outlined a similar situation throughout Europe which prevailed from the time of Christ: the Roman army and its entourage bringing plants, texts, physicians, the conquered people picking up some of this knowledge and adding to their own healing lore, then being themselves trained and combining old knowledge with new and passing it on. It would have been the same with the medieval monks and their medicine. In fact Stoll describes how medical training occurred in the monasteries, and it is markedly similar to today's *curandero's* apprenticeship:

> With regard to the multiplicity of remedies, the imprecision of the nomenclature, and the uncertainty in measurements, the question arises concerning the scientific and practical knowledge of the monks who were responsible for preparing the medications. The practical skills and experience could only have been gained during a long period in a monastic pharmacy (where medicines are prepared), such as the pharmacies shown in the plans for monasteries during the Carolingian period. *This knowledge would have been transmitted personally from one monk to another.* Above all, the itinerant Irish monks, for whom the monasteries on the Continent served as havens, for example St. Gall, Lorsch, or Reichenau, spread that kind of knowledge from their home monasteries.
>
> *emphasis added in author's translation*[59]

The person-to-person distribution of medical knowledge that existed in colonial New Spain persists in New Mexico (to cite one instance of how this tradition was kept alive). About the tradition, Michael Moore, a recognized specialist in the herbal tradition of the Southwest, writes:

> The New Mexican, either indio, primo, or anglo, is surrounded by plants whose medicinal uses are known and systematized by hundreds and thousands of years of usage. The remedios in this little book are a complete hybrid of two cultures. The spanish primos brought their traditional herbs, such as Manzanilla and Alhucema; the pueblo indians introduced them to Inmortal and Osha. Present usage is the result of nearly four hundred years of Spanish and over a thousand years of Indian pragmatism. ... What I have compiled

in this book is what I have learned, observed and used as of 1977, a frozen cross-section of a moving stream.[60]

In his book, similar to medieval medical texts, Moore lists the Spanish, Latin, and English names for the plants and their primary and secondary uses.

Moore's observations were validated during a week-long seminar "Medicinal Plants of the Southwest" held at Ghost Ranch, New Mexico, in June 1997, taught by three practicing herbalists who gathered their plants in the wild and obtained them from commercial sources. As the workshop leaders pointed out, for anyone, yesterday and today, who collects plants in the wild, as opposed to growing or obtaining them from another, a difficult part of the task is simply being able to identify the plants in the field. Even armed with a modern field guide to herbs and with photos and drawings, identification is often only made possible by familiarity with the plant itself. Sometimes only a slight difference is crucial; for example, the slightly sticky feel of a true cleavers (clivers), which has medicinal properties, is all that distinguishes it from a non-medicinal and similar-looking brother growing nearby. All three of the workshop leaders operated from a similar body of knowledge about herbs and plants and ingredients used in preparing them, but each one had slight variations on what might be prescribed for a given condition, or differed in opinion on the best remedy for another. A strategy of starting with a small dose to see what works and being willing to alter the remedy was the rule, as was the most important ingredient—patience. Unlike pharmaceutical drugs, herbs (poisonous ones excepted) do not usually work immediately.

Familiarity with the flora and familiarity with families of plants is essential to the tradition of gathering plants to use medicinally (or for food, for that matter): texts are only a reminder. Such must have been the case with the medieval medical texts, whose illustrations have long been considered worthless in identifying the plants to which they refer. It is possible, indeed probable, the illustrations were never intended to be any kind of field guide, but served as aids to memory. After all, plants look different at different points in their growing cycle, and a picture (or photo) captures it at one point in its life. Essential is experience in the field with identification, the knowledge when it is best to gather each plant, and the part of parts of the plant to be used.

The possible efficacy of the remedies has been questioned on much the same grounds. Five or six different plants (or more) in several locations throughout the manuscript are suggested to help heal a condition with no accompanying guidelines on which to choose. This is not the way moderns would like things to be, and here, both *curanderismo* and the practice of herbal medicine can help in understanding the medieval text.

Plants may help either alone or with other plants, and experienced healers who know them have their own preferences and do not require detailed instructions to administer them. Writing about preparation of such medicines in the medieval world, C. Stoll[61] said:

To the almost countless numbers of simples [remedies using one plant], early medieval medicine added a large choice of composites [remedies using several plants]. Here, the monks served to organize and collect the texts that had been scattered and then they made them useful for and accessible to the monasteries. . . . The early medieval monks took antidotes and remedies from classical works and often adapted them to local and personal needs, for which reason hardly any of the anonymous collections of remedies agrees fully with another.

"Arznei," 175–6

Illuminating to the topic here is Stoll's point that many of the preparations differ ever so slightly from one compilation to another, even though they use similar ingredients for similar treatments. And particularly significant is the fact that substitutions were commonly made using a plant or other ingredient with similar properties, a trend seen in the later Middle Ages in extensive lists of possible *quid pro quo* substitutions. This same practice was seen to be alive and well in the classes and workshops on herbalism I attended.

The situation in New Mexico, with its mingling of cultures and a sharing of information in whatever form available, written or from memory, does not differ appreciably from what is written about early-medieval Europe. The difficulty on this level—person to person, often both unlettered—is that no record remains of any of their transactions and conversations. The outcome, years later, of these transactions may be the only witness to their having occurred. The slight changes in copies and versions of medieval medical texts witness to much unrecorded information altered by human interactions over the course of many years in many countries, and help explain how the common reservoir of knowledge about healing and plants was spread both by texts and in person.

In "Theory and Practice in Medieval Medicine," John Riddle wrote:

Although speculative medical theory was almost totally abandoned, fifth-century through tenth-century records show that medical progress was not solely dependent on written language. Instead this evidence shows that a medical practice existed based upon a pharmacy that not only preserved the older practical knowledge but also recognized and used new drugs.

"Theory," 159

Particularly relevant here is his argument that oral as well as written transmission of knowledge occurred over many years in medieval Europe:

When one particular part of an herb, say a root, was found as being effective for some specific action, this information was orally transmitted whenever and wherever men communicated and one generation taught the other. This process takes place independently of literary transmission. There was a continuous practice of medicine which was independent of loss, attrition, or,

> eventually, the recovery of classical medical theory. Far from being a gray
> science in a gray, confused period, early medieval medicine was a partly
> empirical skill. … The assumption that one can know early medieval medi-
> cine simply in identifying the texts is faulty.
>
> *"Theory,"* 165

New World *curanderismo* suggests that Riddle's theory can be validated through a
living tradition.

It appears, then, that an important aspect of early-medieval medical writings
awaits additional attention. Source studies, philological studies, isolation of supposed
barbaric from classical elements, and similar research have immense value to demonstrate what happened **in the texts**. However such careful evidence captures only
part of any healing tradition; technical texts by their nature have both written and
unwritten aspects, i.e., explicit and tacit knowledge. On a much simpler lever, it's
like exploring the sources and variants of very old cooking recipes and never trying
to follow the directions in practice. Reasons for changes in medical manuscripts as
they were translated or copied may have stemmed at least in part from unwritten
shared knowledge and/or the monks and other practitioners' interpreting rather
than blindly translating.

The *Old English Herbarium* as a practical text

Like work in the United Kingdom by the National Institute of Medical Herbalists,
the American Herbalists Guild promotes the legitimacy of its profession in regular
scientific reports in the publications of the American Botanical Council.[62] Its
publications and Website and similar sources provide a wealth of verified scientific information about medical herbalism and herbs to the public and the medical
profession. However, the warning with which historian Duffin begins her medical
history applies to research into the efficacy of medical herbs and medical herbalism;
the initial questions that guide research goals tend to determine the outcomes. The
humanities are no different from the sciences in this regard, and the questions we
ask of history often determine the answers we obtain from research into the past.

In the twenty-first century, the first question about herbal medicine, ancient or
modern, is usually, "Does it work?" Since at least the nineteenth century, the answer
has been a resounding "no," absent any proof. Currently, what is said to *work* in
terms of evidence-based medicine may not mean the same thing as it does in other
healing systems. *To work* can mean to *cure* but it can also denote *improve symptoms* or
simply *make a person feel better*. Semantics aside, evidence-based medicine requires
experimental proof that a treatment or drug works in effecting a defined result;
what is not always calculated in its working is at what cost and the impact of related
side effects.

Modern experiments are in fact demonstrating the effectiveness of individual
medicinal plants and even of certain Old English remedies. One of the earliest such
studies was "A drynke þat men callen dwale to make a man to slepe whyle men

kerven him: A surgical anesthetic from late Medieval England." Here, Linda Voigts and Robert Hudson sought evidence in numerous Middle English manuscripts that surgical anesthetics were used and, when they were found, the ingredients they contained. The authors found recipes for an anesthetic called *dwale* in at least 27 different manuscripts, and theirs was one of the first scientific approaches to the contents of early herbals and recipe books. About their approach, they wrote:

> We also think it helpful to draw on the resources of twentieth-century pharmacological knowledge to analyze the recipe [for *dwale*]. It must be understood, however, that the use of current pharmacological literature has distinct limitations when applied to texts like *dwale*. Pharmacology today involves a high degree of accuracy in identification and quantification that cannot exist for medieval medicinal compounds. Indeed, nineteenth-century dispensatories are more useful for studying medieval medicine than are today's textbooks of pharmacology. Older dispensatories provide details of pharma-cognosy, medical indications, methods of preparation, warnings, dosages, and so on that no longer appear in current descriptions of highly standardized, often synthetic medicaments.[63]

Ingredients were analyzed in turn, including what each was mixed with, to find out whether such a recipe would work in producing sleep, and if so why. The authors cite a similar approach by M.L. Cameron, who had examined a text long thought to be magic because it prohibited the use of iron. Cameron looked at the recipe not as a magical text, but from the standpoint of a scientist, questioning whether using an iron container would have affected the ingredients in any way. The answer was yes, and the recipe was found to be based on observation and experience.

Such was Voigts's and Hudson's approach. A careful study of the ingredients and the instructions on how to administer the drink as well as the details about how to awaken the patient (use vinegar and salt on the temples, 37) led them to the con-clusion that this Middle English *stupefactive*, as it was called, did work and that the ingredients were carefully prescribed and thought out. An interesting conclusion they reached was that *dwale* may have been an English invention; soporific sponges were the rule on the continent and *dwale* was the only native English name for a medicinal recipe found in Middle English texts.

Voigts and Hudson's study also suggests that imprecision is actually not a nega-tive aspect of traditional herbal remedies, medieval or modern; they draw their strength from the healer's knowledge about the patient and the observed symptoms, and about the available plants and recipes that might help. Again from the article on *dwale*:

> What we cannot know, of course, is the dosage. The recipe, which says the patient should drink until he falls asleep, is vague on that point, but that vagueness may be deliberate. Even if we assume that the names in the recipe correspond to current terminology, several factors underscore the possible

variations in a medieval recipe. We cannot identify the plant species with certainty, and the time and method of collection and the preparation all result in variations in the amount of active ingredient present. It is almost certain that large differences in amounts of active ingredients were the rule, a situation that is emphasized repeatedly in the twentieth century. Adding to these uncertainties are the idiosyncratic reactions to drugs and anesthetics that still vex medicine today. … All these variables, over which the medieval medical practitioner has no control, suggest that the practice of giving *dwale* until the patient fell asleep was undoubtedly safer than giving some prescribed amount.

Dwale, 42

An early advocate for studying scientifically the possible efficacy of medieval remedies, botanist M.L. Cameron wrote that a quarter of the drugs used in medicine are from flowering plants or are synthetic and copy products made from plants, adding the farsighted remark:

Much evaluation of plants and their medicinal value is now in progress in pharmaceutical laboratories and the results are often of much interest. The greater part of the identifiable ingredients of the Anglo-Saxon pharmacopoeia are still to be found in herbal collections and are used for the same purposes, so that we may say that Anglo-Saxon remedies were probably as good as those recommended by herbalists today. Moreover, a surprisingly large number of their ingredients are known from recent investigation to contain substances of real therapeutic value and to have been used by them for conditions where their therapeutic value should have had beneficial effects … as good as anything available up to the end of the nineteenth century.[64]

In addition, also in an early study, John Mann, professor of organic chemistry at Reading, demonstrated the scientific basis for many folk remedies, a number of which are herbal. He wrote,

The remedies that we buy are often the same as those which were prescribed 5000 years ago. The same can be said for many of the medicines we use, and the aim of this book is to demonstrate how at least some of the substances used for murder, magic, and folk medicine have been successfully transformed into clinically acceptable drugs.[65]

Unlike when these studies were published, research into the effectiveness of individual medicinal plants can now be found with easy Internet searches and is reported in many books and journals on herbalism.[66] Yet most medieval remedies employ more than one plant. At issue is whether the preparations with multiple ingredients can also be shown to be effective. A matter of continuing debate is whether a remedy must be replicated as described in the old text using plants or parts of them, or whether the modern approach of determining and then using only their active components will give the same results. Many herbalists side with using real plants to duplicate the original remedy.

In 2015, media across the globe spread the news of a startling discovery from the University of Nottingham: that an eye salve in the Old English *Leechbooks* was more effective against staph infection than many modern drugs.[67] The results and a study of medieval remedies generally by the interdisciplinary team that investigated the salve are summarized in "Could Medieval Medicine Help the Fight Against Antimicrobial Resistance," available open access as part of a book titled *Making the Medieval Relevant*.[68] The remedy came from *Bald's Leechbook* and was made using a species of allium, garlic, wine, and oxgall all mixed in a copper bowl. The many sources listed in this study indicate that investigations into the possible efficacy of early-medieval remedies had been afoot for some time, such as Frances Watkins's 2013 dissertation on antimicrobials from native British plants.[69] Such scientific studies are becoming more common as interest in medicinal herbs and herbalism grows. These studies and readily available information about the effectiveness of medicinal herbs are helping to reestablish the reputation of this ancient tradition.[70]

Evaluating remedies in the *Old English Herbarium*

Whether a remedy in the *Old English Herbarium* can be proved scientifically to work is a matter for specialist and pharmaceutical researchers to determine, such as those mentioned above. However, it can be shown that the plants in the *Herbarium* could have been grown, obtained, and used in early-medieval England, and the work should not be deemed useless for its time. It does not represent some kind of higher medical knowledge beyond the reach of the monks, midwives, and leeches. The majority of the remedies in the *Herbarium* could have been prepared with no eso-teric ingredients or equipment, and they, like those in Dioscorides, like those in the sixteenth-century Culpepper's *Herbal*, and like those in scores of twentieth-century publications, are based on simple methods of preparation and generally on a plant or plants and a few other fairly common ingredients. Granted, however, medieval ingredients may not always be common in our modern urban environment.

The preparations in the *Old English Herbarium* are on the surface quite simple. The numbers following each excerpt below refer to chapters in the *Herbarium*, standard in every edition. The translations here are the author's:

> For liver disturbances, pick some vervain on Midsummer's day, and crush it into a powder; take five spoonfuls of the powder and three draughts of good wine; mix them together and give to the patient to drink.
>
> *4*

> For a headache, take some basil, crush it with rose or myrtle juice [probably the essence of these plants] or vinegar and put it on the forehead.
>
> *119*

[Rue] Soak the leaves in old wine, then put the extract into a glass container; afterwards apply it. [Dioscorides has a whole chapter on wines used in medicines.] Pound the rue in a wooden bowl, then pick up as much as you can grasp with three fingers, put it into a container and add a draught of wine mixed with two draughts of water, then give it as a drink.

117

[Take leek] ... lard, bread, and coriander. Pound them together as you would to make a poultice and lay this on ...

125

The reference to Midsummer's day in remedy 4 has been said to be a bit of magic, but most probably it indicates when the plant is best to harvest.

The remedies call for seething, boiling, and mixing plants with fats and waxes, crushing and chopping them, drying them, and making decoctions and teas, to name but a few of the procedures. In the twentieth century, M. Grieve's *A Modern Herbal* gives the following quite similar directions for medicinal remedies:

An infusion may be made by pouring a pint of boiling water on an ounce of the bruised root [of angelica] and two tablespoonfuls of this should be given three or four times a day, or the powdered root administered in doses of 10 to 30 grains.

Grieve, 38

Black Bryony is a popular remedy for removing discoloration caused by bruises and black eyes, etc. The fresh root is scraped to a pulp and applied in the form of a poultice. For sores, old writers recommend it being made into a ointment with hog's grease or wax, or other convenient ointment.

Grieve, 131[71]

And they are the same as found in works written about Southwestern herbal medicine as practiced by the *curanderas*:

[Hediondilla or Chaparal Bush] Primary: a poultice for rheumatism. Method A: Slowly pan fry the leaves in lard, cool, and apply. Method B: Grind with Osha and Tobacco, mix with beeswax or Trementina, warm and apply. A pint of the leaves can be boiled in a gallon of water for an hour and used in a bath. Remain until the water is cool; not recommended more than once every several months.

Moore, 10

[Moradilla or Dakota Vervain] ... the powdered tops can be mixed with lard or vaseline and applied to the back of the neck for pain.[72]

Yet the examples cited are in works written for an interested general public and what might be termed popular herbalists. On the surface, they are quite similar to the medieval medical texts, and are based on the same ancient tradition with the same types of preparations. What differs over time are the practitioners who use them and the medical expertise with which they read and use their texts.

A comparison of Grieve and Moore's instructions with the three-to-four-page essays on individual plants and how to use them in more recent works by trained medical herbalists Tobyn, Denham and Whitelegg, and the methodologies in Brice-Ytsma and Watkins is telling. The latter two books are aimed at well-trained herbalists, but written in a style accessible to all. The ancient tradition to which the *Old English Herbarium* and other such works belong is in new and competent hands, whose shared expertise could help textual scholars decipher what is in the early-medieval medical texts, both said and unsaid. The difference between all of these modern works highlights how far medical herbalism has come in being reestablished and (re-) accepted as a legitimate practice in the modern world. Modern herbalism in all its forms offers translators of older medical texts the possibility to recapture at least some of the tacit information buried in the written words of their manuscripts.

The preface to the *Old English Herbarium* that Cockayne wrote in the 1860s for the Rolls Series paints a Dark Age picture of medieval medicine generally and casts doubts about the usefulness of the *Herbarium* to early-medieval England. In contrast, this study documents that the *Herbarium* and the Latin works on which it was based were important and useful texts. Specifically within the narrower pantheon of Old English medical texts, classifying the *Herbarium* as a purely classical/rational work, thus by inference or stated as having existed largely in the world of books, does not do it justice. Evidence points to its having been part of a rich, varied, and unique early-medieval tradition, monastic medicine, that was similar throughout Europe. The preparations are not difficult or esoteric, and many ingredients could have been grown, collected, or imported.

Lay and monastic practitioners were part of this tradition, with some of the information transmitted in texts, some orally. This kind of transmission is markedly similar to the practice of *curanderismo* the Southwest, a healing tradition that began in medieval Spain and came to the New World, where it mingled with First Nation practices. It is also the way practical wisdom is transmitted in any kind of technical field, even applied nuclear physics, where written instructions can only make up part of knowledge transmission.

Read as a guide to medicinal plants recommended for given conditions accompanied by advice on how to make remedies using them, the *Old English Herbarium* could—in the right hands—serve as a sort of a primer on herbal medicine as practiced a thousand years ago. It is part of a very long historical chain of such works. However, without the tacit (unwritten) knowledge only an experienced practitioner has, the remedies as written in this work may seem imprecise, incomplete, and useless. Teams are now investigating their efficacy and individual studies are being made on the medicinal values of the plants often with a great amount of success. The *Old English Herbarium* and many of its medieval kin are finally transcending the dark cloud cast upon them in the nineteenth century and showing their vivid colors.

Notes

1 Jacalyn Duffin, *History of Medicine: A Scandalously Short Introduction* (Toronto: University of Toronto Press, third edition, 2021), ix, is widely used in medical schools today. Duffin breaks modern Western medicine into its specialties and looks back through the history of each. This division suggests that the specialization begun in the nineteenth century makes it difficult today to write about the history of medicine as a whole. In the West, we see medicine in terms of specialties rather than as a monolith, and this way of thinking affects how older medical systems are assessed.

2 The components include *Pseudo-Apulei Herbarius*, the longest, which is a fourth/fifth century herbal from the Mediterranean area; *De herba vettonica* attributed to (pseudo) Antonius Musa and is material about betony that became the entire first section of the Old English work; the *Liber medicinae ex herbis femininis* and *Curae herbarum*, both herbals attributed to Dioscorides, but popular works on their own.

3 For the Latin and other sources, consult Niles and D'Aronco 2023, which will update long-standing authority, Hubert Jan De Vriend, *The Old English Herbarium and Medicina de Quadrupedibus*, EETS, O.S. 286 (London: Oxford University Press, 1984), lv–lxviii; also Ernst Howald and Henry E. Sigerist, *Antonii Musae de Herba Vettonica Liber, Pseudo-Apulei Herbarius, Anonymi de Taxone Liber, etc.* in *Corpus Medicorum Latinorum*, Vol. 4 (Leipzig, 1927).

4 Doyle, dissertation "Anglo-Saxon Medicine," 33–4, also stresses the need in any study of the Old English medical writings, to take into account all the Latin medical texts available in England before 1000 and his is primarily a philological study. Yet many remain unedited, untranslated, and hard to access.

5 A detailed study of the medical manuscripts from this early period, including authors and scribes, is in Florence Eliza Glaze, "The Perforated Wall: The Ownership and Circulation of Medical Books in Medieval Europe, ca. 800–1200," Ph.D. dissertation, Department of History, Duke University, 2000.

6 For a discussion of the title and its author; Linda Ehrsam Voigts, "The Significance of the Name Apuleius to the Herbarium Apulei," *Bulletin of the History of Medicine*, Vol. 52 (1978): 214–27 and M.A. D'Aronco and M.L. Cameron, *The Old English Illustrated Pharmacopoeia* (Copenhagen: Rosenkilde and Bagger, 1998).

7 Augusto Beccaria, *I Codici di Medicina del Periodo Presalernitano (Secoli Ix, X e XI)* (Roma: Edisioni de Storia e Letteratura, 1956) remains the major source for medical manuscripts before Salerno.

8 The most recent translation is Dioscorides, *De Materia Medica*, transl., Lily Y. Beck, third rev. ed., (Hildesheim; New York: Olms-Weidmann, 2017). Latin translations were made soon after Dioscorides completed his work in Greek and they circulated throughout Europe, discussed in John A. Riddle, "The Textual Tradition of Dioscorides in the Latin West" in *Catalogus Translationum et Commentanorum*, ed., F. Edward Cranz Vol. IV (1980): 1–143.

9 Pliny the Elder, *Natural History*, transl., H. Rackham, Vols. 10 (London: Heinemann, 1938–62).

10 For example, studies such as Nicholas Everett, *The Alphabet of Galen: Pharmacy from Antiquity to the Middle Ages* (Toronto; Buffalo: University of Toronto Press, 2012); Rudolph E. Siegel, *Galen's System of Physiology and Medicine* (Basel: S. Karger, 1968).

11 Jerry Stannard, "Botanical Data and Late Mediaeval 'Rezeptliteratur'" in *Fachprosa-Studien: Beiträge zur mittelalterlichen Wissenschafts- und Geistesgeschichte*, ed., Gundolf Keil (Berlin: E. Schmidt, 1982), 390. The German word *Rezept* might be translated as recipe, prescription, or remedy. It simply means the directions for preparing a medication out of plants and other (mostly) natural substances as given in the medieval herbals and other medical texts. *Rezeptliteratur* is a specific term for the literature containing this lore, a genre discussed later in this chapter.

12 A thought-provoking reconsideration of the period is found in Bryan Ward-Perkins, *The Fall of Rome and the End of Civilization* (Oxford: Oxford University Press, 2005). Note that the "fall of civilization" here does not have its customary meaning. The concept of late antiquity was originally promoted by Peter Brown, *The World of Late Antiquity* (London: Harcourt Brace Jovanovich, 1971).

13 A detailed discussion of other authors whose medical writings are known to have circulated throughout the early-medieval period either in whole or in part is found in the Glaze and the Doyle dissertations.

14 Debby Banham, "Dun, Oxa and Pliny the Great Physician: Attribution and Authority in Old English Medical Texts," *Social History of Medicine*, Vol. 24, No. 1 (2011): 57–73. The volume has a number of informative articles.

15 Meaney, "Extra-Medical Elements," 56.

16 Peregrine Horden, "What's Wrong with Early Medieval Medicine," in *Cultures of Healing-Medieval and after: Collected Studies* (London: Routledge, Variorum Series, 2019): 146.

17 MacKinney, 28–9.

18 Jerry Stannard, "Marcellus of Bordeaux and the Beginnings of Medieval Materia Medica," *Pharmacy in History*, Vol. 15, No. 2 (1973): 47. Also, Max Niedermann, ed., *Marcellus Über Heilmittel*, 2nd ed., Vols. 2, (Berlin: Akademie Verlag, 1968).

19 D'Aronco and Cameron "Pharmacopoeia," 45.

20 John M. Riddle, "Theory and Practice in Medieval Medicine," *Viator: Medieval and Renaissance Studies*, Vol. V (1974): 157–84.

21 Discussed in Anne Van Arsdall, "The Transmission of Knowledge in Early-Medieval Medical Texts: An Exploration," in *Between Text and Patient: The Medieval Enterprise in Medieval and Early Modern Europe*, eds. Florence L. Glaze and Brian K. Nance (Firenze: SISMEL, 2011): 201–15. Its premise is that many early medical writings contain instructions that only become fully comprehensible when the unwritten "how to" part can somehow be supplied.

22 In a related event, in 1985 AVISTA was created as an organization devoted to the study of medieval science, technology, and art and it later added medicine to its scope, but not to its name. See www.avista.org. (Association Villard de Honnecourt for the Interdisciplinary Study of Technology, Science, and Art.)

23 Crossgrove, 50. By analogy, in future histories of twenty-first century medicine, how much space will be devoted to medicine outside mainstream Western practice, although "alternative medicines" serve a good deal of the global population.

24 Riddle, "Theory and Practice," 160–1.

25 Moreno Olalla, 12.

26 Examples are the articles in Jansen-Sieben, ed., *Artes Mechanicae en Europe médiévale/en middeleeuws Europa* (Bruxelles: Archives et Bibliothèques de Belgique, 1989), in particular Julius Jörimann, "Frühmittelalterliche Rezeptarien," Robert Halleux, "Recettes D'Artisan, Recettes D'Alchimiste," Gundolf Keil, "Die Medizinische Literatur des Mittelalters," and Carmélia Opsomer et Marc Binard, "Materiaux pour une Histoire Quantitative de la Pharmacopée Présalernitaine." Also consult the citations in D'Aronco and Cameron.

27 Henry E. Sigerist, *Studien und Texte zur frühmittelalterlichen Rezeptliteratur* (Leipzig: Verlag von J.A. Barth, 1923): 185–6. (transl., *Studies and texts for early-medieval Rezeptliteratur*) "Der gemeinsame Grundstock, den die [the Salernitan texts] haben, ist nichts anderes als gerade das Rezeptmaterial des 6/7. Jahrhunderts, zu dem im Laufe der Zeit gelegentlich neue Rezepte hinzukamen oder alte in modernisierter Form."

28 "So glaube ich denn auch, daß wir in den meisten Fällen originale Kompilationen vor uns haben, Sammelungen, die sich der Schreiber für seine klosterärztlichen Bedürfnisse zusammenstellte."

29 Ulrich Stoll, "Das Lorscher Arzneibuch: Ein Überblick über Herkunft, Inhalt und Anspruch des ältesten Arzneibuchs deutscher Provenienz," (transl., The Lorsch remedy book; overview of the origins, contents, and treatments in the oldest remedy book of Germany) in Keil and Schnitzer, 73 cited immediately following.

30 Gundolf Keil und Paul Schnitzer, eds., *Das Lorscher Arzneibuch und die Frühmittelalterliche Medizin: Verhandlungen des Medizinhistorischen Symposiums im September 1989 in Lorsch* (Lorsch: Verlag Laurissa, 1991). (transl., The Lorsch monastery remedy book and early-medieval medicine; proceedings of a symposium in 1989 at Lorsch.) The introduction has a brief overview of the manuscript, its relationship to the Carolingian reforms, and its place in medical history. *Bald's Leechbook* is a similar compilation, although one is in Latin and the other in Old English, but both used a variety of similar sources, only a few of which are in the vernacular.

31 Sigerist's writings are fundamental to this viewpoint. It is noteworthy that Singer often echoed Sigerist, who wrote earlier than he, but seldom cited Sigerist by name.

32 "Klöster stellten sich als Siedlungsmittelpunkte die medizinische Versorgung, und Klöster sind es gewesen, die als Schaltstellen der Wissenvermittlung über Umfang und Auswahl des medizinischen Traditionsangebotes entschieden." Gundolf Keil, "Möglichkeiten und Grenzen frühmittelalterlicher Medizin" (transl., The possibilities and limitations of early-medieval medicine) in Keil and Schnitzer, 225.

33 Max Neuburger, *History of Medicine*, transl., E. Playfair, Vol. II (London: Oxford University Press, 1915), originally published in German in 1905. Neuburger praises Alcuin (735–804 CE) as a "highly gifted Anglo-Saxon" who "disseminated the scientific traditions of the schools of York, Winchester, and Canterbury upon the continent. … " Sadly, Alcuin's name appears rarely in writings in English on Anglo-Saxon medicine.

34 Karl-Heinz Leven, *Geschichte der Medizin: von der Antike bis zur Gegenwart* (München: C.H. Beck, 2017): 33. (transl., History of medicine from classical times to the present) "Entscheidend neu war der Caritas-Gedanken, der im Neuen Testament (Mt 25, 36–40) formuliert war."

35 Ibid., 33.

> Periodisierungsversuche sind auch im Hinblick auf die Medizin schwierig. Die Medizin des Mittelalters gründete weitgehend auf der antiken Tradition, so dass keine deutliche Trennung auszumachen ist. Zahlreiche Züge der vormodernen Medizin waren bis gegen 1800 "mittelalterlich," so dass auch diese Abgrenzung unscharf ist.

36 Roger Dachez, *Histoire de la médecine: De l'Antiquité à nos jours* (Paris: Éditions Tallandier, 2021): 282.

> De cette fondation jaillirent de nombreuses autres un peu partout en Europe, mais d'abord en Italie, près de Pavie, puis dans les pays germaniques, comme à Saint-Gall ou Cologne, enfin en Angleterre, à Oxford, York ou Canterbury. Plus tard d'autres ordres naquirent, notamment en France avec Cluny, Clairvaux ou Cîteaux.

37
  Die Klostermedizin ist in erster Linie eine medizinhistorische Epoche und keine Therapierichtung. Deshalb finden Sie auf diesen Seiten keine Informationen zur sogenannten "Hildegard-Medizin", wohl aber zur historischen Person und zum Werk der Hildegard von Bingen. Die Forschergruppe versteht ihre Arbeit als pharmazie- und medizinhistorische Grundlagenforschung im Dialog mit pharmazeutisch-klinischen Studien.

38 For more information: Michael Lapidge, "The School of Theodore and Hadrian," *Anglo-Saxon England*, Vol. 15 (1986): 45–72.

39 Covered in M.A. D'Aronco, "The Benedictine Rule and the Care of the Sick: the Plan of St Gall and Anglo-Saxon England," in *The Medieval Hospital and Medical Practice*, AVISTA Studies in the History of Medieval Technology, Science, and Art, ed., B. Bowers (Aldershot: Ashgate, 2007): 235–51; and "How English is 'Anglo-Saxon' Medicine? The Latin Sources for Anglo-Saxon Medical Texts," in *Britannia Latina. Latin in the Culture of Great Britain from the Middle Ages to the Twentieth Century*, eds., Charles Burnett and Nicholas Mann (London: the Warburg Institute/Turin: Nino Aragano, 2005): 27–41.

40 Several papers on the role of monasteries in the early development of hospitals are in Peregrine Horden's *Cultures of Healing: Medieval and After* (New York: Routledge, 2019), a collection of the historian's papers over several decades. Though he acknowledges the role of monasteries in medicine, Horden is not especially confident that their practice had much medical value. On the other hand, Professor James Palmer, the person behind on-line "The Merovingean World" is one of the few current academics putting the intersection of science, culture, and religion in the early-medieval word as the center of his studies: https://merovingianworld.com/about/

41 For an in depth study of this topic, see the monumental work by Peter Brown, *The Rise of Western Christendom: Triumph and Diversity, A.D. 200–1000* (Chichester: Wiley-Blackwell, 2013). It is an insightful guide to the growth and spread of Christianity in the several regions of the West where it was shaped differently in each region in response to local needs and political situations. The papers in Horden's *Cultures of Healing* cited earlier in many ways complement Brown, but from a different point of view.

42 Victoria Sweet, *God's Hotel: A Doctor, a Hospital, and a Pilgrimage to the Heart of Medicine* (New York: Riverhead Books, 2012) and *Slow Medicine: The Way to Healing* (New York: Riverhead Books, 2017), both popular best-sellers.

43 Private discussion with practicing UK medical herbalist Vicki Pitman.

44 Peter Biller and Joseph Ziegler, eds., *Religion and Medicine in the Middle Ages* (Woodbridge: York Medieval Press, 2001).

45 Book review of Biller and Ziegler by Linda Voigts in *Social History of Medicine* (2003): 135–7; Monica Green's review in *Bulletin of the History of Medicine*, Vol. 78 (2004): 709–10, who optimistically wrote, "This extraordinary collection demonstrates the new approach to the pairing of 'religion and medicine' with new eyes."; and M.K.K. Yearl's review in *Journal of the History of Medicine*, Vol. 58 (Jan. 2003): 90–3, noting the absence of monastic medicine, but hoping the book may be a "springboard for other studies" showing science and faith not at odds but intertwined.

46 Arthur Ciaran, '*Charms*', *Liturgies, and Secret Rites in Early-Medieval England*, Anglo-Saxon Studies 32 (Woodbridge: Boydell Press, 2018).

47 Claire Burridge, "Healing Body and Soul in Early-Medieval Europe: Medical Remedies with Christian Elements," *Studies in Church History*, Vol. 58 (June 2022): 46–67: open access at https://doi.org/10.1017/stc.2022.3

48 Roy Flechner, and Maire NiMhaonaigh, eds., *The Introduction of Christianity into the Early-Medieval Insular World: Converting the Isles I* (Turnhout: Brepols, 2016).

49 Faith Wallis and Robert Wisnovsky, eds., *Medieval Textual Cultures: Agents of Transmission, Translation and Transformation* (Berlin/Boston: DeGruyter, 2016): 1. The papers here study translations/transmissions of primarily technical writings.

50 For more detail, read Anne Van Arsdall, "Medical Training in Anglo-Saxon England: An Evaluation of the Evidence," in *Form and Content of Instruction in Anglo-Saxon England in the Light of Contemporary Manuscript Evidence*, eds., Patrizia Lendinara, Loredana Lazzari, and M.A. D'Aronco (Turnhout: Brepols, 2007): 415–34.

51 Lesser, "Book in Britain," 14. In chapter one, the term "textual communities" is attributed to Brian Stock in *Implications of Literacy* (Princeton, 1983): 88.

52 Emily Kesling, *Medical Texts in Anglo-Saxon Literary Culture* (Cambridge: D.S. Brewer, 2020).

53 One, "The Foundations of Herbalism," was a class taught over nine months, involving lectures and practical experience with herbal medicine; December 1998–August 1999. The North American College of Botanical Medicine in Albuquerque, NM offered a three-year program leading to a Bachelor of Science degree and aimed to qualify graduates to practice. Because of funding issues and difficulties in obtaining accreditation in the United States, it had to close its doors only a few years later. Its former Webspace has been appropriated by others.

54 Begun in 2010, the network continues to thrive. Its website provides information on the network and the history of herbalism, as well as providing many papers and on-line seminars on related topics. www.herbalhistory.org

55 A comprehensive yet intimate look into the practice of modern medical herbalism is in Brice-Ytsma and Watkins, "Herbal Exchanges," 2014. I am indebted to several HHRN members for their discussions with me, in particular Frances Watkins, Anne Stobart, Alison Denham, and Vicki Pitman.

56 Contemporary medical herbalists are engaged in a serious effort to document the history of their profession apart from that of medicine and/or pharmacy, under which it is often placed (or excluded from). See Susan Francia and Anne Stobart, eds., *Critical Approaches to the History of Western Herbal Medicine: From Classical Antiquity to the Early Modern Period* (London: Bloomsbury, 2014). Chapter One, "The Fragmentation of Herbal History" is of particular interest here.

57 The way in which historic texts about native plants in the New World, such as the *Rerum*, have been studied is remarkably similar to studies of the Old English medical texts that seek native, non-Christian, magical elements, discussed in Anne Van Arsdall, "An Old World Herbal in the New World: the Badianus Manuscript," in ... *un tuo serto di fiori in man recando; scritto in onore di M.A. D'Aronco*, ed., Patrizia Lendinara (Udine: Forum, 2007): 29–41.

58 The history of New Mexico is covered in Thomas E. Chavez, *An Illustrated History of New Mexico* (Albuquerque: University of New Mexico Press, 2004); Joseph P. Sanchez, Robert L. Spude, and Art Gomez, *New Mexico: A History* (Norman: University of Oklahoma Press, 2013).

59 C. Stoll, 178.

> In Betracht der Vielfalt der Rezepturen, der Ungenauigkeit der Nomenklatur und der Unsicherheit der Gewichtsumrechnung stellt sich in besonderer Weise die Frage nach den entsprechenden wissenschaftlichen und praktischen Kenntnissen der für die Arzneibereitung verantwortlichen Mönche. Die praktischen Fertigkeiten und Erfahrungen konnten nur durch einen längeren Aufenthalt in einem "armarium pigmentorum," wie die "Apotheke" im karolingischen Klosterplan bezeighnet wird, erworben werden. *Diese Kentnisse wurden also auf ganz persönliche Art von Mönch zu Mönch weitergegeben.* Vor allem die irischen Wandermönche, denen die Klöster auf dem Kontinent, zum Beispiel St. Gallen, Lorsch oder Reichenau als

Herberge dienten, vermittelten entsprechende Kentnisse aus ihren Heimatklöstern [emphasis added].

60 Michael Moore. *Los Remedios de la Gente: A compilation of Traditional New Mexican Herbal Medicines and Their Use* (Santa Fe, 1977): 2.

61

Neben der fast unübersehbaren Anzahl von Simplicia verfügte die frühmittelalterliche Medizin über eine große Auswahl von Composita. Die Mönche wirkten auch hier sammelnd und ordnend, indem die meist in den überlieferten Schriften verstreut aufgefunden Vorschriften dem gezielten Gebrauch in den Klöstern zugänglich machten. ... [Antidotaren and Rezepten] waren von den Mönchen des frühen Mittelalters aus den Werken der Antike übernommen und jedoch teilweise dem örtlichen und persönlichen Bedarf angepaßt worden, weshalb kaum eine der anonymen Rezeptsammlungen völlig mit den anderen übereinstimmt.

62 For more information: https://nimh.org.uk/ for the herbalists' institute in the United Kingdom; www.americanherbalistsguild.com for the herbalists' guild in the United States; .com; and www.herbalgram.com for the journal of the botanical council.

63 L.E. Voigts and Robert P. Hudson, "A drynke þat men callen dwale to make a man to slepe whyle men kerven him: A Surgical Anesthetic from Late Medieval England," in *Health, Disease and Healing in Medieval Culture*, eds., Sheila Campbell, Bert Hall, and David Klausner (New York: St. Martin's Press, 1992): 36.

64 M.L. Cameron, "Anglo-Saxon medicine and magic," *Anglo-Saxon England*, Vol. 17 (1988): 118. See also D'Aronco and Cameron "Pharmacopoeia."

65 John Mann, *Murder, Magic, and Medicine* (New York: Oxford University Press, 1992): 3.

66 See, for example, the quarterly journal *Herbalgram* and more scholarly *Fitoterapia*, and Tobyn, Denham, Whitelegg "Western Herbal Tradition." It has a succinct overview of herbalism, 25 chapters devoted to individual medicinal herbs regarded from several angles, historic and practical, and includes useful bibliography. Its approach is in stark contrast to long beloved and much cited M. Grieve, *A Modern Herbal* (1931; New York: Dover Publications, 1971).

67 For example, on 30 March 2015, BBC News on-line posted an article with the headline "1,000-year-old onion and garlic eye remedy kills MRSA" (still available on line).

68 Freya Harrison and Erin Connelly, "Could Medieval Medicine Help the Fight Against Antimicrobial Resistance?" in *Making the Medieval Relevant* (Berlin: DeGruyter, 2020) available through DeGruyter Open Access by searching the Internet for the chapter title.

69 Frances Watkins, "Investigation of Antimicrobials From Native British Plants Used in 10th Century Anglo-Saxon Wound Healing Formulation" Ph.D. diss., University of East London, 2013.

70 Outside the scope of this study is the long-standing controversy in the United States over whether the U.S. Food and Drug Administration should test and legislate standards for herbal medicines (which the National Institutes of Health (NIH) call "supplements," with medicinal plants used by herbalists and over-the-counter bottled products apparently considered co-equal). The NIH operates a National Center for Complementary and Integrative Health www.nccih.nih, earlier called complementary and alternative medicine (CAM), with a Website offering definitions of recognized healing practices that are outside the mainstream of American medicine and a wealth of other information. Herbalism is not listed as a health topic (unlike aromatherapy and homeopathy). Certain medicinal plants are listed there and discussed as herbal supplements.

71 M. Grieve, *A Modern Herbal* (1931; New York: Dover Publications, 1971).

72 Moore, "Remedios," 12.

4

ABOUT THE *OLD ENGLISH HERBARIUM*

Manuscripts, illustrations, and need for an alternative to Cockayne's translation

The manuscripts, their dates, and editions

The *Old English Herbarium* and a book of medicinal remedies made from animal parts and products (the *Medicina de Quadrupedibus*) are found together in several manuscripts written in Old English. Philologist M.A. D'Aronco, an authority on these texts, describes them as "… translations of a group of medical documents in Latin, which together can be considered to form the common pharmacopoeia of the early Middle Ages."[1] These and several other Old English medical texts mentioned in previous chapters are the earliest examples of such works in any vernacular of Europe.

The *Old English Herbarium* is made up of 185 short chapters that were taken from several late-antique Latin works, combined into one larger work, then translated into Old English. Each chapter features a different plant and uses for it. Betony is the topic of chapter 1 and is actually a treatise on betony (*de Vettonica*) attributed to first-century botanist Antonius Musa; chapters 2–132 are from the *Herbarius of Pseudo-Apuleius*, a fourth/fifth-century work that lists medicinal plants and their uses. The final chapters, 133–185, are from other sources, including *Liber medicinae ex herbis femininis* and *Curae herbarum*, both wrongly attributed to Dioscorides, and other as-yet unidentified sources. (De Vriend discusses them at length on pages lv–lx; and John M. Riddle, "Pseudo-Dioscorides' *Ex herbis feminis* and Early Medieval Medical Botany," *Journal of the History of Biology* 14 [1981]: 43–81 gives a history of this work and its long association with the *Herbarium*.)

Another work, *Medicina de Quadrupedibus* (Medicines from Animals) is often found with it in the manuscripts. It too has several sources: a treatise on uses for badger, a treatise about uses for mulberry tree, and a selection from Sextus Placitus Papiriensis's treatise on medicinal remedies from animals.

DOI: 10.4324/9781003162285-4

The *Herbarium* (as well as *Quadrupedibus*) survives in four manuscripts, three at the British Library: Cotton Vitellius C. iii, Harley 585, and Harley 6258B (in early Middle English). The fourth, MS Hatton 76, is at the Bodleian Library, Oxford. The British Library's extensive website makes available digital images of its manuscripts, detailed information about them, and selected bibliography listing relevant studies. (Directions for use are on its website: bl.uk/manuscripts.) The Digital Bodleian (digital.Bodleian.ox.ac.uk) makes Hatton 76 readily available.

A facsimile edition of Cotton Vitellius C iii was printed in 1998, as noted earlier, edited by D'Aronco and Cameron; in addition, the Cotton MS is available in microfiche.[2] Neil Ker's *Catalogue of Manuscripts Containing Anglo-Saxon* discusses the manuscripts in some detail (items 218, 231, 264, and 328), but omits the early Middle English Harley 6258B.[3] For information on these and many other medieval manuscripts containing medical and scientific content, see the (US) National Library of Medicine's website (nlm.nih.gov/hmd/indexcat/aboutetkevk2.html). There, a searchable database called the *eTK/eVK2 Project* is found, created using the Latin, Old and Middle English manuscripts listed in Thorndike and Kibre's (TK) *Catalog of Incipits* and in an updated and enlarged *Scientific and Medical Writings* (eVK) by Voigts and Kurtz.[4]

The most recent edition of the *Old English Herbarium* was published in 1984 by Jan De Vriend for the Early English Text Society Series. It offers Latin parallels to the Old English text as well as detailed information about each of the manuscripts in which the *Herbarium* appears.[5] The profusely illustrated Cotton Vitellius C. iii was De Vriend's main text, as it was for Cockayne. De Vriend replaced earlier editions by Hugo Berberich[6] and Aaltje Johanna Geertruida Hilbelink.[7] In addition, Dumbarton Oaks Medieval Library is preparing new editions and translations of all the Old English medical texts through Harvard University Press, expected to begin publication in 2023 (see http://domedieval.org/). The *Herbarium*, *Quadrupedibus*, and another work, *Lacnunga* (remedies), are to appear together in volume one; i.e., Niles and D'Aronco 2023.

An annotated bibliography for the *Herbarium* and other medical (and magical) texts appeared in 1992,[8] and the 1998 facsimile edition by D'Aronco and Cameron not only updates this bibliography but also includes Continental scholars not generally mentioned in publications on Old English. Studies since that time specifically on the *Herbarium* have been relatively few (see D'Aronco 2003 for works to 2002), the other medical texts with their non-medical aspects drawing more interest for reasons suggested in two earlier chapters here.[9]

Considerable discussion about the dating for each manuscript can be found in many publications, and the websites where they can be viewed also list dates. All of the manuscripts date to near the early eleventh century. However, it is essential to remember that the discussion on their dating concerns the year when each individual manuscript was copied out, not when the works in them were first translated from Latin into Old English (and whether that was first orally as needed for medical practice or in writing as formal documents). Of course, when the original translation(s) was made is part of every discussion. However, determining when and how that happened is much harder than determining when the translations were first written down, a date that is necessarily based on evidence in manuscripts that survived.

None of the four manuscripts is believed to be the first version of a translation/compilation in Old English; all are believed to be later copies of as-yet unknown originals. Those originals are surmised to have existed in at least two different manuscript families in places where manuscripts are known to have been created and copied, such as Winchester and Cambridge. However, developing a vernacular vocabulary to convey technical Latin concepts and correct plant names obviously takes time and requires people who understand the technology both in principle and in practice. How long that process took and when it began is not yet known, because the clues tend to exist in places outside the extant medical manuscripts (such as in glossaries and other kinds of writings).

About when Old English was first used to transmit medical information, D'Aronco[10] said:

> On occasion, the [medical] texts evince similarities of form and substance such as to lead us to suppose that at least as early as the late ninth century there had grown up a sort of corpus of remedies in Old English.
>
> *"Dating," 12*

D'Aronco links the creation of the *Herbarium* to that of the *Leechbook* (the compiler of *Lacnunga* is known to have used the *Herbarium*, thus postdating it).

> It is clear that when the *Læceboc* was compiled, the translations of the Herbal and the *Medicina de Quadrupedibus* were not yet available in the form in which they have come down to us. They were only to come into circulation later on and could only subsequently have been consulted for the compilation of other books of remedies.
>
> *"Dating," 13*

To reinforce her findings, D'Aronco used considerable evidence from extant glossaries containing the specialized vocabulary of the medical texts, finding that their compilers did not have texts such as the *Herbarium* available at an early time, and demonstrating their relatively late composition. D'Aronco dates the creation of an original *Herbarium* to "before the end of the tenth century" (16). Earlier, in the introduction to his edition, De Vriend conceded that it was hard to prove the original translation dated to earlier than the tenth century, but argued it made sense to link its creation to study of herbal medicine in the Northumbrian monasteries during the seventh or eighth century (De Vriend, xliii).

The only certainty is that at some point before the eleventh century, the need for such translations became pressing for reasons we can only surmise. One theory often cited is King Alfred's well-known cultural renaissance (CE 878–892) when the king instigated a program of translations into Old English; yet medical works do not seem to have been part of it. If most practitioners, lay and monastic, read and orally transmitted information about medicine in Latin, a vernacular vocabulary for how to identify plants, make medications, and use them would not have been needed. Perhaps literate Old English speakers (possibly healers themselves) who read Latin made the translations with or for healers, creating instructions in the vernacular that could be read aloud and memorized by users who did not read. The illustrations could have been shown and discussed. D'Aronco went so far as to say that the *Herbarium* translation

> seems not to have been targeted at the educated (and Latin-speaking) world of the monasteries so much as at a wider public that was not entirely made up of specialists. The Herbal is not presented as a medical treatise and requires no special knowledge of physiology. … The Herbal is more similar to a first-aid manual.
> *"Dating,"* 16

Work is still needed to determine who the users were, whether they were lay or religious, and how the Old English texts figured into medical treatment and knowledge transmission, both verbal and written. The four extant manuscripts can only supply pieces of a much larger story that awaits discovery. And too many Latin medical texts are known to have been available and used in England at the same time. When they are edited and made available for study in parallel with the Old English texts, a much more complete picture of health care in early-medieval England will emerge. Eventually, other information too will supplement the manuscripts; for example, outlines of monastery buildings showing infirmaries and gardens, evidence from excavations and trash heaps, and descriptions of health issues in other genres (legal codes, saints' lives, for example, and manuscript illustrations). Interactions between townspeople and monasteries are subjects needing increased study. In addition, modern practitioners of healing practices that sprang from the same sources can be consulted for their insight into these technical texts, which outline a skilled profession.

To summarize, the *Old English Herbarium* exists in three eleventh-century manuscripts, one of them illustrated, as well as in one from the twelfth century.

> **Cotton Vitellius C. iii** (British Library: bl.uk/search) includes an illustrated *Herbarium* (and *Quadrupedibus*) the text used in Cockayne 1961 and 1965, Vol. 1, and called MS V by Cockayne and De Vriend (listed as Ker 218). The British Library website suggests the work dates to the third quarter of the ninth century, but dates this manuscript to the early eleventh century.

> **Hatton 76** (Bodleian Library, Oxford: digital.bodleian.ox.ac.uk/search) contains the *Herbarium* with spaces left for illustrations but none in place (as well as *Quadrupedibus*); it is called MS B in Cockayne and De Vriend, who used it for comparison with V (listed as Ker 328). The Bodleian has a tentative date of twelfth century for the manuscript.

Harley 585 (British Library: bl.uk/search) has the *Herbarium* (and a partial *Quadrupedibus*), called MS H in Cockayne and De Vriend; both used it for comparison with MS V. This manuscript also contains the collection of recipes and charms known as *Lacnunga*, printed in Cockayne's Vol. 3, as well as parts of the *Quadrupedibus*, and the *Lorica* of Gildas in Latin with Old English glosses. De Vriend notes there are a few marginal sketches in the *Herbarium* section, mainly of serpents (listed as Ker 231). The British Library website dates the manuscript to the late tenth/early eleventh century and calls it a medical miscellany.

Harley 6258B (British Library: bl.uk/search) contains the *Herbarium*, and was called MS O by Cockayne and De Vriend. De Vriend pointed out that its organization differs from all the others (not listed in Ker). It also contains the Old English *Quadrupedibus*, and a translation of *Peri didaxeon*, a Latin collection of recipes. The British Library website dates it to the twelfth century and calls it a medical miscellany.

Though the *Herbarium* is not in the following manuscript, another important Old English medical text mentioned often in this study, *Bald's Leechbook*, is found here:

Royal MS 12 D XVII (British Library: bl.uk/search) contains medical recipes, charms, and the Old English work that Cockayne called *Bald's Leechbook*, which is in Cockayne Vol. 2. See Marilyn Deegan, "A Critical Edition of MS. B.L. Royal 12. D. XVII: Bald's 'Leechbook'Vols. 1 and 2," diss., University of Manchester, 1988; Conan T. Doyle, "Anglo-Saxon Medicine and Disease: A Semantic Approach." 2 Vols. Ph.D. dissertation, Corpus Christi College, Cambridge, 2011. Vol. 2, "Appendix: Bald's Leechbook" 2017, available open access: https://doi.org/10.17863/CAM.1443. The British Library website dates it to the mid-tenth century with the title "Bald's Leechbook."

Cotton Vitellius C. iii has always been the preferred manuscript to study because of its illustrations and generally good condition, despite its having been damaged in a fire in 1731 at Ashburnham House where it was housed. Brightly painted drawings of plants and animals throughout the *Herbarium* portion distinguish this manuscript from all others.

Illustrations in the Cotton *Old English Herbarium*

Among the manuscripts containing the *Herbarium*, Cotton Vitellius C. iii is unique because of its illustrations. They have been the subject of several specialized studies concerning their style and antecedents in earlier manuscripts, seldom to try to understand the purpose they served for those who used the texts in context of healing. Following the argument presented in Chapter 3, from the standpoint of their value to the user, the plant drawings might be considered aids to memory, schematics to assist someone who already knew the plants fresh or dried. The three title pages of human figures at the beginning of the manuscript helped establish the authority of the work for the medieval reader as coming from ancient and accepted sources, but even without them, the work was so very well known, such illustrations were unnecessary. The authority figures simply added to the value and usefulness of this codex. That all the illustrations can be linked to European Continental sources bolsters the thesis advanced earlier that early-medieval English medicine can be closely linked to a pan-European tradition.

The illustrations in the Cotton manuscript consist of (1) three title pages on 11v, 19r, and 19v, (2) plant illustrations that are placed near the beginning of every entry in the body of the herbal and exist for every plant but the last one, (3) snakes, spiders, and scorpions, which appear near the remedies in the *Herbarium* that are useful in healing their bites, and (4) animals that were used in preparing the remedies in the *Medicina de Quadrupedibus*, a work not discussed here.

The three illuminated title pages have been the subject of discussion, in fact more so than the numerous drawings of plants, animals, and snakes in the remedy portion. On 19r is a framed image with a large central figure holding plants in his hands, a centaur to his left, and a figure in classical robes to his right; below the frame are the names Aesculapius, Plato, and Centaurus. Above and below the human figures are animals and snakes. On 19v is the title of the work—*Herbarium Apulei Platonici Quod Acceptit Ab Escolapio et Alchirone Centauro Magistro Achillis*—encircled in a frame. Linda Voigts, who has studied the illustrations in this manuscript extensively, interpreted these folios together as being author portraits, examples of a standard type of illustration present in herbals from classical times through the Middle Ages:

> This author portrait is found between the table of contents and the first chapter of the herbal; it depicts the source of and the authority for the remedy book. Portrayed in this miniature are Aesculapius, Chiron, and, in the center, the putative author of the herbal, Apuleius Platonicus, often designated in herbals as Plato or Plato Apoliensis.[11]

Voigts suggested that the title on the reverse explained that the Plato/Apuleius figure was receiving the book from the two patrons of medicine.

D'Aronco, who wrote the section on codicology and paleography for the facsimile edition, interprets the drawing differently. She believes that the scene illustrates the contents of the manuscript (the herbal portion by the plants in Plato's hands and the *Medicina de Quadrupedibus* by the animals in the background). She suggests that Aesculapius and Chiron's handing the herbal to the mortal author Plato was "a symbolic act, representing the passage of medical knowledge from the gods to mortals, while at the same time attributing the paternity of the work to an undisputed authority who confers on it legitimacy and status" (D'Aronco and Cameron, 26). In the opinion of both Voigts and D'Aronco, these title page illustrations can be traced in content and style to late classical types.

Less conclusive are their discussions about the illustration on folio 11v, which begins the herbal portion of the Cotton manuscript, coming before the table of contents. Here is found a large central figure who is standing on what appears to be a lion, holding a spear in his right hand and a book in his left. The lion appears to be biting the spear. To his right is a tonsured figure holding out a book to him, and at the bottom left is a Roman soldier. Cockayne thought that this was a dedicatory page to begin the manuscript, and that one of the figures "depicts the church dignitary for whom the work was copied, one a tonsured priest presenting a volume, and one is soldier with a roman air" (Cockayne, 1965, 1: lxxvii). However, no inscription is present to aid in identifying any of the figures.

Voigts said that a dedication page such as this one, like the author/portrait page on 19r, was a classical genre, and she linked it in style to the monastery of Saint-Bertin in French Flanders (Voigts, 1976). Further, she identified the central figure with early-English tomb sculpture, concluding that the codex was dedicated to a bishop or abbot-saint "of particular importance to the house which produced or commissioned the work" (Voigts, 1976, 54). Here, she again pointed to northern France for similar depictions, but conceded that the identity of the figure might never be known. About the other two figures, Voigts said only that one was a monk, the other a "non-royal lay donor, a phenomenon rare in Anglo-Saxon manuscripts," and observed generally about the dedication page that it was "highly irregular among Anglo-Saxon dedication pages" (Voigts, 1976, 55).

D'Aronco, on the other hand, questioned whether this page really depicts a dedication scene, arguing that it "ought to be viewed as a composition with a semantic structure of its own that can be read only in the context of the work it is intended to illustrate, that is within the traditional iconography of herbals" (D'Aronco and Cameron, 29). Her conclusion was that this page "could be the result of the conflation of single author-portraits modernized according to contemporary canons" (D'Aronco and Cameron, 30). She suggested that the central figure depicts the author of the text, Aesculapius or Apollo/Apuleius, and that the other two figures bring up to date a discussion scene of two figures associated with healing, Antonius Musa and Marcus Agrippa (who are transformed, respectively, into a monk and a Roman soldier holding a scroll).

Studies of the plant illustrations have also tended to focus on who copied which model, thus helping establish manuscript stemma. Attention is generally called only to those few illustrations that clearly do not depict the plant called out in the text, yet it is remarkable how closely many illustrations capture the essential appearance of the plants, albeit in almost cartoon fashion. The most up-to-date study of the illustrations in all the known manuscripts of the Pseudo-Apuleius herbal is a 1977 study by Heide Grape-Albers, cited in Chapter 3 here, which traces the history of illustrated Pseudo-Apuleius manuscripts from late-classical times through the Middle Ages.[12] She uses the illustrations to help establish that the manuscript families proposed long ago by Howald and Sigerist for the *Herbarium of Pseudo-Apuleius* were essentially correct and also argued that in every instance, the texts (even when excerpted) and their plant illustrations remained together through the centuries the manuscripts of this work circulated and were recopied (Grape-Albers, 13–21 and 164–6; D'Aronco and Cameron, 31–8, base their discussion on this study).

In the present work, the drawings continue an ancient tradition of copying from an existing manuscript. They are hand-drawn from the D'Aronco-Cameron facsimile (see Introduction, "About the Drawings") and serve to emphasize the central role medicinal plants play in the remedies, indeed in medicine then. The plants are a constant reminder of the major components of these medicinal remedies, i.e., plants whose identity and use is important. After the plants themselves, the next in importance is the ability to find help quickly when someone has an adverse reaction to a poisonous drink or bite; for this, the scorpions and snakes of course stand out on the page. The images in the translation only give a suggestion of how the original looks: the books and websites cited here are recommended to anyone interested.

Outside the scope of the present study, but an interesting question, is the possible relationship between the Cotton manuscript and one at Montecassino Monastery from about the same period whose illustrations appear remarkably similar. Grape-Albers puts them in the same manuscript family. In her dissertation, Voigts does not agree, finding that the Old English manuscript may have been the source for the Italian manuscript (Voigts, 1973, 56 ff.). (The many illustrated versions of the *Herbarium* are also discussed in Minta Collins's work, cited earlier.)

The snake and scorpion paintings in the manuscript are an interesting side issue. Cockayne believed these illustrations, prominent throughout the *Herbarium*, were entirely fanciful. It must be said they have received little attention, the plants being the main interest. However, German scholar Arthur Gross connected snakes that are called out by name in Wolfram von Eschenbach's thirteenth-century *Parzifal* directly to the *Herbarium of Pseudo-Apuleius*. Gross also pointed out that remedies for snakebite and for wounds caused by weapons poisoned with snake venom, and drawings of snakes were always an important part of the *Herbarium* and remained a constant part of its transmission.[13]

There is no doubt that the snakes, spiders, and scorpions were important to this work: remedies for bites from such creatures outnumber those for any other single complaint, numbering about 48 instances. In terms of their frequency, the next most common conditions addressed are stomach/abdominal pain and swelling (43) and various kinds of wounds and sores (45), which are often described with considerable detail so the healer can decide whether the remedy offered is appropriate to use. Although no real conclusions can be drawn from the frequency of conditions cited, they are informative. Numbering far fewer than the three types mentioned, but fairly frequently called out are eye conditions (24), constipation and diarrhea (10 each), inability to urinate (20), bladder stones and pain (15), fever (17), headache (20), worms (10), aching joints (11), pain in the spleen (13), swellings (18), gout (15), antidotes to poison (10), and dropsy (8). Conditions specific to women are mentioned in 16 instances, and some of the remedies may have been intended to produce miscarriages/abortions though they do not say so specifically.

D'Aronco notes that the reptiles and insects can in some instances be recognized. Snakes and serpents in Vitellius C. iii are depicted in such lavish detail that the species portrayed is sometimes recognizable, as, for example, the snake on fol. 32v, col. 2, whose head is adorned with horns and wattles. This is clearly *Cerastes cerastes* (= *C. Cornutus*), the sand viper, and we note a similar care for detail in the snake on fol. 49r, col. 1, in which we can recognize a water snake (*chersydros*) (D'Aronco and Cameron, 41).

The illustrations of plants, animals, reptiles, and snakes served to make a book of remedies such as the *Herbarium* and its major source, the *Herbarium of Pseudo-Apuleius*, even more useful. But even without illustrations, the work was popular and used. The title pages may have had meaning to the medieval user that is not entirely clear to us, but they were obviously of some importance because of their continuation in use from late antique times into the Renaissance.

Need for alternatives to Cockayne's translation

Cockayne's translations of the Old English medical texts in the 1860s were the only ones available for nearly 150 years. Readers of his versions, in particular of the *Old English Herbarium*, were easily misled (1) about the intended use for the herbal—the remedies appear to be only for men because of the personal pronouns used, (2) about the seeming absence of complaints specific to women—Cockayne translates many of them into Latin or Greek, not English, and (3) about the seriousness of the text—his arcane style casts doubt immediately on the serious nature of the remedies.

Cockayne chose to translate medical remedies in this style: "If a mans head be broken, … In case a mans inwards be too costive, … In case blood gush up through a mans mouth, … In case a carbuncle is going to settle on a man" (Cockayne, 1965, 1: 3; note that he uses "mans" for man's, a customary style at the time). The Old English word he was translating is the indefinite *man*, which means "one" or "a person," just like the modern German word *man*. Even in the English of Cockayne's day, "a man" was a gender-specific term. There was no linguistic reason to use "a man" in the translation, particularly in such frequent formulas as *Wiþ þæt man … sy* (if a person is …), which Cockayne invariably translates as "In case a man be …" Translating Old English *man* as "a person" or "one" is not only closer to the original, but correct. The Latin originals avoided pronouns in remedies, preferring passive constructions and such wording as "for headache take this plant," or "this plant is used for headache."

The following excerpts from the first entry in the *Herbarium* concerning uses for betony illustrate the subtle shift that occurs in going from Latin to Old English to Cockayne (and to Grattan-Singer as well):

> **Latin** text: *Ad alvum concitandum, … ad sanguinem qui per os reiciunt et purulentum, … ad carbunculos* (i.e., for this condition take …)
>
> *De Vriend, 1984, 33–5*

Old English text: *Gif mannes innod to faest sy* ... , *wiþ þe men blod up welle,* ... *Gif man wylle spring on gisittan* (If a person's abdomen is ...) **Cockayne**'s translation: In case a mans inwards be too costive, ... in case blood gush up through a mans mouth, ... in case a pustule is going to settle on a man.

Cockayne, 1965, 1: 3

An understandably coy practice of Cockayne's, in view of his being an ordained minister in Victorian England, was his habit of often lapsing into Latin and Greek instead of straightforward English when he encountered a remedy dealing with female functions. However Victorian this avoidance might be, it is misleading for a reader who cannot understand the Latin or Old English originals and is depending on Cockayne for information. Such a reader might be left with the impression that medieval people did not deal in a straightforward manner with "delicate" subjects, when in fact they did.

An example is in chapter 178, which lists seven uses for nettle. Item 6 in the Old English version begins, *Wið wifes flewsan genim ðas yclan wyrte on mortere wel gepunude* (literally: For a woman's periods take the same plant thoroughly pounded in a mortar ...). Without explanation, following the five remedies he translates into English, here at item 6, Cockayne translates the entire entry into Latin, beginning *Ad mulieris fluxus, herbam hanc in mortario tusam, ita ut omnino lenta fiat* ... (Cockayne, 1965, 1: 312–13).

However, the misconception Cockayne created that had the most widespread effect was that medieval medicine is not to be taken seriously. By using antiquated and contorted turns of phrase, Cockayne may have sought to give his translations a flavor of the old language, but, as discussed in Chapter 2, they came across as ridiculous even in the nineteenth century. Language style very much affects how information is received. "Worts, wambs, ill runnings of the inwards, head breaches, swart roots, and a sun that upgoeth" (all taken from Cockayne's *Leechdoms*) are not terms that connote serious medicine. Curious choices of words and phrases in the translations coupled with the prefaces Cockayne supplied to each volume of the *Leechdoms* created a long-lasting, negative image of medieval medicine.

More than a century and a half has passed since Cockayne's works first appeared, and English language usage has been changing, as has scholarship on older systems of medicine. The philosophy guiding my translation was always that this was a text written to transmit information on the healing properties of plants, to provide instructions on making remedies using them, and often also how to administer them. The *Old English Herbarium* is a key late-antique/early-medieval medical text from Western Europe; a modern translation allows it to be clearly understood by many audiences.

Notwithstanding the need to provide alternatives to almost all of Cockayne's work, these remarks are not intended to diminish his contribution to scholarship. In fact, he alone transcribed, translated, and thus made available nearly all the known Old English medical texts, while his colleagues worked on the more popular Old English histories and poetry. Any discussion of Old English medicine or magic will necessarily and always begin with Cockayne, whose life story outlined in the first chapter helps in understanding his mindset and approach to things Old English.

In the original *Leechdoms* volumes, Cockayne's transcriptions are printed on pages facing his translations so the reader can easily compare them. (All three volumes are available free through Google Books.) The typeface for his transcriptions must have been designed specifically for the Rolls Series editions; it replicates manuscript letters. A great deal of effort went into designing the typeface and ensuring the printer could correctly copy his hand-written transcriptions. Cockayne refers to his work as a "facsimile" in Vol. 1 of the *Leechdoms* (lxxv), and he notes that he did not normalize the Old English, deferring to the original manuscripts. As he explains:

> The text has been printed in the form, as regards the shape of the characters, which they take in the original MSS. Besides the objection to printing in the character of our own day, which arises in the heart of every man who dislikes to dress up antiquity in modern clothes, there is one which is not sentimental at all; by a change in levelling we lose all the chronological characteristics of a manuscript arising from the form of the letters.
>
> *Cockayne, 1965, 1: xc*

He often mentions the importance of not standardizing but keeping variations when editing Old English writings because through them, the evolution of the English language could be traced. On this topic, Cockayne discusses what he considers dangerous consequences of establishing a standard version of Old English and normalizing an edition to that standard. His main reason, as he stated above, was that the forms of the letters give a clue as to the age of the manuscript, and he thought it important to preserve in print the form of the letters in the manuscript he was using. Known always as an extremely exact and careful scholar, in his preface Cockayne established Cotton Vitellius C iii as his main text for the *Herbarium*. In the printed version, he refers to variant readings in other manuscripts at the bottom of each page. In spot checks with De Vriend's edition and with D'Aronco and Cameron, it must be said Cockayne's transcriptions are exact (perhaps with a nod to the women in his family as well, as noted in Chapter 1).

In keeping with his desire to provide a facsimile, rather than an edition, Cockayne did not punctuate the Old English, as most editors are inclined to do, De Vriend included. Imitating the original, Cockayne provided capital letters at the beginning of paragraphs and then printed the remainder of the paragraph without added punctuation. His editorial decisions were limited to deciphering letters that were nearly impossible to distinguish clearly and in separating some words that were run together in the manuscript. The points Cockayne raised about editing and printing Old English works are still valid. He was justifiably concerned about the effect editors have on the interpretation and reception of a given work; concerns that apply equally to translators. Cockayne's rather lengthy remarks are in the preface to vol. 1 of the *Leechdoms* (Cockayne, 1965, 1: xc–cv) and outline his philosophy of editing Old English texts.

Sources used for the present translation

In the first edition, my translation of the *Old English Herbarium* was based primarily on De Vriend's 1984 edition, Cockayne's translation, and D'Aronco and Cameron's facsimile. That remains true for this revised second edition, with the bonus of having the digital versions of the manuscripts available at the British Library and Bodleian websites to consult when needed. In addition, Professor M.A. D'Aronco has very kindly discussed with me various possible alternative translations and interpretations while she worked on her own new editions and translations for the Dumbarton Oaks Medieval Library.

Cockayne's translation was both a source and in some instances a hurdle to overcome. I note where my translation differs appreciably from his. However, I do not address all the issues connected with his translation. For example, I do not point out the several places where Cockayne uses Greek names, Greek spellings, and Greek letters for some of the plants and sometimes the conditions (see Cockayne, 1961 and 1965 to see where he uses Greek in the *Herbarium* translation). In the original manuscripts, Greek words were written in the same style as the Old English words, but as a good philologist of his day, Cockayne wrote them using Greek letters, at times even correcting the name as it was written there.

We do not know what names were commonly used for plants in various segments of society in early-medieval England; it may well have been a Latin or Greek name, as is the case today for people who use Latin binomials when talking about plants. It is noteworthy that Latin plant names prevail in the original Old English translation, the vernacular name appearing most often only once toward the beginning of a chapter. When more is known about the users of these manuscripts, such fine points of language may well be significant. Little is known about who actually taught medicine and remedy making, in what language, and where (monastery or village or both); such studies are just beginning and generally involve interdisciplinary teams.

References for Old English plant names in the first edition were Cockayne, De Vriend's edition of the *Old English Herbarium, The Old English Illustrated Pharmacopoeia* by D'Aronco and Cameron, Peter Bierbaumer's three volume *Der botanische Wortschatz des Altenglishen* (Frankfurt/M: Peter Lang, 1975), and Tony Hunt's *Plant Names of Medieval England* (Cambridge: D.S. Brewer, 1989).[14] When the first edition appeared, D'Aronco and Cameron was the most complete published study of the *Old English Herbarium*; they consulted all available earlier sources to identify the plants in the *Herbarium*. For that reason, theirs were the plant names I used and continue to use except where noted.

In revising my translation, I consulted the recently available on-line version of the *Dictionary of Old English (DOE)*, which goes through the letter "i"; the *DOE Corpus*, which lists all the works in which nearly every word in OE can be found; and the useful on-line *Dictionary of Old English Plant Names*, which is based on Bierbaumer's book, with much of the information continually updated (http://old english-plantnames.org/).

Cockayne gave few sources for his botanical knowledge. Immediately preceding his Glossary in Vol. 3 of the *Leechdoms*, he states that his work

> relies almost entirely upon original authorities; upon a collation of the manuscript ancient extant glossaries with their printed editions, which have been falsified by ignorant conjectures; and upon a careful examination of many Saxon volumes never yet published. No reliance has been placed on modern productions, in the way of dictionaries; they will be found full of errors.
>
> *Cockayne, 1965, 3: 363*

The last statement recalls his 1864 attack on Bosworth's *Anglo-Saxon Dictionary*, and Cockayne here footnotes his own publication with reference to the slur on modern dictionaries: the *Shrine* of 1864. (It is extremely difficult to identify Cockayne's sources from the notes he provides in all his works.) While seeking additional details about Cockayne's puzzling death some years after the first edition of this book was published, it was bittersweet to learn that on his final day alive, he was still interested in the subject, avidly inquiring into the names of local plants near St. Ives.

For the first edition, supplemental information on herbs and plants came from M. Grieve's *A Modern Herbal*, Culpepper's *Culpepper's Herbal, The Greek Herbal of Dioscorides*, ed. Robert Gunther (see bibliography for complete citations; however, the 2017 Dioscorides *De Materia Medica*, transl. Beck replaces Gunther in this edition), Malcolm Stuart, *Encyclopedia of Herbs and Herbalism* (London: Orbis Books, 1979), and from the several classes and workshops previously mentioned.

Many newer works about medicinal plants are now available, such as previously mentioned Tobyn, Denham, and Whiteleg's *Western Herbal Tradition*; James A. Duke, *Handbook of Medicinal Herbs* (Boca Raton: CRC Press, 2002), and for the United Kingdom, Stace's authoritative *New Flora of the British Isles* and the Collins Flower Guides. In addition, the Internet is now an inexhaustible source of information about medicinal plants and their use. All sites usually include photographs and details about the plants' habitats and efficacy. However, the efficacy of remedies and/ or of medicinal plants is a focus I leave to others more qualified than I in botany and phytotherapy. For those interested, such information is much more abundant and more easily accessible at the present time, particularly on-line, than it was when the original edition of this book appeared.

D'Aronco and Cameron discuss the issues involved in trying to correctly identify plants in medieval texts, as does Tony Hunt in his *Plant Names of Medieval England* (Cambridge: D.S. Brewer, 1989). D'Aronco and Cameron use J. André, *Lexique des termes de botanique en latin* (Paris: Klincksieck, 1956), which De Vriend does not cite, though it was available when his edition was made. In addition, D'Aronco and Cameron use G. Maggiulli and M.F. Buffa Giolito, *L'altro Apuleio. Problemi aperti per una nuova edisione dell'Herbarius* (Naples, 1996), cited as "*Nomenclatura della piante.*" All of them use Bierbaumer's three volumes on Old English plant names (1975–79). The on-line Anglo-Saxon Plant Name Survey at the University of Glasgow mentioned in the first edition of this book ceased to exist in 2016. Much of its work and current studies on Old English plant names are found in the on-line "Dictionary of Old English Plant Names," eds. Peter Bierbaumer and Hans Sauer with Helmut W. Klug and Ulrike Krischke at http://oldenglish-plantnames.org/. It builds upon and enlarges Bierbaumer's 1975 volumes.

Units of measure in medieval texts are generally regarded with despair, either because their meaning is not known with any certainty, as in the case of jar or pitcher, or because the weight or size of something such as a penny's weight or a spoonful is also not clear. My theory is that the intended users of this work knew how to follow the instructions as written, that the *Herbarium* and works like it were general guidebooks and references, not detailed manuals on how to pre-scribe and make herbal remedies. They are early examples of technical writings, intended for knowledgeable users. De Vriend discusses in detail the modern equivalents of Old English and Roman weights and measures, and I very gen-erally use his equivalents to convert the measures into modern terms. However, an ideal approach would be to work with a medical herbalist who uses standard modern quantities to study individual medieval remedies. Together, a more real-istic idea could be had for how these remedies were made and administered, and what standard was behind them.

As to the challenge of being able to identify correctly the 185 plants in the *Herbarium*, a small number may never be identified to everyone's satisfaction. However, it is remarkable that a very large number of them have been identified with certainty, given the huge geographic area and the great span of time involved in the long life of this work. Moreover, in practice, healers have always sought var-ieties of plants to help the ill wherever they might be living.[15] The *Herbarium*, albeit originally existing as several separate works, was used in medieval Europe over many centuries from Italy to England and Scandinavia. Using the remedies would have surely entailed many substitutions of varieties of plants in the same family, and this would have affected how the remedies were transmitted. Merely because **we** cannot identify plants based on the illustrations and descriptions given in this and other manuscripts does not necessarily mean that the writers and illustrators did not know what they were doing. Rather, we need to bring new eyes and new sens-ibilities to the texts. Tobyn, Denham, and Whitelegg's *Western Herbal Tradition* is an example of new eyes on old texts, with its easy-to-follow and detailed discussions of a number of medicinal plants that are mentioned in the old texts and continue to be used.

Notes

1 M.A. D'Aronco, "The Old English Pharmacopoeia: A Proposed Dating for the Translation," *AVISTA Forum Journal* 13/2 (2003): 9. Information on sources is largely based on this and Hubert Jan de Vriend, ed., *The Old English Herbarium and Medicina de Quadrupedibus* (London: Oxford University Press, 1984). More recent work on sources is in Doyle 2011 and Kesling 2020.

2 Cotton Vitellius C. iii is in Vol. 1 of the *Anglo-Saxon Manuscripts in Microfiche Facsimile* (Binghamton, NY: Medieval & Renaissance Texts & Studies, 1994), in D'Aronco and Cameron 1998, and in the on-line access mentioned.

3 Neil R. Ker, *Catalogue of Manuscripts Containing Anglo-Saxon* (Oxford: Clarendon Press, 1957).

4 TK refers to the printed version of Lynn Thorndike and Pearl Kibre, *Catalog of Incipits of Medieval Scientific Writings in Latin*. eVK refers to the electronic Linda Voigts and Patricia Derry Kurtz, *Scientific and Medical Writings in Old and Middle English*, on CD-ROM; the Web version expands and updates the information on CD-ROM.

5 De Vriend discusses the manuscripts in detail, including sources, dating, language, and interrelationship with each other (xi–lxxv), as does Kesling 2020.

6 Hugo Berberich, ed., *Das Herbarium Apulei nach einer früh-mittelenglischen Fassung* (1901; Amsterdam: Swets und Zeitlinger NV Nachgedruckt, 1966). This is Harley 6258B, the MS O. Cockayne did not use. Berberich's study contains 12 pages about the MS and the script, "Lautlehre" on pages 14–30, grammar on pages 33–6, and the text makes up pages 65–138. The edition contains no commentary or glossary.

7 Aaltje Johanna Geertruida Hilbelink, *Cotton MS Vitellius C. iii of the Herbarium Apulei* (Amsterdam: NV Swets und Zeitlanger, 1930). This dissertation has a very general two-page introduction and only cites Cockayne. After the edited text is a short study of forms by grammatical class.

8 Stephanie Hollis and Michael Wright, *Old English Prose of Secular Learning* (Cambridge: D.S. Brewer, 1992).

9 Exceptions are the publications by D'Aronco cited here; as well as Kesling 2020. Also of interest is Stephanie Hollis, "Scientific and Medical Writings," in *A Companion to Anglo-Saxon Literature*, eds. Phillip Pulsiano and Elaine Treharne, (London: Blackwell Publishers, 2001); and to some extent, Doyle 2000.

10 References are to page numbers in D'Aronco 2003.

11 Linda Ehrsam Voigts, "A New Look at the Manuscript Containing the Old English Translation of the *Herbarium Apulei*," *Manuscripta* 20 (1976): 42. See also her 1978 article on the name Apuleius.

12 Grape-Albers issued a new facsimile of Vienna 93, the focus of her earlier study; see her *Medicina Antiqua: Codex Vindobonensis 93* (London: Harvey Miller, 1999) with an introduction by Peter Murray Jones. See also Collins 2000 for a discussion of the illustrative traditions in Greek, Arabic, and Latin herbals through the fifteenth century. Of related interest is Peter Murray Jones, *Medieval Medicine in Illuminated Manuscripts* (London: British Library, 1998).

13 Arthur Gross, "Wolframs Schlangenliste (*Parzifal* 481) und Pseudo-Apuleius," in *Licht der Natur: Medizin in Fachliteratur und Dichtung*, eds. J. Domes, W. Gerabek, B. Haage, C. Weißer und V. Zimmermann (Göppingen: Kümmerle Verlag, 1994), 128–48. Gross based some of his arguments on Grape-Albers.

14 For those primarily interested in the linguistic aspects of the vocabulary in this and other medical writings in Old English (word formation and so forth), see Hans Sauer's articles "Towards a Linguistic Description and Classification of the Old English Plant Names," in *Words, Texts and Manuscripts: Studies in Anglo-Saxon Culture Presented to Helmut Gneuss*, ed. Michael Korhammer et al. (Cambridge: D.S. Brewer, 1992), 381–408; "On the Analysis and Structure of Old and Middle English Plant Names," *The History of English* No.3 (1997): 133–61; and "English Plant Names in the Thirteenth Century: The Trilingual Harley Vocabulary," in *Middle English Miscellany*, ed. Jacek Tisiak (Posnan: Motivex, 1996), 135–55. See also M.A. D'Aronco, "The Botanical Lexicon of the *Old English Herbarium*,"

Anglo-Saxon England 17 (1988): 15–33; Janet M. Bately, "Old English Prose Before and during the Reign of Alfred," *Anglo-Saxon England* 17 (1988): 93–138. The most recent comprehensive philological study is Conan Doyle's 2011 dissertation.

15 Concerning substitutions in classical and medieval medical texts, see Alain Touwaide, "Quid Pro Quo: Revisiting the Practice of Substitution in Ancient Pharmacy" in *Herbs and Healers from the Ancient Mediterranean through the Medieval West*, eds. Anne Van Arsdall and Timothy Graham (Farnham: Ashgate, 2012), 19–61; John M. Riddle, *Quid pro quo: Studies in the History of Drugs* (Brookfield, VT: Ashgate, 1992).

5

THE *OLD ENGLISH HERBARIUM*

A modern translation

Author's notes to the translation

Usage and style: The early-medieval translation from Latin to Old English has a direct and even conversational style. The Latin originals are quite terse and generally use the passive voice; thus, the Old English has a style quite different from them, but follows the texts fairly closely. In several remedies, a personal note attests that someone found that the remedy works well. And, yes, philologists have found mistakes in the translation and omissions—nevertheless, this text existed as we see it and it was used despite its flaws.

My translation is not literal, in the sense that Cockayne's is. His work is a more-or-less word-for-word rendition of the Old English, but his choice of words to render it is at best dated and hard to understand today. I make no attempt to mimic the Old English word order, and many filler words (then, and) are omitted, as is some of the repetition (for example, "that same plant"). By not providing a literal translation, some interesting turns of phrase in Old English were unfortunately lost in striving for clarity.

Two major considerations had to be weighed: (1) faithfulness to the Old English and (2) transmitting information accurately to modern readers of English (particularly to those who cannot read Latin or Old English). Verbs such as *cnucian* (*cnocian*) "to pound" pose a challenge, because in making remedies, plants can be bruised, mashed, crushed, pulverized, or chopped, all with the same general action as being pounded. Indeed, healers have long used a mortar and pestle to pound and crush their medicinal plants—today's herbalists might use a blender! The *Herbarium* uses *cnucian* over and over. I retain it for the most part because (1) that is what is in the text and (2) it can be understood by anyone familiar with herbal preparations as a general instruction to break up the plant so it will work readily. Having more knowledge about what to do other than "pound" would come from experience.

DOI: 10.4324/9781003162285-5

Another example is the verb *wyllan* (literally, to boil). At hands-on workshops on making medicinal herbal remedies, the caution was generally given never to boil (truly boil hard) herbs; instead, they are simmered or cooked just below the boiling point (one *curandera* said the water should be "smiling"). To reflect accurately both the verb and customary practice, I usually translate *wyllan* as "gently boil." *Seoðan* (to seethe or simmer) could have meant either simmer or actually to seethe (infuse)—in reality, both produce nearly the same result—and in observing preparations being made, the medieval practitioner would have learned the subtle difference between "simmer" and "seethe," which I use nearly interchangeably.

By its nature, translation is interpretation, not just of the words but of the work itself. The interpretation guiding this work is that the *Herbarium* was not intended to be a step-by-step manual in preparing remedies and treating people. Instead, it has notes for healers to help them determine or remember how to treat medical conditions, similar to a number of contemporary works on medicinal plants. Most of the remedies follow a formula: (1) for this condition, (2) take the plant, (3) prepare it in a certain manner, (4) administer it, (5) this is the result you can expect. Not all parts of the formula are always present, and many actions are not fully explained.

For example, how one "collects" (picks, harvests, digs up, cuts, etc.) the plant is missing, details on the preparation other than seethe or mix are absent, and how to administer it (other than "put it on") is usually omitted. And too, the patient can be missing entirely; the user is directed to seethe the plant in water and give to drink, or, to treat a wound, to pound the plant with fat and put it on. Such terse instructions have usually been retained in this translation, the rationale being that the object is clearly understood from the context and that many remedy books written even today employ such shorthand.

Common is the instruction to pound a plant in wine and give to drink (shorthand for pound the plant until it reaches a certain state of malleability, put it into a certain amount of wine, let it steep in the wine for some length of time depending on the plant and how long it takes for it to infuse into the liquid, then perhaps strain the liquid, and give that liquid to the patient to drink). Quite often the directions say, "give it to drink and lay it on the wound," which could be interpreted as, give the liquid as a beverage, then lay the soaked and softened plant onto the wound. The same is true for the frequent instruction: pound the plant in grease and put it on. Here again, the plant would be pulverized fresh or dry, mixed with grease, the salve would be allowed to rest for some time, and then the salve put on the patient's wound. The instructions are translated as written; certainly, those with specialized knowledge needed to interpret them will know how to unpack them.

Medicine of all types has long required an apprenticeship as part of learning, and it is clear that this text was written for someone who was learning or already knew how to use its abbreviated instructions. What is found here was not for a "student leech," a term coined by Olds (1984), but instead was wisdom transmitted from one healer to another, much of it within the vast network of medieval Benedictine monasteries discussed in Chapter 3. Informed users would have been able to supply missing information from their own store of practical knowledge. Just as in cooking, the recipes one follows benefit from seeing and experiencing what is actually meant by simmer, cook, boil gently, a rolling boil, cook just below the boiling point, and so forth.

If it meets its purpose, this book will provide unbiased information about some of the texts and the practice of early-medieval medicine as well as on the history of medicinal plant use. It is definitely not intended to demonstrate the quaintness of medieval medicine—far from it. Cockayne's three volumes do that extremely well. A primary goal is to provide an accurate and useful version of the *Old English Herbarium* as a witness to an unbroken tradition of herbal medicine from before this millennium, through it, and on to the next.

Structure of the work: The *Herbarium* is both a herbal and a remedy book. It begins with a lengthy contents list made up of 185 chapter headings, each giving the name of one plant in Latin and often in Old English as well. Under each chapter heading is a list of the conditions with which that plant helps. The contents list outlines precisely what is in the *Herbarium* and provides a quick way to locate conditions and plants to treat them. Following the contents list, the body of the *Herbarium* fills out the details of each chapter, providing remedies and directions on what to do. Like the contents list, the body of the herbal uses only plant names as its chapter headings. Neither the contents list nor the chapters are numbered in the original.

Cockayne added a precise numbering system, coordinating the contents list with the text. His numbering system has been adopted in all subsequent editions and translations, with very minor changes, such as in DeVriend's edition, which my work follows. Cockayne used roman numerals everywhere, as does DeVriend; I use arabic.

In this translation, **headings in the contents list** retain the original Latin name as written, and only if there was an Old English name in the original do I add a modern English plant name to the heading. In the **translated text of the original OE Herbarium**, which follows the contents list, the headings for each of its 185 chapters are plant names only, sometimes in Latin, sometimes in Old English, sometimes both. In the Cotton MS, each plant is accompanied by a large illustration showing how it looks, its name a part of the design. Only the final entry has no illustrated chapter heading.

Unlike the brief original chapter headings, in my **translation of the Herbarium** each chapter heading provides (1) a modern English plant name, established more or less certainly, (2) modern Latin binomial, (3) medieval Latin or Greek name as found in the *Herbarium*, and (4) the Old English name if one was in the original.

Below the chapter headings are numbered lists of conditions and remedies; here is where directions for use are found. In my translation, wherever the original used an Old English plant name I translate it directly into modern English. However, wherever a Latin or Greek name is used, it appears exactly as written. My reasoning is that the language used for plant names will be a significant factor in ascertaining how the *Herbarium* was actually used in practice. Note for readers not familiar with Latin: Latin plant names, like all Latin nouns, have case endings that change with their grammatical use in a sentence. Thus, the name in the heading (nominative) and in the text (if other than nominative) will not always be the same; e.g., *Betonica, Betonicam.*

Quirks of the text and how they are reflected in this updated translation

LANGUAGE. **Old English uses "*man*"** to mean "one/a person" followed by "him" in many remedies, an English usage that not too long ago was thought to have no gendered connotation. As noted earlier, Cockayne translated *man* not as "one" but as "a man" and "he/him," making the text sound as though written about men. Unlike in the first edition and bucking formal written English but following widespread spoken English usage, I use "them" for the objective following "one, a person, someone" to avoid gender bias and also the cumbersome "him/her."

Fetus (foetus)/menses/anus/diarrhea/urination/constipation/genitals. To mirror the style of the original as much as possible, I use colloquial English in this medical text—not the more formal Latin terms that are customary today. This style is not intended to diminish the serious intent of this medical text, but rather reflects that Latin or French words became part of vernacular use much later than when the *Herbarium* was translated. Instead, I use child instead of fetus, women's periods for menses, rear for anus and rectum, stopped up intestines for constipation, and private parts for genitals. I shied away from using very colloquial terms for defecation (shit) and urination (piss or pee) and instead use very runny stools for diarrhea and pass water for urination. Fevers that come every third or fourth day replace tertian and quartan fevers.

In the Old English, *cild/cyld* is used for child and for fetus, whether alive or stillborn. Chapters 63.1 and 165.4 use *tudder/tuddor* for child; the first with the modifier "dead," the second without to denote an unborn child. Because in this work, the Old English does not seem to have a unique word for fetus or stillborn, I decided to use child for all these terms, and to modify it only as and where the original does. The word "flux" appears a few times in the translation as a direct translation of the often ambiguous term *flewsa*, literally bodily "flow" of some kind. For a woman's "flow," the meaning is clear. However, when it appears simply as a condition needing treatment but little more information than that, I simply use "flux."

In addition, I have omitted in this edition several notes indicating when a remedy might have implied its use as an abortifacient. Abortion vs. menstrual regulation vs. fertility concerns are topics meriting further study and scrutiny, deserving more than a note insinuating the intent of the remedy. It is clear when menstruation is being discussed, but the reasons why are debatable. For this topic, the interested reader might consult the many publications by John M. Riddle and Monica H. Green; for example, Riddle's *Eve's Herbs* (1999) and Greene's *The Trotula: An English Translation of the Medieval Compendium of Women's Medicine* (2002).

CONDITIONS. **Worms about the navel/worms in the rear** are handled differently in this edition than in the first. The kinds of worms meant in this herbal and where they manifest are not certain; sometimes they seem to be intestinal, sometimes anal, and sometimes, around the navel, which might be a skin condition, such as *molluscum contagiosum* or *cutaneous larva migrans*. In the first edition (pp. 181–2), I explain why I translated OE *nafola*, meaning "navel" as anus. It was primarily because many remedies cure worms with a herbal beverage of some kind to expel them, and that a knot of skin, such as at the anus, can be called an *umbilicum*, the word for navel in Latin. However, it seemed wiser to use the literal meaning of the OE word *nafola* here until more evidence could support the translation I used earlier. Absent archeological evidence for the kinds of worms present in early-medieval times, it is not possible to determine with any certainty the kinds of worms meant here nor where they manifested. The fifth-century physician Marcellus of Bordeaux devoted chapter 28 of his medical treatise to curing various kinds of worms (*lumbrici et tinae*) using remedies similar to those in the *Herbarium*. Many involve drinking an herb or mixture of herbs to kill and expel the worms and/or applying or inserting the herbs (in)to the anus. Worms were a popular topic.

Impetigo/leprosy. In the first edition, I translated OE *teter* as impetigo, a specific condition, but have come to realize that what the condition *teter* actually connotes is not really known. Cockayne correctly translates it as "tetter," an archaic word for skin infections. DeVriend gives ringworm as its meaning. In this edition, I use "skin conditions" for *teter*. Another skin condition, *hreofl* (110.3 and 146.4), can be found translated as leprosy; in fact the online *Dictionary of Old English* (DOE) has it as a real possibility. It means rough, scabby, scaly skin, and more evidence would prove whether such specificity is warranted. For it, I use "bad skin condition." Leprosy was widespread at the time, but questions remain about the Old English terms specific to it.

Fotadle is commonly translated as "gout," which is a specific disease requiring diagnosis by a professional. I used "gout" in the first edition; however, here, I replace it with "foot disease," less specific, awaiting a name when evidence warrants it.

Abbreviations in notes for sources frequently cited (all given fully in bibliography)

C: Cockayne's translation of the *Old English Herbarium*
BT: Bosworth-Toller's *Anglo-Saxon Dictionary*.
D'A: D'Aronco and Cameron. *The Old English Illustrated Pharmacopoeia*.
DeV: DeVriend. *Old English Herbarium*.
DOE: *Dictionary of Old English* (on-line with restricted use)
DOEPN: Dictionary of Old English Plant Names
    Other works are cited by the author's last name.

In notes to the translation to show where mine differs appreciably from Cockayne's, the Old English word in question is cited, then Cockayne's translation is given as C = …

Herbarium

The chapters of the book of medicine begin:

1. The name of the plant is *betonica*, which is **wood betony**
   - (1:1) For dreadful nightmares and for terrifying visions and dreams
   - (1:2) For a shattered skull
   - (1:3) For eye pain
   - (1:4) For earache
   - (1:5) For dimness of the eyes
   - (1:6) For watery eyes
   - (1:7) For flow of blood from the nose
   - (1:8) For toothache
   - (1:9) For a pain in the side
   - (1:10) For pain in the loins
   - (1:11) For stomach pain
   - (1:12) For the intestines being stopped up
   - (1:13) For blood gushing through the mouth
   - (1:14) For not getting drunk
   - (1:15) For a boil on the face
   - (1:16) For an internal rupture
   - (1:17) For fatigue from much riding or walking
   - (1:18) For feeling unwell or nauseous
   - (1:19) For good digestion of food
   - (1:20) For not being able to keep food down
   - (1:21) For abdominal pain or bloating
   - (1:22) For drinking poison
   - (1:23) For snakebite
   - (1:24) For snakebite
   - (1:25) For bite of a mad dog
   - (1:26) For a sore throat or part of the neck
   - (1:27) For sore loins or an ache in the thighs
   - (1:28) For high fever
   - (1:29) For foot disease

2. The *arniglosa* plant, which is **common plantain**
   - (2:1) For headache
   - (2:2) For a sore stomach
   - (2:3) For abdominal pain
   - (2:4) Again, for a swollen stomach
   - (2:5) For bleeding from the rear
   - (2:6) For wounds
   - (2:7) To soften the stomach

(2:8)   For snakebite
(2:9)   Again, for snakebite
(2:10)   For intestinal worms
(2:11)   For a hard place on the body
(2:12)   For fever that returns in four days
(2:13)   For foot disease and sore tendons
(2:14)   For fever that returns in three days
(2:15)   For two-day fever
(2:16)   For inflamed wounds
(2:17)   For swollen feet on a trip
(2:18)   For a sore on the nose or cheek
(2:19)   For strange pimples on the nose
(2:20)   For mouth injuries
(2:21)   For bite of a mad dog
(2:22)   For daily internal weakness

3.   The *pentafilon* plant, which is **cinquefoil**
    (3:1)   For joints that ache or are afflicted by illness
    (3:2)   For stomach pain
    (3:3)   For aching mouth, tongue, and throat
    (3:4)   For headache
    (3:5)   For severe nosebleed
    (3:6)   For aching midriff
    (3:7)   For snakebite
    (3:8)   For burns
    (3:9)   If you want to stop ulcerous sores from spreading

4.   The *uermenaca* plant, which is **vervain**
    (4:1)   For wounds, carbuncles, and swollen glands
    (4:2)   Again, for swollen glands
    (4:3)   For those who have clogged veins so that blood cannot get to the private parts and for those who cannot keep their food down
    (4:4)   For liver pain
    (4:5)   For bladder stones
    (4:6)   For headache
    (4:7)   For snakebite
    (4:8)   For poisonous spider bite
    (4:9)   For bite of a mad dog
    (4:10)   For fresh wounds
    (4:11)   For snakebite

5.   The *sinphoniaca* plant, which is **henbane**
    (5:1)   For earache
    (5:2)   For swollen knees or calves or other swellings on the body
    (5:3)   For toothache

(5:4)   For soreness or swelling of the private parts
(5:5)   For painful breasts
(5:6)   For sore feet
(5:7)   For lung diseases

6. The *uiperina* plant, which is **bistort** or **snakeweed**
    (6:1)   For snakebite

7. The *ueneria* plant, which is **"bee plant"**
    (7:1)   To prevent bees' swarming
    (7:2)   For inability to pass water

8. The plant *pes leonis*, which is **lion's foot** or **lady's mantle**
    (8:1)   For being under an evil spell

9. The *scelerata* plant, which is **celery-leaved crowfoot**
    (9:1)   For wounds and carbuncles
    (9:2)   For swellings and warts

10. The *batracion* plant, which is **buttercup** or **meadow crowfoot**
    (10:1)   For lunacy
    (10:2)   For darkened sores

11. The *artemesia* plant, which is **mugwort**
    (11:1)   For a sore abdomen
    (11:2)   For sore feet

12. The *artemesia tagantes* plant, which is the second kind of mugwort, called **tansy**
    (12:1)   For bladder pain
    (12:2)   For sore thighs
    (12:3)   For sore and swollen tendons
    (12:4)   For severe foot disease
    (12:5)   For fever

13. The *artemesia leptefilos* plant, which is a third kind of mugwort, called **roman wormwood**
    (13:1)   For stomachache
    (13:2)   For trembling tendons

14. The *lapatium* plant, which is **dock**
    (14:1)   For hardened swellings that form on the private parts

15. The *dracontea* plant, which is **dragonwort**
    (15:1)   For snakebite
    (15:2)   For broken bones

16. The *satyrion* plant, which is **orchis** or **wild orchid**
    (16:1)   For painful wounds
    (16:2)   For eye pain

17. The *gentiana* plant, which is **yellow gentian**
    (17:1) For snakebite

18. The *orbicularis* plant, which is **cyclamen** or **sowbread**
    (18:1) For hair loss
    (18:2) For irritable bowels
    (18:3) For pain in the spleen

19. The *proserpinaca* plant, which is **knotgrass**
    (19:1) For spitting blood
    (19:2) For pain in the sides
    (19:3) For sore nipples
    (19:4) For eye pain
    (19:5) For earache
    (19:6) For very loose stools

20. The *aristolochia* plant, which is **heartwort** or **birthwort**
    (20:1) Against strong poison
    (20:2) For bad fevers
    (20:3) For sore nostrils
    (20:4) For a person who is chilled
    (20:5) For snakebite
    (20:6) For an upset child
    (20:7) For a sore growing on the nose

21. The *nasturcium* plant, which is **watercress** or **garden cress**
    (21:1) For hair falling out
    (21:2) For head sores accompanied by dandruff and itching
    (21:3) For soreness in the body
    (21.4) For swellings
    (21:5) For warts

22. The *hieribulbum* plant, which is **meadow saffron** or **autumn crocus**
    (22:1) For sore joints
    (22:2) If pimples grow on a woman's nose

23. The *apollinaris* plant, which is **ashwagandha**
    (23:1) For sore hands

24. The *camemelon* plant, which is **chamomile**
    (24:1) For eye pain

25. The *chamedris* plant, which is **wall germander**
    (25:1) For bruises
    (25:2) For snakebite
    (25:3) For foot disease

26. The *chameælee* plant, which is **wild teasel**
    (26:1) For liver disease
    (26:2) For poison
    (26:3) For dropsy

27. The *chamepithys* plant, which is **ground-pine**
    (27:1) For wounds
    (27:2) For abdominal pain

28. The *chamedafne* plant, which is **figwort** or **lesser celandine**
    (28:1) To stimulate the bowels

29. The *ostriago* plant or **madder**
    (29:1) For bothersome sores

30. The *brittanica* plant, which is **water dock**
    (30:1) For mouth sores
    (30:2) Again, for mouth sores
    (30:3) For toothache
    (30:4) To move clogged bowels
    (30:5) For pain in the side

31. The *lactuca* plant, which is **prickly lettuce**
    (31:1) For dim eyes
    (31:2) Again, for dim eyes

32. The *agrimonia* plant, which is **agrimony**
    (32:1) For sore eyes
    (32:2) For sore abdomen
    (32:3) For ulcerous sores and wounds
    (32:4) For snakebite
    (32:5) For warts
    (32:6) For soreness of the spleen
    (32:7) If you want to cut something from the body
    (32:8) For a blow from iron

33. The *astularegia* plant, which is **asphodel**
    (33:1) For leg-shank pain
    (33:2) For liver pain

34. The *lapatium* plant, which is **sorrel**
    (34:1) If body stiffness occurs

35. The *centauria maior* plant, which is **yellow centaury**
    (35:1) For liver diseases
    (35:2) For wounds and ulcerous sores

36. The *centauria minor* plant, which is **common** or **lesser centaury**
    (36:1)   For snakebite
    (36:2)   For eye pain
    (36:3)   Again, for the same
    (36:4)   For nerve spasms
    (36:5)   For tasting poison
    (36:6)   For worms around the navel

37. The *personacia* plant, which is **beet**
    (37:1)   For wounds and snakebite
    (37:2)   For fevers
    (37:3)   For ulcerous sores on wounds
    (37:4)   For pain in the abdomen
    (37:5)   For bite of a mad dog
    (37:6)   For fresh wounds

38. The *fraga* plant, which is **wild strawberry**
    (38:1)   For pain of the spleen
    (38:2 a) For shortness of breath
    (38:2 b) For abdominal pain

39. The *hibiscus* plant, which is **marsh mallow**
    (39:1)   For foot disease
    (39:2)   For any accumulation of diseased matter growing on the body

40. The *ippirus* plant, which is **horsetail**
    (40:1)   For swollen stomach
    (40:2)   For coughing up blood

41. The *malfa erratica* plant, which is **mallow**
    (41:1)   For bladder pain
    (41:2)   For sore tendons
    (41:3)   For pain in the side
    (41:4)   For fresh wounds

42. The *buglossa* plant, which is **alkanet/bugloss**
    (42:1)   For fever that comes every three or every four days
    (42:2)   For shortness of breath

43. The *bulbiscillitica* plant, which is **sea-onion** or **squill**
    (43:1)   For dropsy
    (43:2)   For painful joints
    (43:3)   For the disease the Greeks call *paranichias*
    (43:4)   If one cannot quench the thirst of a person with dropsy

44. The *cotiledon* plant, which is **navelwort**
    (44:1)   For swellings

45. The *gallicrus* plant, which is **cockspur-grass**
    (45:1) For dog bite

46. The *prassion* plant, which is **horehound**
    (46:1) For a head cold and for violent coughing
    (46:2) For stomachache
    (46:3) For worms around the navel
    (46:4) For sore joints and for swellings
    (46:5) For taking poison
    (46:6) For scabs and skin infections
    (46:7) For lung diseases
    (46:8) For every stiffness in the body

47. The *xifion* plant, which is "**wild gladiolus**"
    (47:1) For strange carbuncles growing on the body
    (47:2) For a fractured skull and poisoned bones

48. The *gallitricus* plant, which is **true maidenhair**
    (48:1) If swellings harm a virgin
    (48:2) For hair loss

49. The *temolus* plant, which is **garlic**
    (49:1) For pain in the womb

50. The *æliotrophus* plant, which is **heliotrope**
    (50:1) For all poisons
    (50:2) For flux

51. The *gryas* plant, which is **madder**
    (51:1) For aching legs and broken bones
    (51:2) For every pain that hurts the body

52. The *politricus* plant or **common maidenhair**
    (52:1) For abdominal pain and to promote hair growth

53. The *malochinagria* plant, which is **asphodel**
    (53:1) For swollen stomach
    (53:2) For loose stools

54. The *metoria* plant, which is **white poppy**
    [(54:1) omitted in the manuscript]
    (54:2) For pain in the temples
    (54:3) For sleeplessness

55. The *oenantes* plant
    (55:1) For inability to pass water
    (55:2) If anyone coughs very strongly

56. The *narcisus* plant, which is **throatwort** or **narcissus**
    (56:1)   For sores that grow on people

57. The *splenion* plant, which is **spleenwort** or **figwort**
    (57:1)   For pain in the spleen

58. The *polion* plant
    (58:1)   For lunacy

59. The *uictoriola* plant, which is **butcher's broom**
    (59:1)   For foot disease and stomachache

60. The *confirma* plant, which is **comfrey**
    (60:1)   For women's periods
    (60:2)   For internal ruptures
    (60:3)   For stomachache

61. The *asterion* plant
    (61:1)   For epilepsy

62. The *leporis pes* plant, which is **hare's foot clover**
    (62:1)   For stopped up intestines

63. The *dictamnus* plant
    (63:1)   If a woman has a dead child inside her
    (63:2)   For wounds
    (63:3)   For snakebite
    (63:4)   For eating something poisonous
    (63:5)   Again, for fresh wounds

64. The *solago maior* plant, which is ***helioscorpion***
    (64:1)   Again, for snakebite

65. The *solago minor* plant, which is ***aeliotropion***
    (65:1)   For worms around the navel

66. The *peonia* plant
    (66:1)   For lunacy
    (66:2)   For aching hip bone

67. The *peristereon* plant, which is **vervain** or **gypsy-wort**
    (67:1)   For dog's barking
    (67:2)   For all poisons

68. The *bryonia* plant, which is **bryony**
    (68:1)   For pain in the spleen

69. The *nymfete* plant
    (69:1a)   For loose bowls
    (69:1b)   Again, for loose stools
    (69:2)   For abdominal pain

70. The *crision* plant, which is **thistle**
    (70:1)   For sore throat

71. The *isatis* plant
    (71:1)   For snakebite

72. The *scordea* plant
    (72:1)   Again, for snakebite
    (72:2)   For sore joints
    (72: 3) For fever

73. The *uerbascus* plant, which is **great mullein**
    How Mercury gave the plant to Ulysses
    (73:1)   Against all bad encounters
    (73:2)   For foot disease

74. The *heraclea* plant
    (74:1)   If a person wants to travel a long way and does not want to fear robbers

75. The *cælidonia* plant, which is **greater celandine**
    (75:1)   For dimness and soreness of the eyes
    (75:2)   Again, for dimming eyesight
    (75:3)   For swellings
    (75:4)   For headache
    (75:5)   If one is burned

76. The *solata* plant, which is **black nightshade**
    (76:1)   For swellings
    (76:2)   For earache
    (76:3)   For toothache
    (76:4)   For a bloody nose

77. The *senecio* plant, which is **common groundsel**
    (77:1)   For wounds, even if they are old
    (77:2)   For a blow from something iron
    (77:3)   For foot disease
    (77:4)   For sore loins

78. The *felix* plant, which is **fern**
    (78:1)   For wounds
    (78:2)   For rupture in a young man

79. The *gramen* plant, which is **couch grass**
    (79:1)   For pain in the spleen

80. The *gladiolum* plant, which is **iris**
    (80:1)   For bladder pain and inability to pass water
    (80:2)   For pain of the spleen
    (80:3)   For abdominal and chest pain

81. The *rosmarinum* plant, which is **rosemary**
    (81:1)   For toothache
    (81:2, 3) For ill people and for itching
    (81:4)   For liver disease and abdominal conditions
    (81:5)   For fresh wounds

82. The *pastinaca siluatica* plant, which is **wild carrot** or **parsnip**
    (82:1)   For difficult childbirth
    (82:2)   For a woman's cleansing

83. The *perdicalis* plant, which is **pellitory of the wall**
    (83:1)   For foot disease and ulcerous sores

84. The *mercurialis* plant, which is **dog's mercury**
    (84:1)   For intestinal blockage
    (84:2)   For pain and swelling of the eyes
    (84:3)   If a great deal of water gets in the ears

85. The *radiola* plant, which is **polypody**
    (85:1)   For headache

86. The *sparagiagrestis* plant, which is **asparagus**
    (86:1)   For pain or swelling of the bladder
    (86:2)   For toothache
    (86:3)   For sore veins
    (86:4)   For a case where one person puts another under a spell by ill will

87. The *sabine* plant, which is **savine**
    (87:1)   For painful joints and foot swelling
    (87:2)   For headache
    (87:3)   For carbuncles

88. The *canis caput*, which is the **small snapdragon**
    (88:1)   For soreness and swelling of the eyes

89. The *erusti* plant, which is **blackberry** or **bramble**
    (89:1)   For earache
    (89:2)   For a woman's periods
    (89:3)   For heart pain
    (89:4)   For fresh wounds
    (89:5)   For pain in the joints
    (89:6)   For snakebite

90. The *millefolium* plant, which is **yarrow**
    (90:1)   For a blow from something iron and that Achilles discovered the plant
    (90:2)   For toothache
    (90:3)   For wounds
    (90:4)   For swellings
    (90:5)   For difficulty in passing water

(90:6)   If a wound has grown cold on a person
(90:7)   If the head breaks out in rashes or for strange swellings on the face
(90:8)   For the same
(90:9)   If the veins are hardened or a person has difficulty digesting food
(90:10)   For intestinal and abdominal pain
(90:11)   If hiccoughs trouble someone
(90:12)   For headache
(90:13)   For bite of the snake called *spalangius*
(90:14)   Again, for snakebite
(90:15)   For bite of a mad dog
(90:16)   For snakebite

91.   The *ruta* plant, which is **rue**
(91:1)   For nosebleed
(91:2)   For swellings
(91:3)   For stomachache
(91:4)   For pain and swelling of the eyes
(91:5)   For forgetfulness
(91:6)   For dimness of the eyes
(91:7)   For headache

92.   The *mentastrus* plant, which is **horsemint**
(92:1)   For earache
(92:2)   For very bad skin conditions

93.   The *ebulus* plant, which is **dwarf elder** or **danewort**
(93:1)   For bladder stones
(93:2)   For snakebite
(93:3)   For dropsy

94.   The *pollegion* plant, which is **pennyroyal**
(94:1)   For abdominal pain
(94:2)   For stomach pain
(94:3)   For itching of the private parts
(94:4)   Again, for abdominal pain
(94:5)   For fever that comes every third day
(94:6)   If a stillborn child is in a woman's abdomen
(94:7)   For sea sickness
(94:8)   For bladder pain and the stones growing there
(94:9)   If anyone suffers from pain around the heart or chest
(94:10)   For a cramp
(94:11)   For stomach and abdominal swelling
(94:12)   For pain of the spleen
(94:13)   For pain of the loins or thighs

95.   The *nepitamon* plant, which is **catmint**
(95:1)   For snakebite

96. The *peucedana* plant, which is **sulphurweed** or **hog's fennel**
    (96:1)   Again, for snakebite
    (96:2)   For witlessness of the mind

97. The *hinnula campana* plant, which is **elecampane**
    (97:1)   For bladder pain
    (97:2)   For toothache and loose teeth
    (97:3)   For worms around the navel

98. The *cynoglossa* plant, which is **ribwort plantain**
    (98:1)   For snakebite
    (98:2)   For fever that comes every fourth day
    (98:3)   For poor hearing

99. The *saxifragia* plant, which is **saxifrage**
    (99:1)   For stones in the bladder

100. The *hedera nigra* plant, which is **ivy**
    (100:1)   Again, for stones in the bladder
    (100:2)   For headache
    (100:3)   For pain in the spleen
    (100:4)   For bite of the critter called *spalangiones*
    (100:5)   Again, to heal wounds
    (100:6)   For evil-smelling nostrils
    (100:7)   For poor hearing
    (100:8)   To prevent headache from sun

101. The *serpillus* plant, which is **wild thyme**
    (101:1)   For headache
    (101:2)   Again, for headache
    (101:3)   For burns

102. The *absinthium* plant, which is **wormwood**
    (102:1)   For removing bruises and other sores
    (102:2)   For ringworm

103. The *salfia* plant
    (103:1)   For itching of the private parts
    (103:2)   Again, for itching of the rear

104. The *coliandra* plant, which is **coriander**
    (104:1)   For worms
    (104:2)   So a woman can give birth quickly

105. The *porclaca* plant
    (105:1)   For excessive flowing of semen

106. The *cerefolia* plant, which is **chervil**
    (106:1)   For stomachache

107. The *sisimbrius* plant
     (107:1) For bladder pain and inability to pass water

108. The *olisatra* plant
     (108:1) Again, for bladder pain and pain when passing water

109. The *lilium* plant, which is **lily**
     (109:1) For snakebite
     (109:2) For swellings

110. The *tytymallus* plant, which is **caper spurge**
     (110:1) For abdominal pain
     (110:2) For warts
     (110:3) For bad skin conditions

111. The *carduus siluaticus* plant, which is **sow-thistle**
     (111:1) For stomachache
     (111:2) So that you will not fear encountering any evil

112. The *lupinus montanus* plant
     (112:1) For worms about the navel
     (112:2) For the same in children

113. The *lactyrida* plant, which is **spurge laurel**
     (113:1) For stopped up intestines

114. The *lactuca leporina* plant, which is **great chondrilla** or **lettuce**
     (114:1) For feverishness

115. The *cucumeris siluatica* plant, which is **squirting cucumber**
     (115:1) For sore joints and foot conditions
     (115:2) If a child is not born right

116. The cannaue silfatica plant
     (116:1) For sore breasts
     (116:2) For chill burns

117. The *ruta montana* plant, which is **wild rue**
     (117:1) For dim eyesight
     (117:2) For a sore chest
     (117:3) For liver pain
     (117:4) For inability to pass water
     (117:5) For snakebite

118. The *eptafilon* plant, which is **tormentil**
     (118:1) For foot disease

119. The *ocimus* plant, which is **basil**
     (119:1) For headache
     (119:2) For eye pain and swelling
     (119:3) For kidney pain

120. The *apium* plant, which is **wild celery**
    (120:1) For eye pain and swelling

121. The *hedera crysocantes* plant, which is **ivy**
    (121:1) For dropsy

122. The *menta* plant, which is **mint**
    (122:1) For skin infections and pimples
    (122:2) For bad scars and wounds

123. The *anetum* plant, which is **dill**
    (123:1) For itching and pain in the private parts
    (123:2) If a woman suffers from the same
    (123:3) For headache

124. The *origanum* plant, which is **wild** or **sweet marjoram**
    (124:1) For foot disease, liver diseases, and shortness of breath
    (124:2) For coughs

125. The *semperuiuus* plant, which is **houseleek**
    (125:1) For accumulations of all bad fluids

126. The *fenuculus* plant, which is **fennel**
    (126:1) For coughs and shortness of breath
    (126:2) For bladder pain

127. The *erifion* plant, which is **rue**
    (127:1) For lung diseases

128. The *sinfitus albus* plant
    (128:1) For women's periods

129. The *petroselinum* plant, which is **parsley**
    (129:1) For snakebite
    (129:2) For nerve pain

130. The *brassica siluatica* plant, which is **cabbage** or **colewort**
    (130:1) For all swellings
    (130:2) For pain in the side
    (130:3) For foot disease

131. The *basilisca* plant, which is **sweet basil**
    (131:1) For all types of snakes

132. The *mandragora* plant
    (132:1) For headache
    (132:2) For earache
    (132:3) For foot disease
    (132:4) For lunacy
    (132:5) Again, for nerve spasms
    (132:6) If anyone sees great evil in the house

133. The *lychanis stephanice* plant, which is **campion**
     (133:1) For all types of snakes

134. The *action* plant
     (134:1) If one coughs up blood and phlegm
     (134:2) For pain in the joints

135. The *abrotanus* plant, which is **southernwood**
     (135:1) For shortness of breath, aching bones, and pain when passing water
     (135:2) For pain in the side
     (135:3) For poison and snakebite
     (135:4) Again, for snakebite
     (135:5) For eye pain

136. The *sion* plant, which is **water parsnip**
     (136:1) For stones in the bladder
     (136:2) For very loose stools and unsettled intestines

137. The *eliotropus* plant, which is **white heliotrope**
     (137:1) For all snakebites
     (137:2) For worms that bother the area around the navel
     (137:3) For warts

138. The *spreritis* plant
     (138:1) For fever chills
     (138:2) For the bite of a mad dog
     (138:3) For pain of the spleen

139. The *aizos minor* plant
     (139:1) For skin infections and eye pain and foot disease
     (139:2) For headache
     (139:3) For bite of the snake named *spalangiones*
     (139:4) For very loose stools and unsettled intestines and if worms trouble
              the intestines
     (139:5) Again, for any disease of the eye

140. The *elleborus* plant, which is **white hellebore**
     (140:1) About the power of this plant
     (140:2) For very loose stools
     (140:3) For diseases and for all evil

141. The *buoptalmon* plant
     (141:1) For any bad boils
     (141:2) For damage to the body

142. The *tribulus* plant, which is **gorse**
     (142:1) For a very hot body
     (142:2) For swelling and foulness of the mouth and throat
     (142:3) For bladder stones

(142:4)   For snakebite
(142:5)   For drinking poison
(142:6)   For fleas

143. The *coniza* plant
    (143:1)   For snakebite, to put gnats, mosquitoes, and fleas to flight, and for wounds
    (143:2, 3) To purify a woman's womb and if a woman cannot give birth
    (143:4)   For fever chills
    (143:5)   For headache

144. The *tricnos manicos* plant, which is **thorn-apple** or **datura**
    (144:1)   For skin conditions
    (144:2)   For a pimply body
    (144:3)   For headache and stomach burn and pimples
    (144:4)   For earache

145. The *glycyrida* plant
    (145:1)   For a dry fever
    (145:2)   For chest, liver, and bladder pain
    (145:3)   For conditions of the mouth

146. The *strutius* plant
    (146:1)   If a person cannot pass water
    (146:2)   For liver diseases, shortness of breath, bad coughs, and loose stools
    (146:3)   For bladder stones
    (146:4)   For bad skin conditions
    (146:5)   For troublesome skin conditions

147. The *aizon* plant
    (147:1)   For erupting sores, festering body, eye pain and heat, and burns
    (147:3)   For snakebite [147:2 is missing]
    (147:4)   For very loose stools, intestinal worms, and terrible chills

148. The *samsuchon* plant, which is **elder**
    (148:1)   For dropsy, inability to pass water, and to move the bowels
    (148:2)   For carbuncles and skin eruptions
    (148:3)   For scorpion sting
    (148:4)   For extremely hot and swollen eyes

149. The *stecas* plant
    (149:1)   For chest pain

150. The *thyaspis* plant
    (150:1)   For all painful intestinal blockage and for women's periods

151. The *polis* plant, which is **wood sage** or **sage-leaved germander**
    (151:1)   For snakebite
    (151:2)   For dropsy

(151:3)   For pain of the spleen, to chase away snakes, and for fresh wounds

152. The *ypericon* plant, which is **St. John's wort**
   (152:1)   To stimulate passing water and monthly periods
   (152:2)   For fever that returns every fourth day
   (152:3)   For swelling and aching of the leg shanks

153. The *acantaleuca* plant
   (153:1)   For coughing up blood and stomach pain
   (153:2)   To stimulate passing water
   (153:3)   For toothache and bad bruises
   (153:4)   For cramps and snakebite

154. The *acanton* plant, which is **Scotch thistle**
   (154:1)   To stimulate passing stools and water
   (154:2)   For lung disease and for intestinal ailments

155. The *guiminon* plant, which is **caraway** or **cumin**
   (155:1)   For stomachache
   (155:2)   For shortness of breath and snakebite
   (155:3)   For tenderness and heat of the abdomen
   (155:4)   For nosebleed

156. The *camelleon alba* plant, which is **carline thistle**
   (156:1)   If intestinal worms trouble one about the navel
   (156:2)   For dropsy and difficulty in passing water

157. The *scolymbos* plant
   (157:1)   For a foul smell in the armpits and anywhere on the body
   (157:2)   For passing foul-smelling water

158. The *iris Yllyrica* plant
   (158:1)   For deep coughs and to move the intestines
   (158:2a)   For snakebite
   (158:2b)   To stimulate a woman's periods
   (158:3)   For boils and painful swellings and all bad swellings
   (158:4)   For headache

159. The *elleborus albus* plant
   (159:1)   For liver diseases and all poisons

160. The *delfinion* plant
   (160:1)   For fever that returns every fourth day

161. The *acios* plant
   (161:1)   For snakebite and sore loins

162. The *centimorbia* plant
   (162:1)   If the back of a horse is injured at the shoulder and the wound
        is open

163. The *scordios* plant
    (163:1, 2) To stimulate passing water, for snakebite, for all poisons, and stomachache
    (163:3)   For phlegm in the chest
    (163:4)   For foot conditions
    (163:5)   For fresh wounds

164. The *ami* plant, which is **bishop's weed**
    (164:1a)   To move the intestines, to stimulate passing water, and for the bite of wild animals
    (164:1b)   For spots on the body
    (164:2)   For discoloration or lack of color on the body

165. The *uiola* plant, which is **wall-flower**
    (165:1)   For pain and inflammation of the womb
    (165:2)   For a variety of disorders in the rear
    (165:3)   For canker sores in the mouth
    (165:4)   To stimulate a woman's periods
    (165:5)   For pain of the spleen

166. The *uiola purpurea* plant
    (166:1)   For fresh wounds and also for old ones
    (166:2)   For hardening of the stomach

167. The *zamalentition* plant
    (167:1)   For all wounds
    (167:2)   For ulcerous sores

168. The *ancusa* plant
    (168:1)   For a bad burn

169. The *psillios* plant
    (169:1)   For hard boils and all bad swellings
    (169:2)   For a headache

170. The *cynosbatus* plant
    (170:1)   For pain of the spleen

171. The *aglaofotis* plant
    (171:1)   For fevers that return every third and every fourth day
    (171:2)   If stormy weather troubles one while rowing
    (171:3)   For cramps and tremors

172. The *capparis* plant, which is **caper**
    (172:1)   For pain of the spleen

173. The *eryngius* plant
    (173:1)   To stimulate passing water, women's periods, and to move the intestines
    (173:2)   For a variety of abdominal conditions

(173:3)   For swollen breasts
(173:4a) For scorpion sting, snakebites, and bites from a mad dog
(173:4b) For skin infections and foot disease

174. The *philanthropos* plant
(174:1)   For snakebites and bite of the serpent called *spalangiones*
(174:2)   For earache

175. The *achillea* plant
(175:1)   For fresh wounds
(175:2)   If a woman suffers from fluid flowing from the sexual organ
(175:3)   For very loose stools

176. The *rincus* plant
(176:1)   To turn away hail and storms

177. The *polloten* plant, which is **black horehound**
(177:1)   For dog bite
(177:2)   For wounds

178. The *urtica* plant, which is **nettle**
(178:1)   For frozen wounds
(178:2)   For swellings
(178:3)   If any part of the body is struck
(178:4)   For pain in the loins
(178:5)   For putrefied wounds
(178:6)   For women's periods
(178:7)   So that the cold will not bother you

179. The *priapisci* plant, which is **greater periwinkle**
For possession by demons, for snakes, wild animals, poisons, for any threats, envy, terror, so you will have blessings, so you will be happy and comfortable

180. The *litosperimon* plant
(180:1)   For bladder stones

181. The *stavesacre* plant
(181:1)   For general bodily discomfort
(181:2)   For scaly skin and scabs
(181:3)   For toothache and sore gums

182. The *gorgonion* plant
(182:1)   For bad swelling of the feet

183. The *milotis* plant
(183:1)   For dimness of the eyes
(183:2)   For muscle spasms

184. The *bulbus* plant
    (184:1)   For swellings and foot disease and any injury
    (184:2a) For dropsy
    (184:2b) For dog bite, if one sweats, for stomachache
    (184:3)   For open sores, scaly skin, and pimples
    (184:4)   For internal tenderness and ruptures

185. The *colocynthisagria* plant, which is **bitter cucumber**
    (185:1)   To move the bowels

Remedies

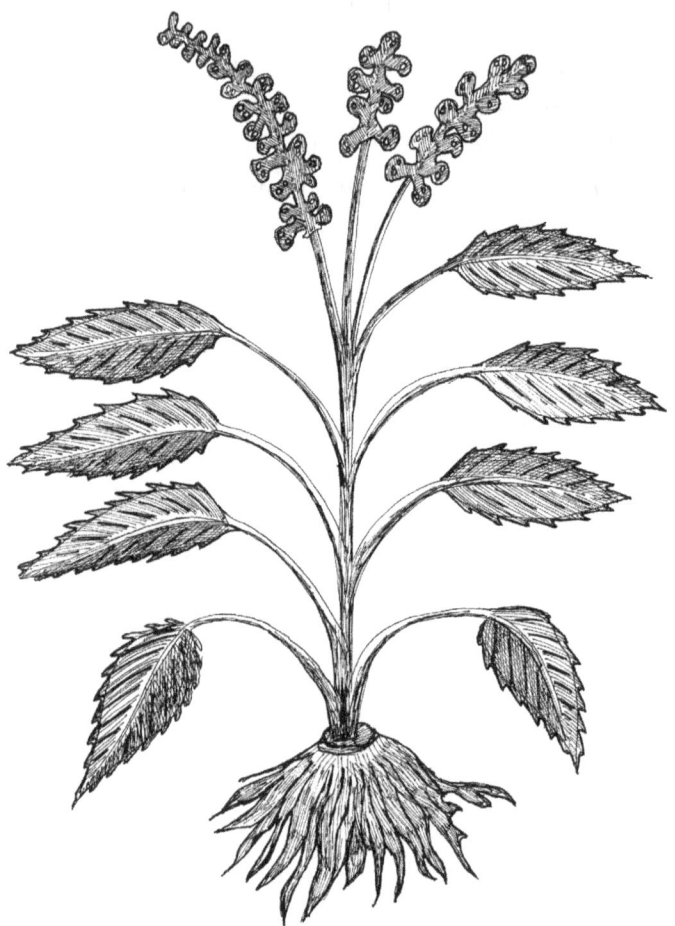

Betony

1. Wood Betony (*Stachys officinalis*), *betonica*, *Biscopwyrt*

    (1:1)   This plant, which is named *betonican*, is grown in meadows, on cleared hilly land,[1] and in sheltered[2] places; it is good both for one's soul and one's body; it protects a person from dreadful nightmares[3] and from terrifying visions and dreams. This plant is very holy and so you must gather it in the month of August without using a tool made of iron; when you have gathered it, shake off the dirt[4] so that none sticks to it and then dry it very thoroughly in the shade. Then, together with its roots, powder it,[5] then use it and taste it when you need to.

(1:2)   If a person's skull is shattered, take the same plant, *betonican*; shred[6] it and pound it to make a fine powder. Then take two coins' weight of it and drink it in hot beer. The skull will heal very quickly after the drink.[7]

(1:3)   For eye pain, take roots of the same plant and simmer them down in water until the liquid is reduced by two-thirds.[8] Bathe the eyes with the water, take the leaves of the same plant, crush them, and lay them on the face over the eyes.

(1:4)   For earache, take the leaves of this same plant when it is greenest, gently boil them in water, and press the juice out,[9] and after it has stood for a time, warm it up again and use a piece of wool to drip it into the ear.

(1:5)   For dimness of the eyes, take one coin's weight of this same plant, *betonican*, and boil gently in water. Give it to drink on an empty stomach, because it dilutes the part of the blood from which the dimness arises.

(1:6)   For watery eyes, take the same plant, *betonican*, and give it to eat. It helps and improves the eyes' sharpness.

(1:7)   For excessive flow of blood from the nose, take the same plant, *betonican*, pound it, and mix with it a bit of salt. Then take as much as you can with two fingers, work it into a ball, and put it into the nostrils.

(1:8)   For toothache, take the same plant, *betonican*, and use a rapid simmer to reduce it down by two-thirds in aged wine. It greatly heals the toothache and swelling.

(1:9)   For pain in the side,[10] take three coins' weight of the same plant; simmer in aged wine. Grind 27 peppercorns and add them to it. Drink three cupfuls at night, on an empty stomach.

(1:10)   For pain in the loins, take the three coins' weight of the same *betonican*, and 17 peppercorns; grind them together and boil gently in aged wine. Give three cupfuls to drink warm at night on an empty stomach.

(1:11)   For stomach pain, take two[11] coins' weight of the same plant, boil gently in water, then give it to drink warm. The stomach pain will diminish and be soothed, so that soon there will not be any pain.

(1:12)   If a person's intestines are blocked,[12] take this same plant in warm water at night on an empty stomach. The person will be well in the space of three nights.

(1:13)   In case blood gushes up through a person's mouth, take three coins' weight of the same plant and three cupfuls of cold goat's milk. They will be healed quickly.

(1:14)   If a person does not want to be drunk, then take the *betonican* plant before drinking.

(1:15)   If a boil appears on the face, take one coin's weight, pound with aged fat, lay on the place where the boil wants to settle, and it will soon be healed.

(1:16)   If a person is ruptured inside or their body is sore, take four coins' weight of the *betonican* plant, boil it gently in wine. Drink it at night on an empty stomach; then their body will soon be relieved.

(1:17)   If a person becomes tired from much riding or much walking, take one coin's weight of the *betonican* plant and simmer it in sweet wine; drink three full cups at night on an empty stomach, then their body will be relieved.

(1:18)   If a person is not feeling well inside or is nauseated, then you take two coins' weight of the *betonican* plant and one ounce of honey. Thoroughly and gently boil this in beer, drink three cupfuls at night on an empty stomach, and their insides will quickly clear up.

(1:19)   If you want your food to digest easily, take three coins' weight of the *betonican* plant and one ounce of honey. Simmer the plant until it thickens, then drink it in two cupfuls of water.

(1:20)   If a person cannot keep down their food and vomits when they swallow, take four coins' weight of the *betonican* plant and boiled honey, then make four little pills from it. Eat one, and take one in hot water and wine together. Then drink three cupfuls of this liquid.

(1:21)   For abdominal pain, or if one is bloated, take the *betonican* plant, crumble it very fine in wine, lay some around the stomach, and eat some of it. That will quickly bring recovery.

(1:22)   If anyone drinks poison, take three coins' weight of that same plant and four cups of wine; gently boil them together, then drink them, and then they will vomit up the poison.

(1:23)   If a snake bites someone, take four coins' weight of the same plant crumbled very small and gently boil in wine. Then do both of these: lay it on the wound and also drink a great deal of it; then you can heal the bite of any snake this way.

(1:24)   Again, for snakebite, take one coin's weight of that same plant, crumble it into red wine (ensure there are three cups of wine), and smear the wound with the plant and the wine; it will soon be healed.

(1:25)   For bite of a mad dog, take the *betonican* plant, pound it very small, and lay it on the wound.

(1:26)   If your throat or any part of your neck is sore, take the same plant, pound it very small, make it into a poultice, and lay it on the neck; it will clean it up both inside and outside.

(1:27)   For sore loins, and if a person's thighs ache, take two coins' weight of the same plant, boil it gently in beer, and give it to them to drink.

(1:28)   If a person is feverish and suffering from being very hot, give the plant in warm water, definitely not in beer. The soreness in the loins and the thighs will get better very quickly.

(1:29) For foot disease, take the same plant, simmer it down in water by two-thirds, pound the plant, lay it on the feet, and rub it on. Drink the juice. You will find recovery and excellent health.

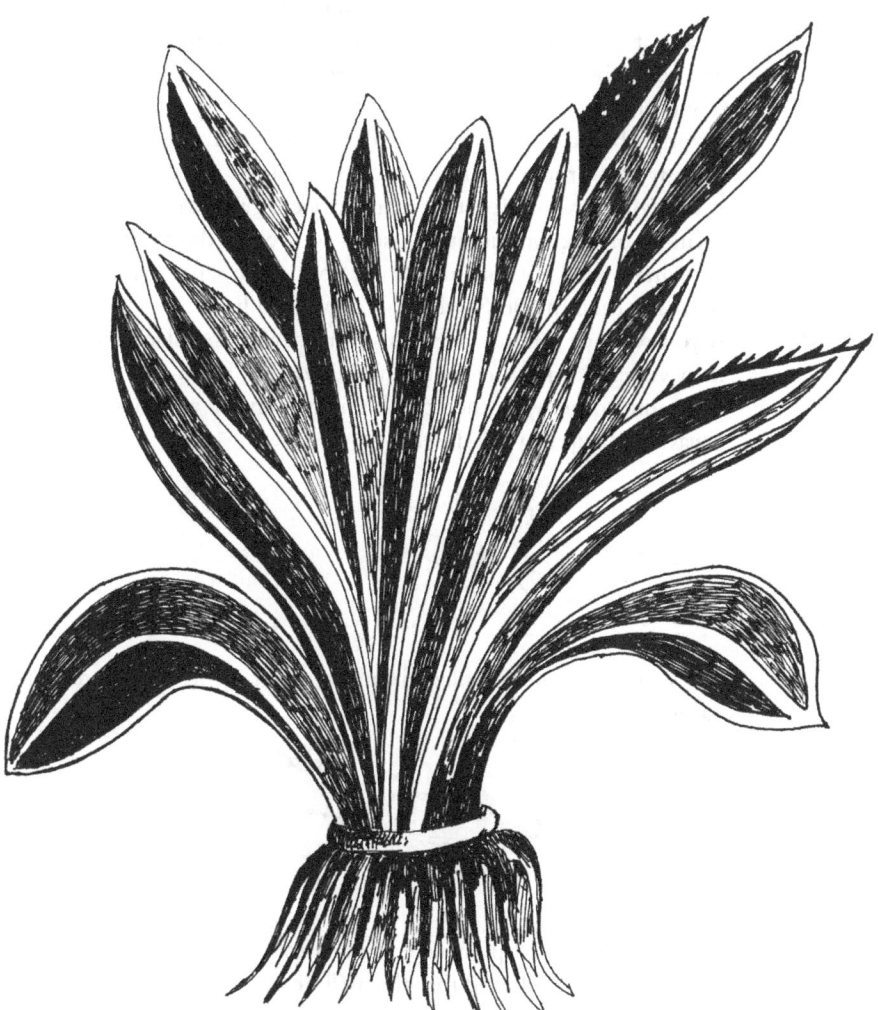

Common Plantain

2. Common Plantain (*Plantago major L.*), *arniglosa, Wægbræde*

(2:1) If the head aches or is sore, take the roots of the common plantain plant and bandage them on the neck; the soreness will leave the head.

(2:2) If a person's stomach is sore, take the juice of the plantain plant, ensure that it is clear,[13] and drink it. Then with a great deal of nausea, the stomach pain will leave. If it happens that the stomach is swollen, shred the plant, lay it on the stomach, and the swelling will go down[14] quickly.

(2:3)　For pain in the abdomen, take plantain juice, put it in some kind of ale,[15] and drink a great deal of it; it heals internally and purges the stomach and the small intestines wondrously well.

(2:4)　Again, if someone has a swollen stomach,[16] simmer the plantain at just below boiling and then eat a great deal of it; the stomach will go down quickly.

(2:5)　Again, if blood is running out of a person's rear, take plantain juice and give it to them to drink; it will soon stop.

(2:6)　If someone is wounded, take plantain seed, grind into a powder, and sprinkle on the wound; it will soon be well. If the body is afflicted anywhere with hot inflammations, pound the same plant and lay it on there; then the body will cool down and heal.

(2:7)　If you want to soften a person's stomach, take the plant and simmer it in vinegar at just below boiling. Pour the liquid and the cooked plant into some wine, then drink this at night on an empty stomach, always one cup as a full dose.[17]

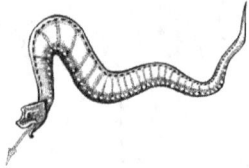

(2:8)　For snakebite, take the plantain plant, crush it into some wine, and eat it.

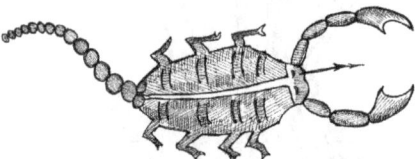

(2:9)　For the bite of a scorpion, take plantain roots and bandage them onto the person; it is believed that this will be of good service.

(2:10)　If intestinal worms trouble a person, take plantain juice (pound and wring the plant [to get the juice]), and give it to the person to drink. Take the same plant, pound it well, lay it on the navel and fasten it there tightly.

(2:11)　If someone's body develops a hard lump,[18] take the plantain plant, mix in unsalted grease, make it into a poultice,[19] and put it onto the hard spot; it will quickly soften and heal.

(2:12)   If someone has fever that returns every four days, take juice from that plant, mix it with water, and give them this to drink two hours before they expect the fever; then hopefully it will help them a lot.

(2:13)   For foot conditions and sore tendons, take the leaves of plantain, mix them with salt, and put this on the feet and the tendons; that is a certain remedy.

(2:14)   For fever that returns every third day, take three plantain roots and mix in water or wine; give them this to drink at night on an empty stomach before the fever comes back.

(2:15)   For fever that returns every other day, pound the same plant very fine and give it to drink in ale; it is believed that this helps.

(2:16)   For inflamed wounds,[20] take the plantain plant and mix it into unsalted grease. Put this onto the wound, and it will heal quickly.

(2:17)   If someone's feet swell during a journey, take the plantain plant and mix it in vinegar. Bathe and smear the feet with it; they will quickly become less swollen.

(2:18)   If a sore develops on someone's nose or cheek, take plantain juice, press it into soft wool, and lay it on the sore. Let it lie there nine nights; it will heal up soon after that.

(2:19)   For any strange pimples that appear on the nose, take plantain seed, dry it, grind, and mix with grease, add a little salt, and soak with wine. Smear this on the nose; it will become smooth and heal.

(2:20)   For injury to the mouth, take plantain leaves and their juice, mix them together, have them in your mouth for a long time, and then eat the root.

(2:21)   If a mad dog bites a person, take the same herb, pound it fine, and apply it; it will quickly heal.

(2:22)   For a person's everyday internal weakness,[21] take plantain, mix it in wine, drink the liquid, and eat the plantain, because it is good for anything that bothers the insides.

3. Cinquefoil (*Potentilla reptans L.*), *pentafolium, Fifleafe*

(3:1)   If a person's joints ache or are attacked by disorders, take the cinquefoil plant, pound it very small with grease and apply it without salt; it will quickly heal.

(3:2)   For a sore stomach, take juice of the cinquefoil plant, press out two spoonfuls, and give to the person to drink; it will clear away all of the soreness.

(3:3)   For an ache in the mouth, tongue, and throat, take cinquefoil roots, boil gently in water, and give it to drink; it will clear the inside of the mouth, and the ache will lessen.

(3:4)   For headache, take hold of a cinquefoil plant, mark around it three times with the little finger and with the thumb,[22] then pull it up from the ground, grind it into small pieces, and bandage it onto the head. The ache will lessen.

(3:5)   If blood runs very fast out of a person's nose, give them cinquefoil to drink in wine and smear the head with it; then the bleeding will quickly stop.

(3:6)   If a person's midriff aches, take the juice of cinquefoil, mix it with wine, and then drink three cupfuls for three mornings and evenings on an empty stomach.

(3:7)   For snakebite, take the cinquefoil plant, mash it in wine and drink a good deal of it; it will bring recovery.[23]

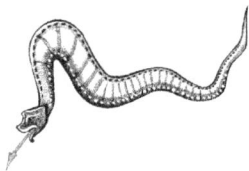

(3:8)   If a person is burned, take the cinquefoil plant, and let them carry it on them; skillful people say[24] that they will recover.

(3:9)   If you want to stop an ulcerous sore from spreading,[25] take the cinquefoil plant, simmer it in wine and in unsalted old barrow-pig's grease. Mix it all together, make into a poultice, and lay it on the sore; then it will quickly heal.

Also, you must prepare [collect and save] the plant in August.[26]

4.   Vervain (*Verbena officinalis* L.), *uermenaca*, *Æscþrote*

This plant, which is called *uermenacam* and another name, vervain, is grown everywhere on flat lands and wet ones.

(4:1)   For wounds, carbuncles, and swollen glands, take the roots of the same plant and fasten them around the neck; it will benefit remarkably.

(4:2)   Again, for swollen glands, take the same plant, *uermenacam*, crush it, and lay it on the swelling; it will heal wonderfully.

(4:3)   For those who have stopped up veins, so that the blood cannot flow to the private parts, and they cannot keep down what they have eaten, take the juice of this same plant and give it to drink. Then take wine, honey, and water and mix them together; it will quickly heal the condition.

(4:4)   For liver pain, gather the same plant on Midsummer's Day and grind it into powder.[27] Then take five spoonfuls of the powder and three cupfuls of good wine, mix them together, and give this to drink. It will be of great benefit and in the same manner will benefit other conditions.

(4:5)   For the condition in which stones develop in the bladder, take the roots of the same plant and pound them. Simmer them in hot wine and give it to drink; it heals the condition in a wonderful way, and not just that one: it also quickly clears away anything that prevents passing water and carries it away.

(4:6)   For headache, take the same plant and bind it on the head; it will lessen the headache.[28]

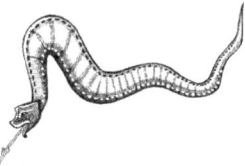

(4:7)   For snakebite: whoever has the *uermenacam* plant with its leaves and roots on them will be safe from all snakes.

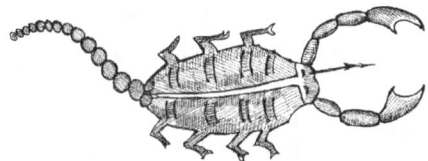

(4:8)   For the bite of a poisonous spider, take the leaves of this same plant, simmer them, bruised, in wine. If there is a swelling where the poison is retained, lay it on there. The swelling will quickly open. After it has opened up, then crush the plant with honey and lay it on there until the place clears up; that will be very quickly.

(4:9)   For bite of a mad dog, take the same plant *uermenacam* and whole grains of wheat.[29] Lay them on the bite so that the grains are softened by the moisture and become swollen; then take the grains and throw them to some hens. If they refuse to eat them, then take other grains and mix with the plant in the same way as you did earlier and lay this on the bite until you feel that the danger is gone and has been drawn out.

(4:10)   For fresh wounds, take the same plant, mix it in butter, and lay it on the wound.

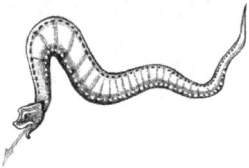

(4:11)   For snakebite, take twigs of the same plant, simmer them in wine, and then pound them. If the location of the bite cannot be seen,[30] and if the swelling has not come to a head, then lay the plant on it and it will quickly open. As soon as it opens, take the same plant, not soaked, and crush it with honey. Lay it on the sore until it has healed; that will be very quickly if one puts it on in this way.

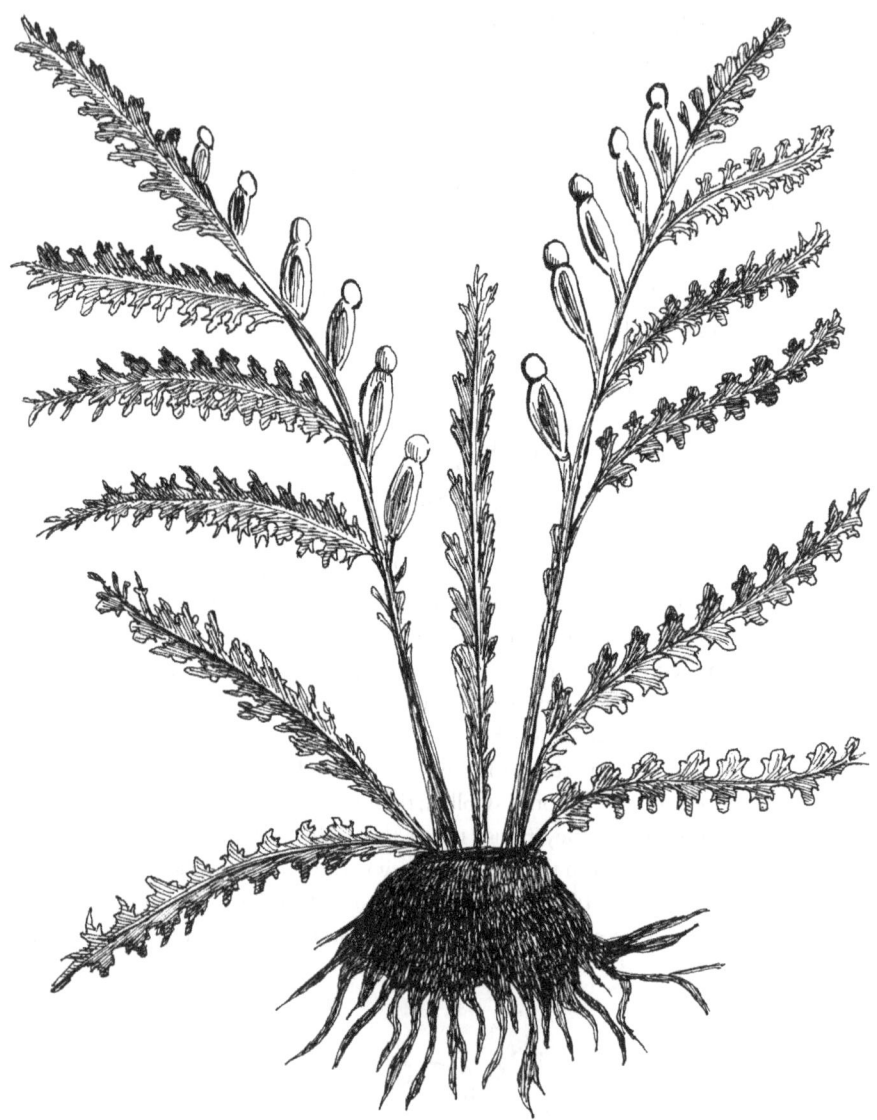

Henbane

5. Henbane (*Hyoscyamus niger L.*), *symphoniaca, hennebelle or belone*
This plant, called *symphoniacum* and another name, *belone*, and some call henbane, grows in cultivated ground, in sandy soil, and in gardens. There is another of this same plant, dark in color[31] and with stronger and poisonous leaves. The former is whiter and it has the following powers:

> (5:1)   For earache, take the juice of this same plant, warm it, and drip it into the ear; it puts the earache to flight in a wonderful way. Likewise, if worms are present, it kills them.

(5:2)   For swollen knees or calves or wherever there is a swelling on the body, take the same plant, *simphonciacan*, crush it, and lay it on; it will take away the swelling.

(5:3)   For toothache, take the roots of this same plant, simmer in strong wine, drink it very warm and hold in the mouth; it will quickly heal the toothache.

(5:4)   For pain or swelling of the private parts, take the roots of the same plant and fasten them to the thigh; it will make both the pain and the swelling of the private parts take flight.

(5:5)   If a woman's breasts hurt, take the juice of this same plant, make it into a drink, give it to her to drink, and smear the breasts with it; she will quickly be better.

(5:6)   For sore feet, take the same plant with its roots and pound them together; lay them on the feet and bind them on; it cures wonderfully and makes the swelling go away.

(5:7)   For lung diseases, take the juice of the same plant and give it to drink; they will be cured remarkably.[32]

6.   Snakeweed (*Polygonum bistorta* L.), *uiperina*, Nædderwyrt

This plant, called *uiperinam* and another name, snakeweed, grows in water and in fields; it has tender leaves and is bitter to the taste.[33]

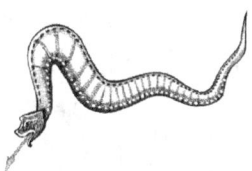

(6:1)   For snakebite, take the same *uiperinam*, pound it, and mix it with wine. Give it to drink; it heals up the bite wonderfully[34] and sends out the poison. You must gather the plant in the month of April.

7.   "Bee Plant" (*Acorus calamus* L.), *ueneria*, Beowyrt

This plant, which is called *ueneriam* in Latin and "bee plant" in our language, is grown in cultivated places, in garden plots, and in meadows; you should gather the plant in the month of August.[35]

(7:1)   So that bees will not swarm, take the same plant we call *ueneriam* and hang it on the hive; they will remain and will never depart, on the contrary, it will please them.[36] This plant is seldom found, and it cannot be recognized except when it grows and blooms.[37]

(7:2)   If someone cannot pass water, and the water has stopped, take the roots of this same plant, simmer them down in clean water by two-thirds, and give this to drink. Within three days, the person will be able to pass water; it cures the condition wonderfully.

8.   Lion's Foot or Lady's Mantle (*Alchemilla vulgaris* L.), *pes leonis*, *Leonfot*
This plant, called *pedem leonis* and another name, lion's foot, grows in fields, in ditches, and in beds of reeds.

(8:1)   If anyone suffers from the condition of being bewitched, you can free them from it[38]: Take five of the plants we call lion's foot without their roots, simmer in water while the moon is waning, and wash them with it. Lead them out of the house in the early evening and fumigate them with the plant called *aristolochiam*. When going outside, they must not look back; in this way, you can undo the condition that binds them.[39]

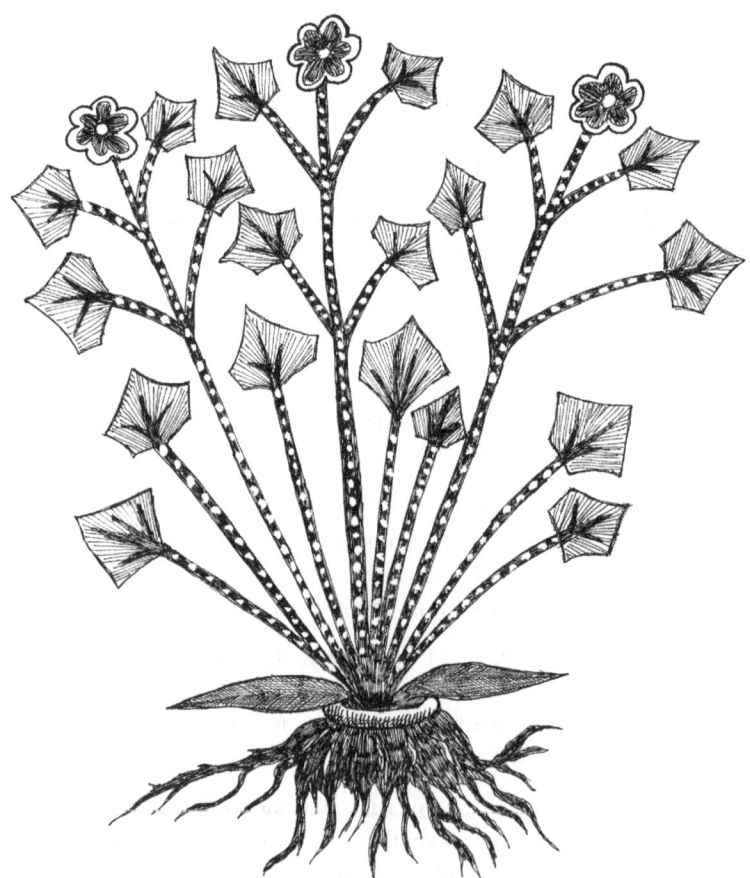

Celery-Leaved Crowfoot

9.   Celery-Leaved Crowfoot (*Ranunculus sceleratus* L.), *scelerata*, *Cluſþunge*[40]
This plant, named *sceleratam* and another name, crowfoot, grows in damp and watery places; whoever eats this plant on an empty stomach will die laughing.

(9:1)   For wounds and for carbuncles, take this same plant, mix it with unsalted grease, put it onto the wound; then it eats and cleans away any pus that is present.[41] However, do not let it stay there longer than necessary, or it will eat into healthy skin. If you want to test this as an experiment, bruise the plant and bind it onto your healthy hand; it will quickly eat into the flesh.

(9:2)   For swellings and for warts, take this same plant, mix it with pig's dung, and put it on the swelling and the wart; within a few hours, it will drive out the pain and draw out the pus.

10. Buttercup (*Ranunculus acris* L.), *batracion, Clufwyrt*

This plant, called *batracion* and another name, buttercup, grows in sandy soil and in fields; it has few leaves, and they are thin.[42]

(10:1)   For lunacy, take the plant and bind it around the person's neck with a piece of red thread when the moon is on the wane in the month of April and in early October; they will be quickly healed.

(10:2)   For wounds that have turned dark,[43] take the same plant with its roots, pound them, mix with vinegar, and put this on the wound; this will quickly heal it up and make it like the rest of the body.

11. Mugwort (*Artemisia vulgaris* L.), *artemesia, Mucgwyrt*

This plant, called *artemesiam* and also mugwort, grows in rocky and sandy places. If someone wants to start out on a journey, they should take some *artemesiam* in hand and keep it with them; then they won't feel the journey's hardship too much. It also chases out possession by the devil; in a house where it is present, it prevents evil remedies; and it also turns away the evil eye.[44]

(11:1)   For a sore abdomen, take the same plant, make it into a powder, mix it with new beer, and give it to drink; it will quickly ease the abdominal pain.

(11:2)   For sore feet, take the same plant, mix it with grease, and put it on the feet; it takes away the soreness of the feet.

12. Mugwort/Tansy (*Tanacetum vulgare* L), *artemesia tagantes, Mucgwyrt*[45]

(12:1)   For bladder pain and when a person cannot pass water, take the juice of this plant, which is also called mugwort (it is, however, another kind) and simmer it in hot water or in wine and give it to drink.

(12:2)   For soreness of the thighs, take the same plant, mix it with grease, and soak it well with vinegar; bandage it on the sore place; on the third day, the person will be better.

(12:3)   For sore tendons and for swelling, take the same plant, *artemesiam*, mix it with oil that has been boiled well; apply it; it heals wonderfully.

(12:4)   If anyone is greatly and heavily tormented with foot disease, take the roots of this same plant and give them in honey to eat. Soon afterward, the person will be cured and cleansed in a way you never suspected it had such great power.

(12:5)   If someone is afflicted by fever, take the juice of this same plant and oil and apply it; the fever will quickly leave them.

13.   Roman Wormwood (*Artemisia pontica* L.), *artemisia leptefilos, Mucgwyrt*
The third plant, which we call *artemesiam leptefilos* and another name, mugwort, grows around ditches and in old dirt mounds; if you break off its blossoms, it has a smell like elder.[46]

(13:1)   For stomachache, take this plant, pound it, and simmer it well in almond oil in the way in which you make a poultice. Then put it on a clean piece of cloth and lay it on the stomach; within five days, the person will be well. If the roots of this plant are hung over the door of a house, then no one may do harm to the house.

(13:2)   For trembling of the tendons, take the juice of this same plant mixed with oil and rub it on there; it quiets the tremors and takes away the entire condition.

Indeed, about the three plants, we call *artemesias,* it is said that Diana found them and gave knowledge of their power and medicinal value to the centaur Chiron. He was the first to prescribe a medicine using this plant and named the plant after Diana, who is called *artemesia.*[47]

14.   Dock (*Rumex* spp. L), *lapatium, Docce*
This plant, called *lapatium* and another name, dock, grows in sandy places and on old dunghills.[48]

(14:1)   For hard swellings that form on the private parts, take the *lapatium* plant and pound it in aged unsalted grease so that there are two parts more of the grease than plant. When it is well mixed, form it into a ball, enfold it in a cabbage leaf, and let it smoke on hot ashes. When it is hot, lay it on the swellings, and fasten it there. This is best for these swellings.

15.   Dragonwort (*Dracunculus vulgaris, Arum dracunculus* L.), *dracontea, Dracentse*[49]
About this plant, which is called *dracontea*[50] and another name, dragonwort, it is said that it should be grown in dragon's blood. It grows at the tops of mountains where there are groves of trees, chiefly in holy places and in the country called Apulia.[51] It grows in stony soil; it is soft to the touch, sweet to the taste, and in smell like green chestnuts, and the root below is like a dragon's head.

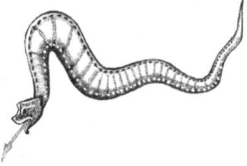

(15:1)   For all snakebites, take the roots of the *dracontea* plant, pound with wine, warm it, and give to drink. It will get rid of all the poison.

(15:2)   For broken bones, take the roots of this same plant and pound them in grease, just like you make a poultice. It will draw the broken bones out of the body.[52]

You should gather the plant in the month called *Iulium* [July].

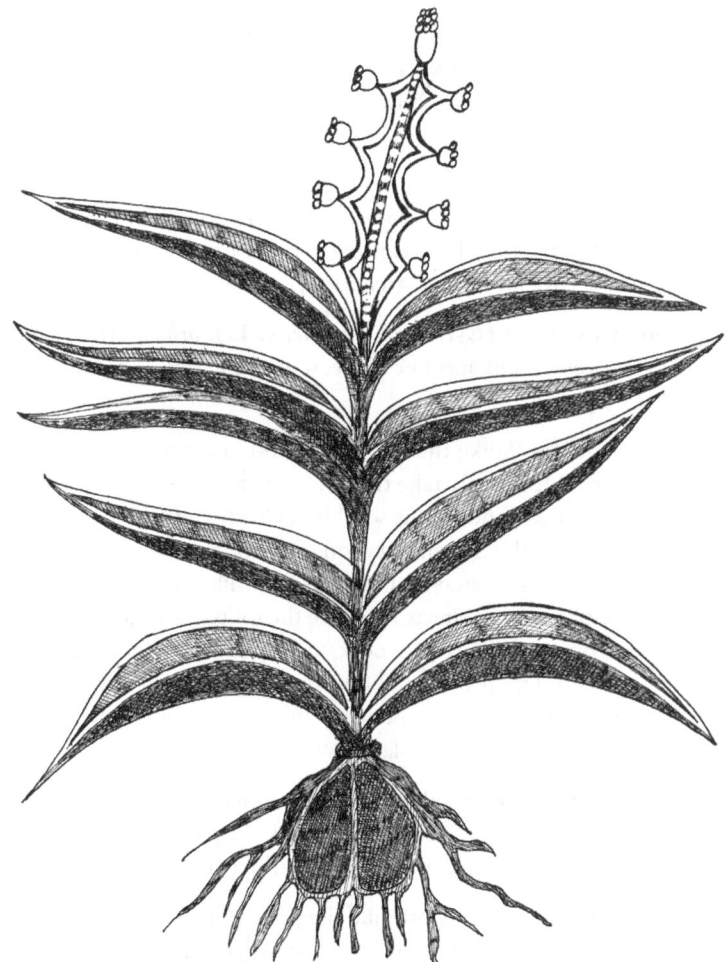

Orchid

16. Orchis, Wild Orchid (*Orchis* spp. L.), *satyrion*, *Hreafnes leac*

This plant, which is called *satyrion* and another name, wild orchid,[53] grows on high mountains, in hard places, sometimes in meadows, and on cultivated and sandy land.

(16:1)   For painful wounds,[54] take the roots of the plant we name *satyrion* and some call *priapisci* and pound them together. It cleanses wounds and is good for scars.

(16:2)   For eye pain, that is, when one is blear-eyed, take the juice of the same plant and apply to the eyes. Without delay, it takes away the pain.

17. Yellow Gentian (*Gentiana lutea* L.), *gentiana*, *Feldwyrt*[55]

This plant, which is called *gentianam* and another name, yellow gentian, grows in the mountains and on hills. It improves all tonics.[56] It is soft to the touch and bitter to the taste.

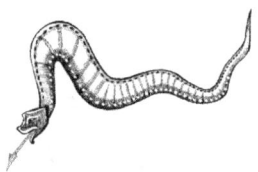

(17:1)   For snakebite, take the roots of the *gentianam* plant, dry them, then pound into a powder weighing about 4 grams; give to drink in three cups of wine. It helps a great deal.

18. Cyclamen, Sowbread (*Cyclamen europaeum* L.), *orbicularis*, *Slite*[57]

This plant, called *orbicularis* and another name, sowbread, grows in cultivated places and on hilly land.

(18:1)   For hair loss,[58] take the same plant and put it in the nostrils.

(18:2)   For irritable bowels, take the same plant, make it into a salve, and put it where the abdomen is sore. It is also beneficial for heartburn.[59]

(18:3)   For pain in the spleen, take one cup of the juice of this plant and five spoonfuls of vinegar. Give this to drink for nine days; you will be surprised about its effects. Also take the roots of the same plant and hang them around the person's neck so that the roots hang in front against the spleen. The person will quickly heal. Whoever drinks the juice of this plant will quickly experience wonderful relief in their abdomen.
   One can gather the plant any time of the year.

19. Knotgrass (*Polygonum aviculare* L.), *proserpinaca*, *Unfortrædde*[60]

This plant, called *proserpinacam* or another name, knotgrass, grows everywhere in cultivated places and on mounds. You should pick the plant in summer.

(19:1)   If a person vomits blood, take the juice of the *proserpinacam* plant and simmer it without letting it steam[61] in good, strong wine. Give it to drink on an empty stomach for nine days. In this time, you will see wonderful effects from it.

(19:2)   For pain in the sides, take the juice of this same plant in oil and rub it on frequently. It will soothe the pain.

(19:3)   For a woman's sore nipples[62] when full of milk and swollen, take the same plant, pound it, soften it in butter, and put it on. It will soothe the swelling and soreness wonderfully.

(19:4)   For eye pain, before the sun rises or just before it fully begins to set, go to the same plant, *proserpinacam*, and mark around it with a golden ring. Say that you want to pick it to make a medicine for the eyes.[63] Three days later, go again before sunrise, pick the plant, and hang it around the person's neck. It will help a great deal.

(19:5)   For earache, take the juice of this same plant made lukewarm and drip it into the ear. It chases away the pain wonderfully. And also, we have found honestly and truly ourselves that it helps. Also, it certainly heals sores on the outside of the ears.

(19:6)   For very loose stools, take the juice of the leaves of this plant and boil gently in water. Give it to drink in the quantity you think suitable, and the person will be well.

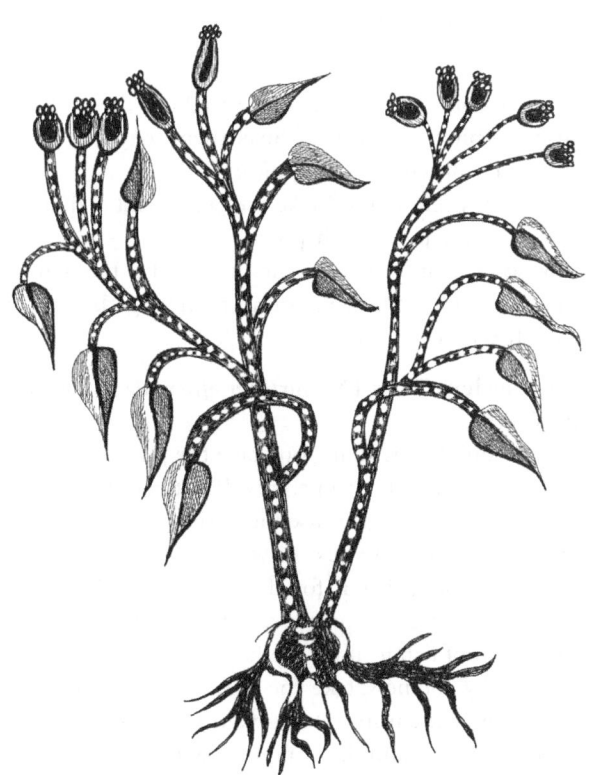

Birthwort

20. **Birthwort, Heartwort (*Aristolochia clematis* L. *or rotunda*), aristolochia, Smerowyrt**

This plant, called *aristolochiam* or another name, birthwort, grows on hilly lands and in firm places.

(20:1)   Against the strength of poison, take the *aristolochiam* plant and pound it. Give it to drink in wine, and it will overcome all the person's strength.

(20:2)   For the most violent of fevers, take the same plant and dry it. Fumigate the person with it; it chases away not only the fever, but also devil-like possession.[64]

(20:3)   For sore nostrils, take the roots of this same plant and put them in the nostrils; it will quickly purge them and lead to healing. In truth, healers cannot cure much without this plant.

(20:4)   If someone is weakened by chills, take the same plant, oil, and pig's grease, and mix them together. It has the strength to warm them.

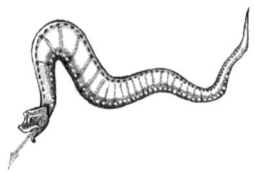

(20:5)   For snakebite, take ten pennies' weight of the roots of the same plant in half a pitcher of wine.[65] Soak them together, and give it to drink often. It will send out the poison.

(20:6)   If a child is very upset,[66] take the same plant and fumigate them with it. You will make them happier.

(20:7)   For sores that grow on the nose, take the same plant, cypress, dragonwort, and honey; pound them together and lay this on the sore. It will soon heal.

21. **Watercress, Garden Cress (*Nasturtium officinale* or *Lepidum sativum* L.), nasturcium, Cærse**

(21:1)   If a person's hair is falling out, take the juice of the plant that is called *nasturcium* or another name, cress. Put it in the nose. The hair will grow.

This plant is not sown, but propagates itself in springs and brooks. It is also written that in some countries it will grow next to walls.

(21:2)   For head sores, that is for dandruff and itching, take the seeds of this plant and goose grease, and pound them together. It draws the whiteness of dandruff off the head.

(21:3)   For bodily soreness, take the same *nasturcium* plant and pennyroyal and simmer them in water; give this to drink. You will improve the body's soreness, and the condition will leave.

(21:4)   For swellings, take the same plant, mix it with oil, and lay it on the swellings. Take the leaves of the same plant and lay them on also.

(21:5)   For warts, take the same plant and yeast, mix them together, lay this on them, and they will soon be taken away.

22. Meadow Saffron, Autumn Crocus (*Colchicum autumnale* L.), *hieribulbum*, Greate wyrt

This plant, called *hieribulbum* and another name, meadow saffron, grows around hedges and in putrid places.[67]

(22:1)   For soreness in the joints, take six ounces of the plant we call *hieribulbum* and the same amount of goat's grease, and one pound plus two ounces of oil from the cypress tree. Pound them together until well mixed. It relieves pain both of the insides and of the limbs.

(22:2)   If pimples grow on a woman's nose, take the roots of the same plant and mix them with oil, then wash with it. It will cleanse away all the pimples.

23. Ashwagandha/Poison Gooseberry (*Withania somnifera*), *apollinaris*, Glofwyrt[68]

About this plant, which is called *apollinarem* and also *glofwyrt*, it is said that Apollo found it first and gave it to the healer Aesculapius.[69] From that, he gave the name to it.

(23:1)   For sore hands, take the same plant, *apollinarem*, pound it with unsalted, aged grease. Add to it one cup of aged wine, and heat it without letting any steam rise (let there be one pound of the grease). Pound together as you would for a poultice and smear it on the hands.

24. Chamomile (*Chamaemelum nobile/Anthemis nobilis* L.), *camemelon*, Mageþe

(24:1)   For eye pain, let a person pick the plant called *camemelon* and another name, chamomile, before sunrise.[70] When picking it, they should say they are picking it for white specks in the eye and for eye pain.[71] Then take the juice and apply it to the eyes.

25. Wall Germander (*Teucrium chamaedrys* L.), *chamedris*, Heortclæfre[72]

This plant, called *chamedris* and another name, germander, grows on hills and in hard soil.

(25:1)   If anyone is bruised, take the plant we call *chamedris*, pound it in a wooden vessel and give it to drink in wine. It also heals a bite or sting.

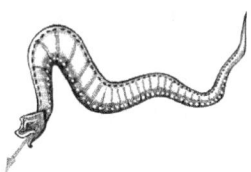

(25:2)   For snakebite, take the same plant, pound it into a powder, and give
to drink in aged wine. It will clear out the poison thoroughly.

(25:3)   For foot disease, take the same plant and give it to drink in warm
wine, just as we said before. It relieves the pain wonderfully and
brings about healing.

You should pick the plant in August.

26. Wild Teasel (*Dipsacus fullonum* L./*Dipsacus silvestris*), *chameælæ*, *Wulfes Camb*

(26:1)   For liver disease, take the plant called *chameaeleæ* and another name,
wild teasel, and give it to drink in wine (for fever in warm water). It
has wonderful benefits.

(26:2)   If anyone has drunk poison, take the same plant, pound it into
a powder, and give it to drink in wine. All the poison will be
cleared out.

(26:3)   For dropsy, take the same plant and the same amount of spurge (figwort), wall germander, and ground-pine, and pound them into a
powder. Give this to drink in wine; five spoonfuls to young men,
three spoonfuls to youngsters, the ill, and to women, and one to little
children.[73] It sends out the fluids very well when passing water.

27. Ground-Pine (*Ajuga chamaepitys* or *Teucrium chamaepitys* L.), *chamepithys*, *Henep*.

(27:1)   For wounds, take the plant that is called *chamepithys* or another name,
ground-pine. Pound it and lay it on the wound. If it is very deep, take
the juice and wring it onto the wound.

(27:2)   For pain in the abdomen, take the same plant and give it to drink. It
alleviates the pain.

28. Figwort/Lesser Celandine (*Ranunculus ficaria* L.), *chamedafne*, *Hræfnesfot*

(28:1)   For stopped up intestines, take the plant the Greeks call *chamedafne*
and the English call figwort or lesser celandine, pound into fine
powder, and give it to drink in warm water. It stimulates the bowels.

29. Madder (*Rubia tinctorum* L.), *ostriago*, *Lyðwort*[74]

This plant, called *ostriago* or another name, madder, grows around graveyards, on
mounds, and on the walls of houses that stand against hills.

(29:1)   For all sorts of bothersome sores, take the plant we call *ostriago*,
pound it, and lay it on the sore. As we said earlier, it will completely
heal every painful thing that develops on the body.

If you want to pick this plant, you should be pure, and you should pick it before
sunrise in the month of July.

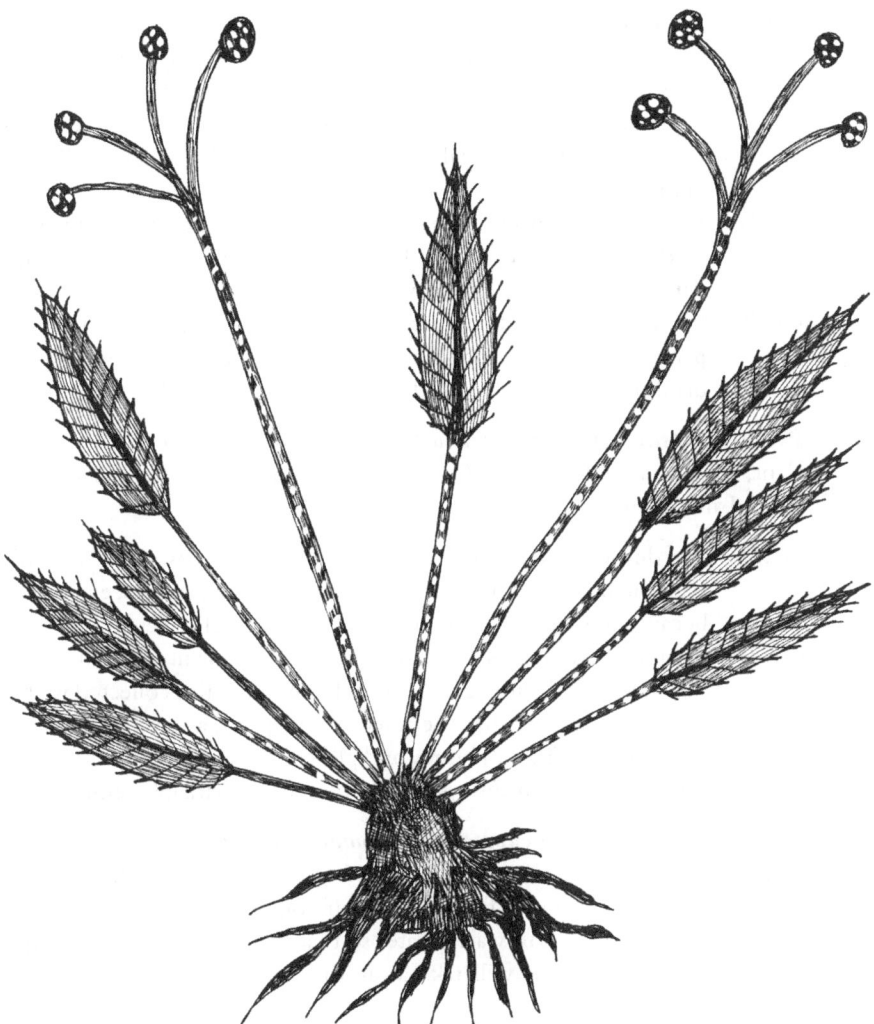

Water Dock

30. Water Dock (*Rumex hydrolapathum* L. or *aquaticus* L.), *brittanica*, *Heawenhnydelu*[75]

(30:1)   For mouth sores, take the plant the Greeks call *brittanice* and the English call water dock, pound it when green, and press out the juice. Give it to drink and to hold in the mouth. Even if some of it is swallowed, it will still help.

(30:2)   Again, for mouth sores, take the same plant, *bryttanicam*. If you do not have it fresh, take it dry and mix with wine to the thickness of honey. Take in the same way as we said earlier; it will have the same healing effects.

(30:3)   For toothache and if they are loose, take the same plant. It helps by using some wonderful power. Save its juice and powdered leaves over winter because it does not grow at all times of the year. You should keep the juice in a ram's horn. Dry the powdered leaves and keep them. Moreover, taken with wine, it also helps very well for the same uses.

(30:4)   For clogged bowels, take the juice of the same plant, and give it to drink undiluted, as much as the person can tolerate.[76] Without danger, it will purge the bowels.

(30:5)   For pain in the side, which the Greeks call *paralisis*, take the same plant fresh with its roots. Pound it and give two or three cupfuls to drink in wine. It is believed that it heals wonderfully.

31.   Prickly Lettuce (*Lactuca scariola* L.), *lactuca*, *Wudulectric*

This plant, which is called *lactucan silfaticam* or another name, prickly lettuce, grows in cultivated and sandy soil.

(31:1)   For dim eyes, it is said that when the eagle wants to fly upward, it will touch and wet its eyes with the juice so that it can see better, and because of that, the eagle obtains the greatest clearness.

(31:2)   Again, for dim eyes, take the juice of the plant we call *lactucam silfaticam* mixed with aged wine and honey, and this collected without smoke.[77] It is best that the juice of this plant, as we said before, be mixed with wine and honey and placed in a glass container for when it is needed. From this, you will observe a remarkable remedy.

32.   Agrimony (*Agrimonia eupatoria*), *agromonia*, *Garclife*

(32:1)   For sore eyes, take the plant called *agrimoniam* and by another name, agrimony. Pound it fresh by itself. If you do not have it fresh, take it dried and dip it in warm water so that you can crush it easily. Apply it, and quickly it will take away the defect and the soreness from the eyes.

(32:2)   For a sore abdomen, take the root of the same plant we call *agrimoniam*, and give it to drink. It helps in a wonderful way.

(32:3)   For ulcerous sores and wounds, pick the fresh plant, bruise it, and lay it on the sore. It will cure the disorder agreeably. If you have the dried plant, dip it in warm water; it is believed that it will heal equally.

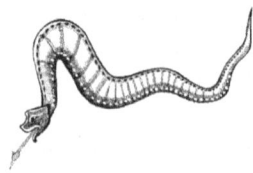

(32:4) For snakebite, take about nine grams of the same plant and two cups of wine. Give this to drink; it clears out the poison in a wonderful way.

(32:5) For warts, take the same plant and pound it in vinegar. Lay it on, and it will make the warts disappear.

(32:6) For soreness of the spleen, take the same plant, and give it to drink in wine. It will take away the soreness from the spleen.

(32:7) If you want to cut anything from the body, and it seems to you that you cannot, take the same plant, bruised, lay it on, and the place will open up and be healed.

(32:8) For a blow from an iron or wooden stake, this same plant is bruised and laid on the wound; it heals in a wonderful manner.

33. **Asphodel (*Asphodelus ramosus* L.), *astularegia*, *Wudurofe*[78]**

(33:1) For pain in the shanks of the legs or in the feet, take the juice of this plant, which is called *asphodel* and another name, woodruff, with almond oil and rub on where it hurts; wonderful relief will ensue. If there is swelling, pound the plant well and lay it on the sore place.

(33:2) For pain in the liver, take the root of this same plant and give it to drink in sweetened water; it will remove the pain in a wonderful manner.

34. **Sorrel (*Rumex acetosa* L.), *lapatium*, *Wududocce***

(34:1) If any part of the body becomes stiff, take the plant that is called *lapatium* and another name, sorrel, some aged pig's grease and crumbs from oven-baked bread. Pound this together in the manner you would make a poultice, lay it on the sore place, and it helps wonderfully.

35. **Greater/Yellow Centaury (*Centaurea centaurium* L.), *centauria maior*, *Eorþgealla or Curmelle seo mare*[79]**

(35:1) For liver disease, take the plant the Greeks call *centauria maior* and the English call greater centaury and some call yellow centaury; simmer it in wine, and give it to drink. It strengthens the liver in a wonderful manner. Do the same for pain in the spleen.

(35:2) For wounds and ulcerous sores, take the same plant, bruise it, and lay it on the sore. It does not allow the sore to spread.

(35:3) This same plant, *centauria*, works very well in healing new and wide wounds so that the wounds quickly close. It also helps the flesh to knit together if one soaks the wound in water containing the plant.

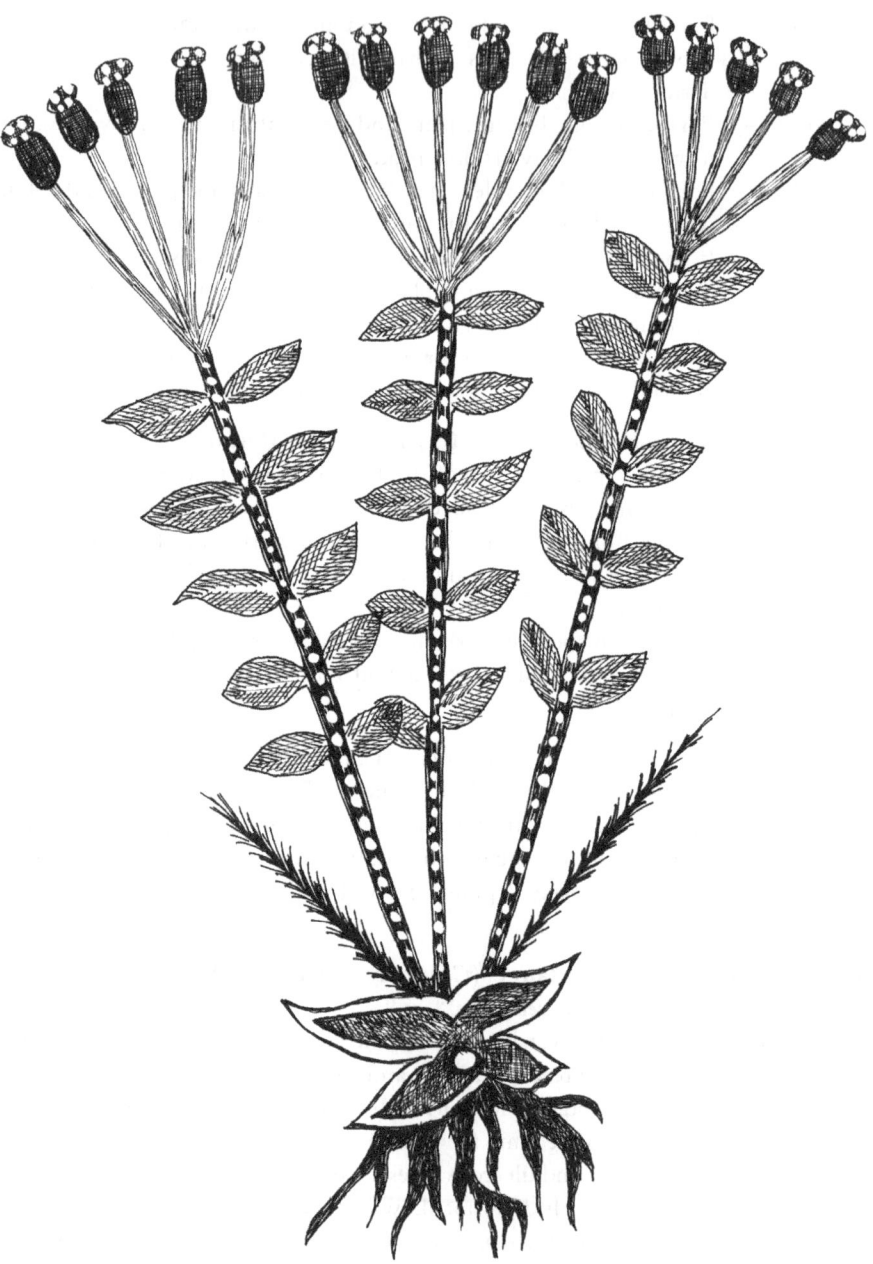

Lesser Centaury

36. Lesser Centaury (*Centaurium umbellatum*), *centauria minor, Feferfuge, Curmelle seo læsse*

This plant, which is called *centauriam minorem* and another name, lesser centaury, and also some call *febrifugam*, grows in solid and sandy earth. It is also said that Chiron the Centaur found the plant that above we called *centurium maiorem* and here *centurium minorem;* for this reason they have the name *centaurias.*[80]

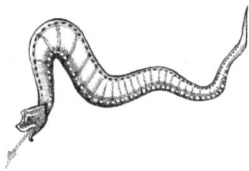

(36:1) For snakebite, take this plant in powdered form, or the plant itself bruised, and give it to drink in aged wine; it works quickly.

(36:2) For eye pain, take the juice of this same plant and apply it to the eyes; it helps poor vision. In addition, mix some honey with it, and it will certainly help dim eyesight, so that sharpness of vision will be restored.

(36:3) If then anyone falls ill,[81] take a good handful of this plant and simmer it in wine or in ale so that there is a jug full of wine. Let it stand for three days. Then take a half a jug full every day as needed mixed with honey. Drink this on an empty stomach.

(36:4) For nerve spasms,[82] take the same plant, simmer it down in water by two-thirds. Give this to drink as much as the person wants and needs to; they will be healed.

(36:5) If poison has been ingested, take the same plant, pound it in vinegar, and give it to drink; it will quickly eliminate the poison. Also, take ten pennies' weight of the roots of this plant, put in wine, and give three cupfuls to drink.

(36:6) In case worms irritate the area around the navel, do as we indicated before for nerve spasms: that is, you take the same plant simmered down in water by two-thirds; it will drive the worms out.

37. Beet (*Beta vulgaris* L.), *personacia, Boete*[83]

(37:1) For all wounds and for snakebite, take the juice of this plant, which is called *personaciam* and another name, beet, and give it to drink in aged wine. It cures all snakebites in a wonderful way.

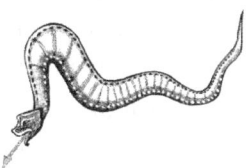

(37:2) For fevers, take the leaves of this same plant and bind them on a feverish person. The fever will quickly disappear.

(37:3) If a cancer sore grows on a wound, take the plant, boil it gently in water, and bathe the wound with it. Then take the plant, soap, and grease; pound them in vinegar. Put this on a cloth and lay it on the wound.

(37:4) For pain in the abdomen, take one cup of the juice of the same plant and two cups of honey. Give this to drink on an empty stomach.

(37:5) For bite of a mad dog, take the roots of this same plant, pound them with coarse salt, and lay this on the bite.

(37:6) For fresh wounds that are oozing,[84] take equal amounts of the roots of the same plant and hawthorn leaves. Pound them together and lay this on the wounds.

38. Wild Strawberry (*Fragaria vesca*), *fraga*, *Streawberge*

This plant, which is called *fraga* and another name, wild strawberry, grows in shady places, in cultivated spots, and on hills.

(38:1) For pain of the spleen, take the juice of the same plant we call *fragan* and honey. Give it to drink, and it will help in a wonderful way.

(38:2) The juice of this same plant helps many who have shortness of breath or abdominal pain when taken mixed with honey and pepper.

39. Marsh Mallow (*Althaea officinalis* L.) *Hibiscus*, *Merscmealuwe*

This plant, called *hibiscum* and another name, marsh mallow, grows in damp places and in fields.

(39:1) For foot disease, take the plant we call *hibiscum* and pound it with aged fat. Lay this on the painful spot, and in three days, it will be healed. Many authorities attest to the efficacy of this plant.

(39:2) For any accumulation of diseased matter on the body, take the same plant, simmer with fenugreek, linseed, and flour. Lay it on the sore, and it will banish all the hardness.

40. Horsetail (*Equisetum* L.), *ippirus*, no OE word

(40:1) If a person has a swollen stomach, take the juice of the plant the Greeks call *ippirum* and the Romans *æquiseiam* in sweetened wine and give two cups of it to drink. It is firmly believed that it helps this condition.

(40:2) If anyone coughs up a lot of blood, take the juice of this same plant, simmer in strong wine without letting steam rise, and drink it on an empty stomach. It will quickly staunch the blood.

41. Mallow (*Malva silvestris* L.), *malua eratica*, *Hocleaf*

This plant, which is called *malue erratice* and another name, mallow, grows everywhere in cultivated places.

(41:1) For bladder pain, take one pound of the plant that we call *maluam erraticam* with its roots, simmer it down in water by one half or until the water measures two cupfuls or more. It should be simmered down by half within three days, as we said before.[85] Give it to drink on an empty stomach; it will cure them.

(41:2) For sore tendons, take the same plant, pound it with aged grease. It soothes the tendons' pain wonderfully.

(41:3) For a pain in the side, take the same plant, simmer it in ale, and after you have simmered it, place it in a mortar together with its leaves and pound it. Put it in a cloth and lay it onto the side, and do not take it off for three days. You will alleviate the pain.

(41:4) For fresh wounds, take the roots of this same plant and burn them into powder, then put this onto the wounds.

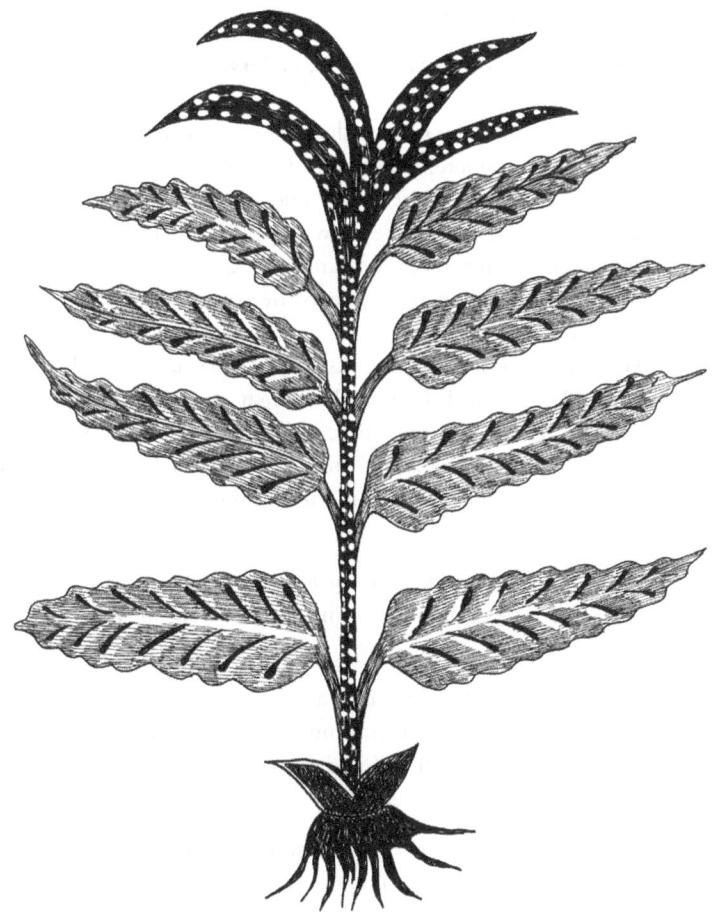

Alkanet

42. Alkanet/Bugloss (*Anchusa officinalis* L.), *buglossa*, *Hundes Tunge*, (*Glofwyrt*)[86]

This plant, which the Greeks call *buglossam* and the Romans *lingua bubula* and the English "glofwyrt" and another name, alkanet or bugloss, grows in cultivated places and in sandy soil.

(42:1)   If anyone has a fever that returns every three days or every four days, take the roots of this plant when it has three pods of seeds. Simmer the roots in water and give to drink; you will cure them.

Plants that have four pods of seeds cure exactly like we said above. Another plant is similar to this one; it has somewhat smaller leaves than dock; its roots taken in water act against toads and snakes.

(42:2)   For shortness of breath, take the same plant, honey, and bread that has been baked using grease, just like you make a poultice. It takes away the pain in a wonderful way.

43. Sea-Onion, Squill (*Scilla maritima* L. or *Urgina maritima*), *bulbiscillitica*, *Glædene*

(43:1)   For dropsy, take the plant called *bulbiscillitici* and another name, squill, and dry it completely. Take its inner part and simmer in water. When it is warm, mix with it honey and vinegar. Give three cupfuls, and quickly the illness will be drawn out when passing water.

(43:2)   For painful joints, take the same plant, as we said earlier, the inside part, and simmer it in ale. Rub the sore place with this and it will heal quickly.

(43:3)   For the condition the Greeks call *paronichias*,[87] take the roots of this same plant, pound them with vinegar and some bread, and then lay this on the sore. It cures the condition in a wonderful way.

(43:4)   If you cannot quench the thirst of a person with dropsy, take a leaf from this same plant and put it under the tongue. Soon it will restrain their thirst.

44. Navelwort (*Cotyledon umbilicus*), *cotiledon*, no OE word

This plant, which the Greeks call *cotiledon* and the Romans *umbilicum uereris*, grows on roofs and on mounds.

(44:1)   For swellings, take this plant and pig's grease (however, for women, unsalted) each in equal amounts by weight and pound them together. Lay this on the swellings, and it will remove them. You should pick the plant in wintertime.

45. Cockspur-Grass (*Panicum crus galli*), *gallicrus*, *Attorlaðe*

This plant, called *gallicrus* and another name, cockspur-grass, grows in firm soil and along roadways.

(45:1)   For dog bite, take the plant and pound it with grease and bread baked on the hearth. Lay this on the bite, and it will quickly be healed. This also helps cure hard swellings, and it removes them.

46. Horehound (*Marrubium vulgare*), *prassion*, *Harehune*

(46:1)   For a cold in the head and if someone is coughing heavily, take the plant the Greeks call *prassion*, the Romans *marubium*, and the English horehound, and simmer it in water. Give it to drink whenever they are coughing heavily, and it will help them wonderfully.

(46:2)   For a stomachache, take the juice of this same plant and give it to drink. It takes stomachache away. If fever bothers them, give the same plant diluted well in water, and it will restore health.

(46:3)   For worms [*rengwyrmas*] around the navel, take equal amounts by weight of the *maribium* plant, wormwood, and lupin, and simmer them in sweetened water and wine. Put this on the navel two or three times, and it will kill the worms.

(46:4)   For painful and swollen joints, take the same plant, burn it to ashes, put it on the sore, and it will quickly heal.

(46:5)   If anyone has taken poison, take the juice of this plant, simmer it in aged wine, and drink it. Quickly it will be better.

(46:6)   For scabs and skin infections, take the same plant, simmer it in water, and wash the body with it where there are sores. It removes the scabs and skin infections.

(46:7)   For lung diseases, take the same plant and simmer it in honey. Give it to eat, and they will be cured in a wonderful manner.

(46:8)   For all stiffness in the body, take the same plant and pound it well with grease. Put this on the soreness, and it will cure it in a wonderful way.

47. "Wild Gladiolus" (*Gladiolus italicus* Mill.), *xifion*, *Foxes fot*[88]

(47:1)   For strange carbuncles that form on the body; take three ounces of the root of this plant, which is called *xifion* and another name, "wild gladiolus," six ounces of fine flour, two cups of vinegar, and three ounces of fox's fat. Pound together with wine, daub a cloth with it, lay it on the sore, and you will be amazed at how the medicine heals.

(47:2)   For a fractured skull, take the upper part of the same plant, dry it, and pound it. Then take the same amount by weight of wine, mix them together, lay it on the sore, and it will pull the broken bone out. Also, if anything on the body is injured, it will heal that, or if anyone steps on something poisonous with their feet; this same plant works very well against poison.

48. True Maidenhair (*Adiantum capillus-veneris* L.), *gallitricus*, *Wæterwyrt*[89]

(48:1)   For swellings that are painful for virgins, take the plant called *gallitricus* and another name, true maidenhair, pound it by itself, lay it on the swelling, and it will heal it.

(48:2)   If someone's hair is falling out, take the same plant, mix it with oil, rub it on the hair, and it will soon stay put.

49.   Garlic (*Allium nigrum* L.), *temolus, Syngrene*[90]
This plant is called *temolum* and another name, garlic. Homer said it was most splendid and that Mercury discovered it. The juice of this plant is extremely beneficial, and its root is round and dark, and also the same size as a leek.

(49.1)   For pain in the womb, take this plant, pound it, and lay it on; it relieves the pain.

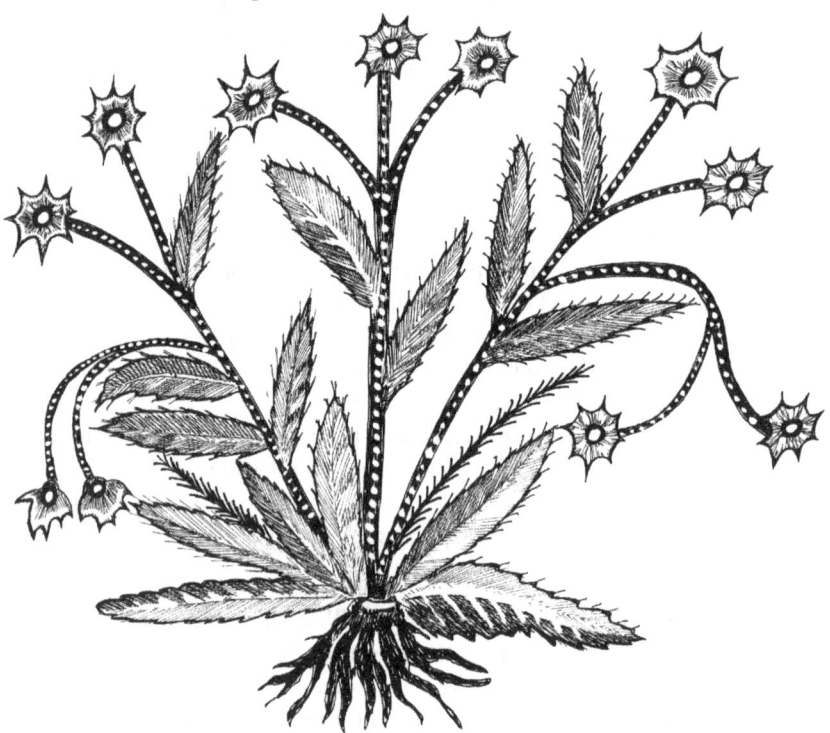

Heliotrope

50.   Heliotrope (*Heliotropium europaeum* L.), *æliotropus, Sigelhweorfa*[91]
This plant, which the Greeks call *æliotrophus*, the Romans *uertamnum*, and the English heliotrope, grows everywhere in cultivated, cleared soil, and in meadows. The plant has a wonderful, divine property; namely, its blossoms turn to follow the sun's course, so that when the sun sets, they close themselves, and when it rises, they open and spread themselves wide. The plant helps in the following remedies, which we have written down.

(50:1)   For all poisons, take the same plant and pound it into fine powder, or give its juice to drink in good wine. In a wonderful way, it will disperse the poison.

(50:2)   For flux, take the leaves of this same plant, pound them, and lay them on the soreness. It is believed that it heals most effectively.

51. Madder (*Rubia tinctorum* L.), *gryas*, *Mæddre*
This plant, which is called *gryas* and another name, madder, grew first in Lucania, has the color of white marble, and is adorned with four red stalks.

(51.1)   For aching bones and for broken bones, take the same plant, pound it, and lay it on the bone. Three days later, the person will be much better, as though a poultice had been put there.

(51:2)   Also, the roots of this same plant help heal any pain that afflicts the body; that is, when one pounds the roots and lays them on the painful place, it will heal all the soreness.

52. Common Maidenhair (*Asplenium trichomanes* L.), *politricus*, *Hymele*[92]
This plant, called *politricum* and another name, common maidenhair, grows on old ruins[93] and also in moist places.

(52:1)   For abdominal pain, take the leaves of this plant we call *politricum*—its twigs are like the bristles on a pig—pound the leaves together with nine peppercorns and nine coriander seeds. Give this to drink in good wine just before taking a bath. Also this plant is effective in making either a man's or woman's hair grow.

53. Asphodel (*Aspherula odorata*), *malochin agria*, *Wuduhrofe*[94]
(53.1)   For a swollen stomach, take the roots of this plant, which the Greeks call *malochin agria*, the Romans *astula regia*, and the English asphodel, and pound them with wine. Give this to drink, and soon you will perceive its benefits.

(53:2)   For loose stools take the seeds of the same plant we call *astula regia* mixed with strong vinegar. Give this to drink, and it will bind the insides.

54. White Poppy (*Papaver somniferum* L.), *metoria*, *(Hwit) Popig*
(54:1)   For eye pain, which we call being blear-eyed, take the juice of the plant that the Greeks call *moetorias*, the Romans *papaver album*, and the English white poppy, or the stem of the plant with the fruit, and lay it on the eyes.

(54:2)   For pain in the temples or in the head, take the juice of this same plant, pound it with vinegar, put it on the face, and it will relieve the pain.

(54:3)   For sleeplessness, take the juice of the same plant, rub it on the person, and you will quickly send them to sleep.

55. Dropwort (*Spiraea filipendula* L.), *oenantes*, *curmealle*[95]
(55:1)   If a person cannot pass water, take the powdered roots of this plant, which is called *oennantes* or ..., give it to drink in two cupfuls of wine. It helps remarkably.

(55:2)   For very bad coughs, take the roots of this same plant; take exactly as we said earlier. It relieves the coughing.

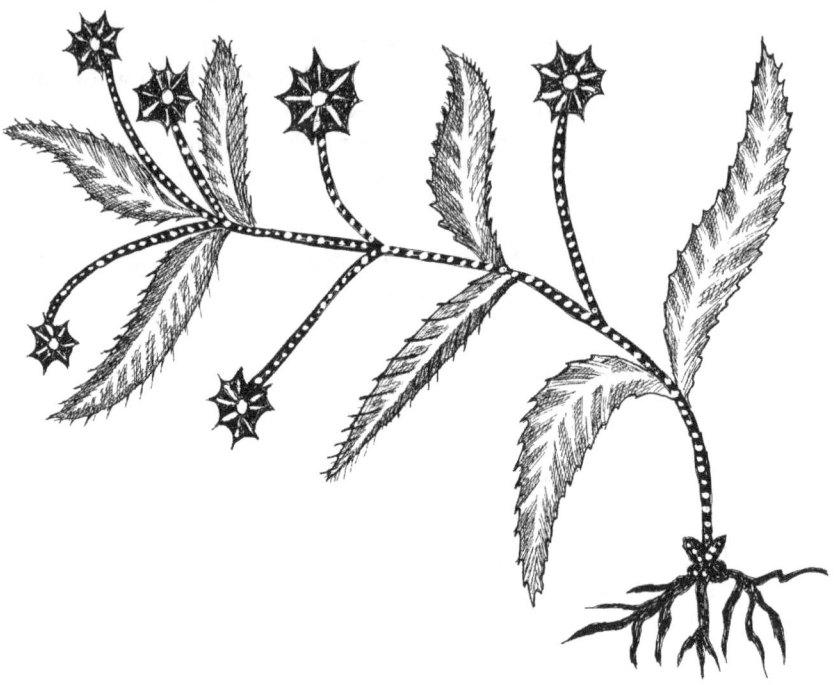

Narcissus

56.   Throatwort, Narcissus, or Nettle-Leaved Bellflower (*Narcissus poeticus* L.), *narcisus*, Halswyrt[96]

(56:1)   For sores that grow on a person, take the roots of the plant that is called *narcisum* and another name, throatwort, pounded with oil and flour just as you would make a poultice. Lay this on the sore, and it will heal wonderfully.

57.   Spleenwort (*Ceterach officinarum* or *Scrophularia nodosa or aquatica*), *splenion*, Brunewyrt[97]

(57:1)   For pain in the spleen, take the roots of the plant the Greeks call *splenion*, the Romans *teucerion*, and the English spleenwort, pound them into a fine powder and give this to drink in a light wine. You will experience something remarkable with it. In addition, it is said that the plant was discovered in this way: it happened that someone threw[98] some intestines, including the spleen, on this plant. The spleen quickly adhered to the plant, and the plant immediately took in the spleen, and because of this, some people called it *splenion*—spleenwort in our language. For that reason, some say that pigs that eat the roots are found not to have a spleen.

Some also say that it has a stalk with branches like hyssop and leaves like beans, and some people call this hyssop for that reason. Gather this plant when it is in full bloom. It is famous chiefly in the mountainous lands named Cilicia and Pisidia.

58. Woodland or Sage-Leaved Germander, Wood Sage, Halwort, Cat-Thyme, Polygermander (*Teucrium scorodonia or polium* L.), *polion*, no OE word

This plant called *polion* and another name ... grows in rough places.

For lunacy, take the juice of the plant we call *polion*, mix it with vinegar, and rub it on the person who is afflicted with the evil condition before it attacks them. Put its leaves and roots in a clean cloth and fasten this around the neck of the person who suffers from the ailment; it proves itself effective.

59. Butcher's Broom or Knee-Holly (*Ruscus aculeatus* L.), *uictoriola*, *Cneowholen*

(59:1)   For foot disease[99] and for the stomach, take two cups of the juice of this plant, which is called *uictoriala* or butcher's broom, and give to drink mixed with honey on an empty stomach. It will quickly reduce the foot disease.

60. Comfrey (*Symphytum officinale* L.), *confirma*, *Galluc*

This plant, called *confirman* and another name, comfrey, grows on the moors, in fields, and in meadows.

(60:1)   For a woman's periods, take the *confirmam* plant, pound it into fine powder, and give it to drink in wine. The flow will quickly stop.

(60:2)   If someone has an internal rupture, take the roots of this same plant and roast them in hot ashes, eat this on an empty stomach with some honey. They will be healed, and it also completely cleans out the stomach.

(60:3)   For stomachache, take the same plant and mix it with honey and vinegar. You will experience the most beneficial effects.

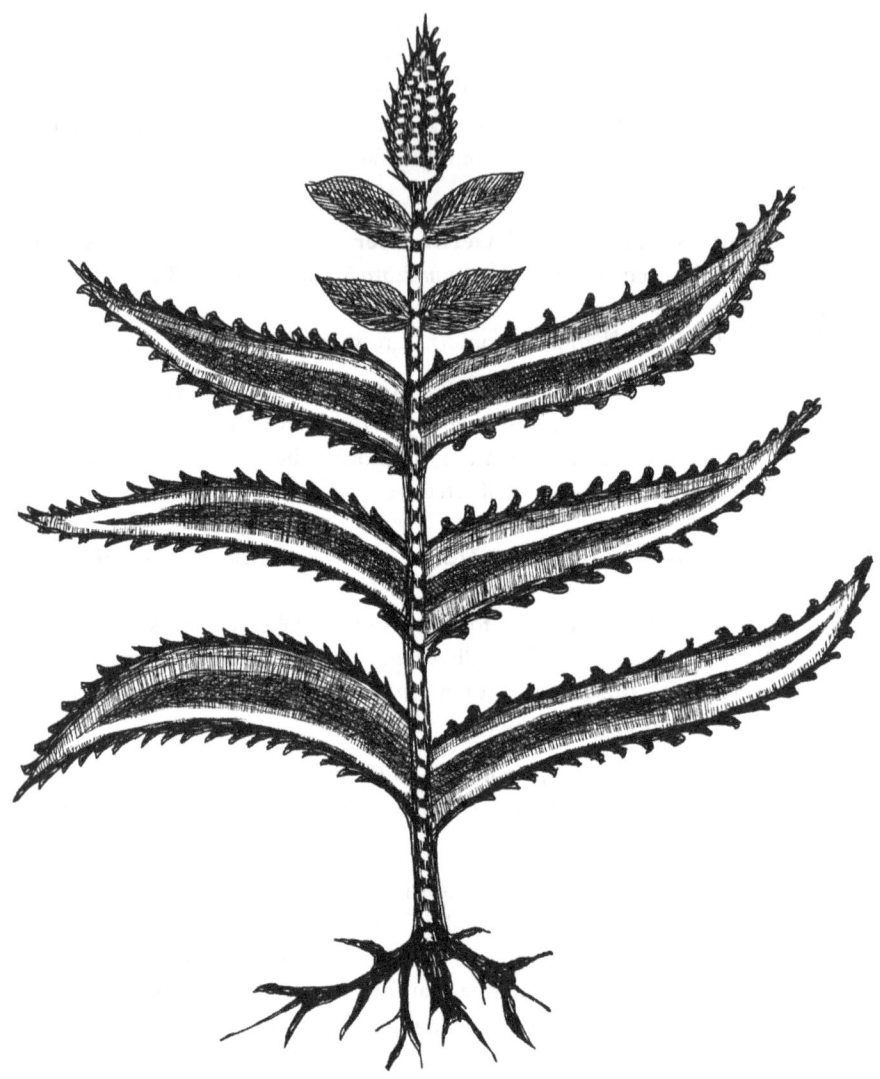

Aster

61. Aster (*Aster amellus* L.), or chickweed, asterion, no OE word[100]
This plant, called *asterion* or …, grows between stones and in rough places.

This plant shines at night like the stars in the skies, and those who see it without knowing that, say they have seen an apparition, and, thus frightened, they are ridiculed by shepherds and those who know more about the power of the plant.

> (61:1)   For epilepsy, take the berries of this plant we call *asterion* and give
>   them to eat when the moon is waning and when the sun is in the

sign of Virgo, which is in the month called August. Hang the same plant around the neck; the person will be healed.

62.   Hare's-Foot Clover (*Trifolium arvense* L.), *leporis pes*, *Haran Hyge*

(62.1)   For stopped up intestines, take the plant called *leporis pes* and another name, hare's-foot clover; dry it, make it into a powder, and give it to drink in wine if they do not have a fever. If they have a fever, give it to drink in water. The blockage will soon be dislodged.

63.   Dittany of Crete (*Dictamnus albus* L., *Origanum dictamnus* L.), *dictamnus*, no OE word

This plant, which is called *dictamnum* or another name ..., grows on the island named Crete and on the mountain named Ida.

(63:1)   If a woman is carrying a dead child inside her, take the juice of the plant we call *dictamnum*; if she does not have a fever, give it to drink in wine. If she suffers from fever, give it to drink in warm water. Quickly it will send out the child without danger.

(63:2)   Again, for wounds, whether caused by iron or a pole or a snake, take the juice of this plant and put it on the wounds and give it to drink. Soon the person will be well.

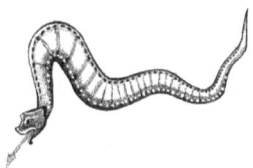

(63:3)   Again, for snakebite, take the juice of this plant and give it to drink in wine. It will quickly drive out the poison.

(63:4)   If anyone eats something poisonous, take the juice of this same plant and drink it in wine. In fact, this plant is so powerful that not only does it kill snakes with its power but also any that are near it, because of the smell. When the wind spreads the smell, wherever snakes are and smell the plant's odor, they are said to die.

It is also said about this same plant that if a roebuck or roe deer is hurt by an arrow or other weapon during a hunt, they will eat the plant as soon as they come upon it, and that it quickly ejects the arrow and heals the wound.

(63:5)   For fresh wounds, take the same plant with stichwort and water germander, pound them with butter, and lay this on the wound. You will be amazed at all the things this plant benefits.

64.   Heliotrope (*Heliotropium* spp. L.), *solago maior*, no OE name

(64:1)   For snakebite and for scorpion's sting, take the plant called *solago maior* and *helioscorpion*, dry it, and then pound it into a fine powder. Give it to drink in wine, and take the pounded plant and put it on the wound.

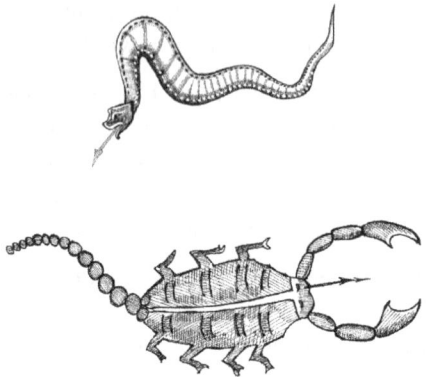

65. **Croton (*Croton tiglium*), *solago minor*, no OE name**[101]

(65:1)   If worms [rængcwyrmas] irritate the area around the navel, take the plant that is called *solago minor* and another name *æliotropion* in a dried form, make it into a fine powder, and give it to drink in warm water. It will kill the worms.

66. **Peony (*Paeonia officinalis* L.), *peonia*, *Peonia***

This plant, which is called *peonian*, was discovered by Prince Peonio, and it gets its name from him. It grows principally in Greece, as the famous authority Homer records in his books. It is found mainly by shepherds, it has seeds the size of *maligranati*, and it shines at night like a lantern. Also, its seed is like a cockle's,[102] and as we said earlier, it is most often found and gathered at night by shepherds.

(66:1)   For lunacy[103]: if one lays the peony plant over someone suffering from lunacy when they are lying down, they will quickly raise themselves up healthy, and if they have it with them, the illness will never again come near them.

(66:2)   For aching hip bone, take a part of the root of this plant and tie it onto the sore place with a clean linen cloth; this will heal it.

67. **Vervain or Gypsywort (*Verbena officinalis* or *Lycopus europaeus*),**[104] **_peristereon_, *Berbene***

This plant, called *peristereon* and another name, vervain, is so much like the color of doves that some people also call it *columbinam*.

(67:1)   If anyone has the plant with them that we call *peristereon*, dogs will not bark at them.

(67:2)   For all kinds of poisons, take this plant powdered, give it to drink, and it will drive away the poison. It is also said that sorcerers use it for their crafts.

68. **Bryony (*Bryonia* L.), *bryonia*, *Hymele***[105]

(68:1)   For pain in the spleen, take the plant called *brionia* and another name, bryony, and give it to eat mixed in food. The pain will gently go away by passing water. This plant is agreeable enough that one can mix it with whatever they customarily drink.

69.   White Water Lily (*Nymfaea alba* L.), Nimpheta, no OE word

(69:1a)   For a bloated stomach, take the seeds of this plant, which is called *nymfeta* or …, pound them with wine, and give this to drink.

(69:1b)   For the same, use the roots and give them to the person who is sick to eat for ten days.

(69:2)   Also, if you give the plant to drink in strong wine, it stops loose stools.[106]

70.   Thistle (*Carduus* supp. L.), *crision*, Claefre[107]

(70:1)   For sore throat: if someone has roots of the plant called *crision* and another name, thistle, and wears it tied about their neck, their throat will never trouble them.

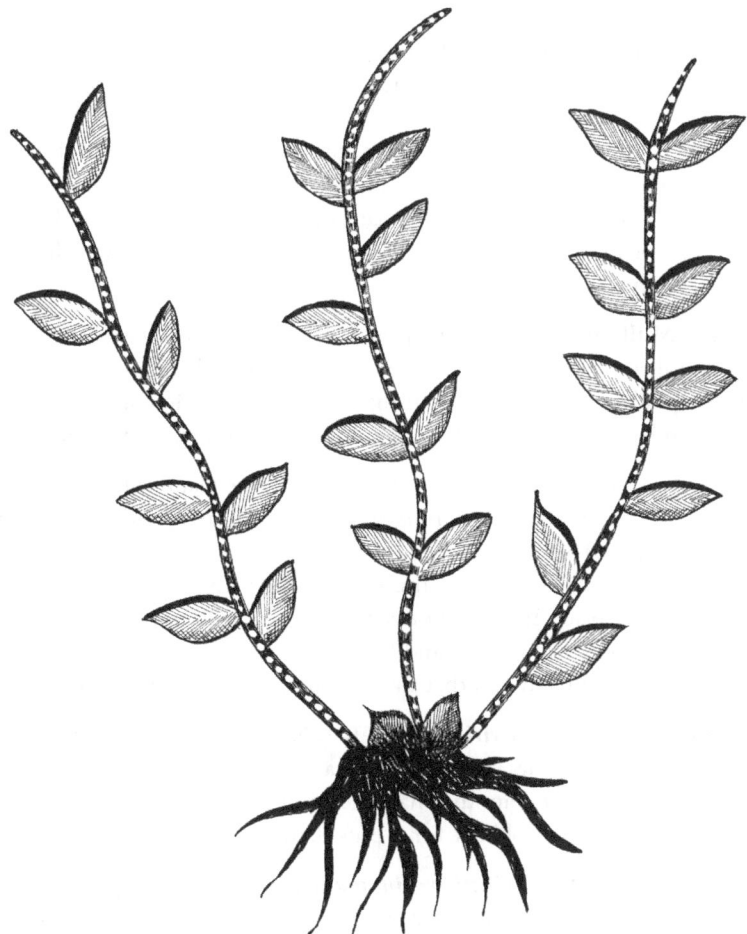

Woad

71.   Woad (*Isatis tinctoria* L.), *isatis*, *Wad*

The Greeks call this plant *isatis*, the Romans *alutam*, and the English *ad serpentis morsum*.[108]

(71:1)   For snakebite, take the leaves of the plant the Greeks call *isatis* and pound them with water. Lay them on the bite. It will be of benefit and will take the soreness away.

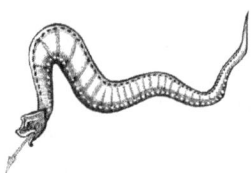

72.   Water Germander (*Teucrium scordium* L.), *scordea*, no OE word

(72:1)   For snakebite, take the plant called *scordean* and another name, …, and simmer it in wine. Give it to drink. Then mash the plant and lay it on the wound.

(72:2)   For soreness of the joints, take the same plant, pound it, and gently boil it with the oil from a laurel tree. It will alleviate the pain.

(72:3)   For daily fever or one that comes every three days, take the same plant and fasten it on the person's body. It takes away the daily and third-day kinds of fever.

73.   Great Mullein (*Verbascum thapsus* L.), *uerbascus*, *Feltwyrt*[109]

This plant, called *uerbascum* and another name, great mullein, grows in sandy soils and on dunghills. Concerning this plant, it is said that Mercury gave it to Lord Ulysses when he met Circe, and because of it, he did not fear any of her evil deeds.

(73:1)   If anyone carries even one twig of this plant with them, no terror will frighten them, no wild beast will scare them, nor will any evil approach them.

(73:2)   For foot disease, take this same plant, *uerbascum*, bruised. Lay it on the sore place. In a few hours, the soreness will heal to the point that the patient will dare to and be able to walk. In addition, our authorities declared and said that this preparation helps remarkably.

74.   Herba Heraclea (*Sideritis romana* L.), *heraclea*, no OE name[110]

(74:1)   Anyone who wants to travel a long way and takes the plant called *heraclean* and another name … with them on the trip does not have to fear any robbers, for it puts them to flight.

75.   Greater Celandine (*Chelidonuim maius*), *caelidonia*, *cylepenie*

(75:1)   For dimness, pain, and film in the eyes, take the juice of the plant called *celidoniam* and another name that is similar to it, greater celandine, and take the roots pounded with aged wine, honey, and pepper. When it is thoroughly mixed, apply to inner corners of the eyes.

Also we found out that some people applied the milk of this plant to their eyes, and they got better from it.

(75:2)   Also, for dimness of the eyes, take the juice of this same plant, or the blossoms pressed and mixed with honey. Mix in gently boiling ashes with this, and simmer together in a brass pot. This is an extremely good remedy for dimness of the eyes.

It is also certain that some people just use the juice, as we said earlier.

(75:3)   For hardened swellings, take the same plant, pound it with grease, and lay it on the swellings; bathe the swellings first with water.

(75:4)   For headache, take the same plant, pound it with vinegar, and rub it on the face and the head.

(75:5)   For burns, take the same plant, pound it with goat's grease, and lay it on the burn.

76.   Black Nightshade (*Solanum nigrum* L.), *solata*, *Solsequia*[111]

(76:1)   For swellings, take this plant called *solate* and another name, black nightshade, pounded and mixed with oil. Lay it on the swelling, and it will help.

(76:2)   For earache, take the juice of this same plant, mix it with cypress oil,[112] and warm it. Drip it into the ear lukewarm.

(76:3)   For toothache, give the berries of this plant to eat.

(76:4)   For a bloody nose, take the juice of this same plant, dip a linen cloth into it, and stop up the nostrils with it. The blood will soon stop.

77.   Common Groundsel (*Senecio vulgaris* L.), *senecio*, *Grundeswylge*

This plant, which is called *senecio* and another name, groundsel, grows on roofs and along walls.

(77:1)   For wounds, even if they are quite old, take the plant that we call *senecio*, pound it with aged lard, lay it on the wounds, and they will heal quickly.

(77:2)   If anyone is struck by something iron, pick the same plant in early morning or the middle of the day, pound it, as we said earlier, with aged lard, lay it on the cut, and quickly it opens and cleanses the wound.

(77:3)   For foot disease, take the same plant, pound it with lard, put it on the foot, and it will relieve the pain. Also, this helps a great deal for painful joints.

(77:4)   For sore loins, take this same plant, pound it with salt just as you would for a poultice, and put it on the loins. The same thing helps for sore feet.

78.   Fern (*Felix* L.), *felix*, *Fearn*

(78:1)   For wounds, take the pounded roots of the plant we call *felix* and another name, fern, and lay them on the wound. Also give about nine grams of stitchwort to drink in wine.

(78:2)   If a young man is ruptured, take the same plant (one growing in the roots of a beech tree), pound it with grease, spread a cloth with it, and fasten this to the sore so that the cloth is always turned upward. On the fifth day, he will be healed.

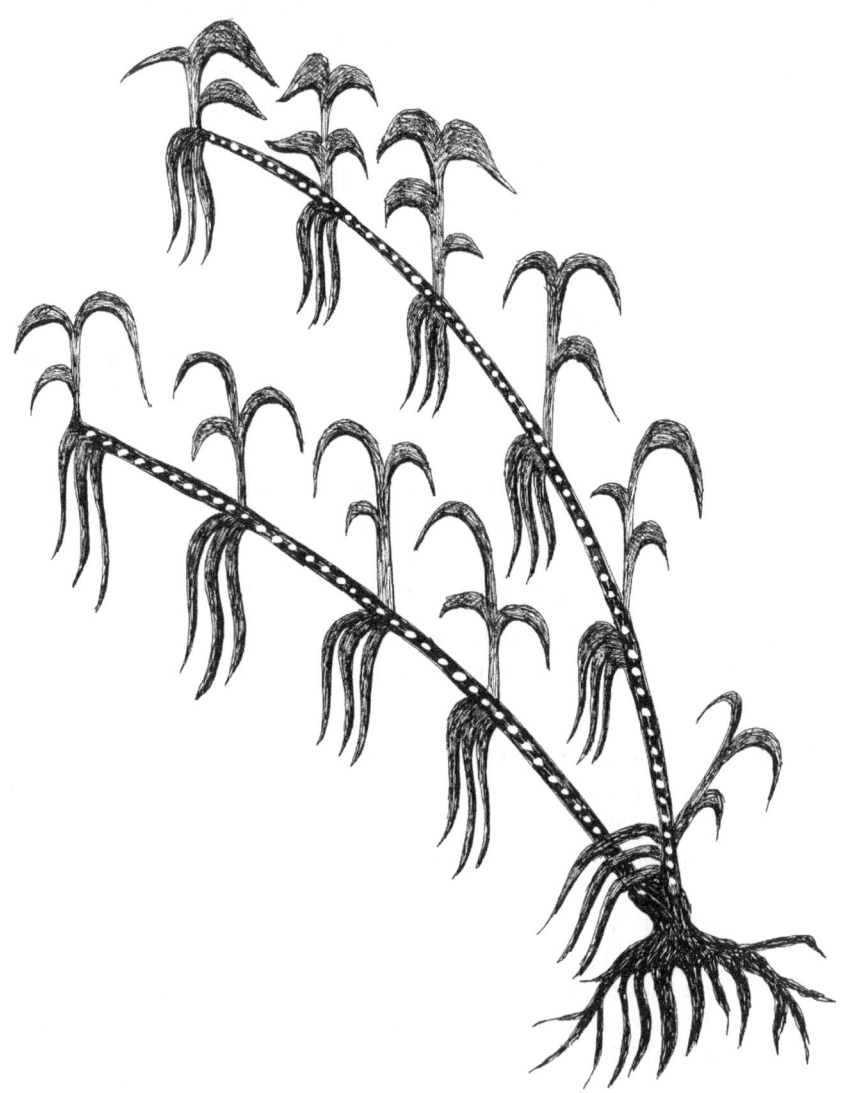

Couch Grass

79.   Couch Grass (*Cynodon dactylon*), gramen, *Cwice*[113]
(79:1)   For pain of the spleen, take the leaves of the plant called *gramen* and another name, couch grass, and simmer them. Apply them to a cloth and lay it on the spleen. You will perceive benefit from this.

80. Iris (*Iris* L. or *Pseudacorus* L.), gladiolus, Glædene

(80:1)   For bladder pain and if someone cannot pass water, take the outer part of the roots of the plant called *gladiolum* and another name, iris, dry it, pound it, and mix with it two cups of wine and three cups of water. Give this to drink.

(80:2)   For pain of the spleen, take the same plant *gladiolum* when it is young, dry it and pound it into powder. Give this to drink in light wine. It is believed that it will heal the spleen in a wonderful manner.

(80:3)   For abdominal and chest[114] pain, take the pounded berries of this plant and give them to drink in goat's milk or better in lukewarm wine. The soreness will go away.

81. Rosemary (*Rosmarinus officinalis* L.), rosmarinum, Boþen

This plant, called *rosmarim* and another name, rosemary, grows in sandy soil and in gardens.[115]

(81:1)   For toothache, take the root of the plant we call *rosmarim* and give it to eat. Without delay, it will relieve the toothache. If the juice is held in the mouth, it will quickly heal the teeth.

(81:2)   For the sickly, take the plant *rosmarinum*, pound it with oil, and rub it on the person. You will heal them wonderfully.

(81:3)   For itching, take the same plant, pound it, and mix its juice with aged wine and warm water. Give it to drink for three days.

(81:4)   For liver disease and abdominal conditions, take a handful of this same plant, pound it in water, and mix it with two handfuls of spikenard and some stalks of rue. Simmer together in water and give to drink. The person will get better.

(81:5)   For fresh wounds, take the same plant we call *rosmarim*, pound it with grease, and lay it onto the wound.

82. Wild Carrot or Parsnip (*Daucus carota* L. or *Pastinaca sativa* L.), pastinaca siluatica, Feldmoru

This plant, which is called *pastinace siluatice* and another name, wild carrot, grows in sandy soils and on hills.

(82:1)   For women having difficulty giving birth, take the plant we call *pastinace siluatice*, simmer it in water, and give it so that she can bathe herself with it. She will be helped.

(82:2)   For women's cleansing, take the same plant, *pastinacam*, simmer it in water, and when it is soft, mix it well and give it to drink. They will be cleansed.

83. Pellitory of the Wall (*Parietaria officinalis* L.), perdicalis, dolhrune

This plant, called *perdicalis* and another name, pellitory of the wall, grows along roads, against walls, and on hills.

(83:1)   For foot disease and ulcerous sores, take this plant that we call *perdicalis* and simmer it in water. Bathe the feet and the knees with it. Then pound the plant with lard, make it into a poultice, and lay it onto the feet and the knees. You will heal them well.

84. **Dog's Mercury (*Mercurialis perennis* L.), *mercurialis*, *Cedelc***

(84:1) For intestinal blockage, take the plant people call *mercurialis* and another name, dog's mercury, crumbled in water. Give this to the sufferer and quickly the blockage will be driven out, and the stomach will be purged. The seed cures in the same manner.

(84:2) For pain and swelling of the eyes, take the pounded leaves of this same plant in old wine and lay them on the swollen eyes.

(84:3) If water gets into the ears, take lukewarm juice of this plant and drip it into the ear. Soon the water will go away.

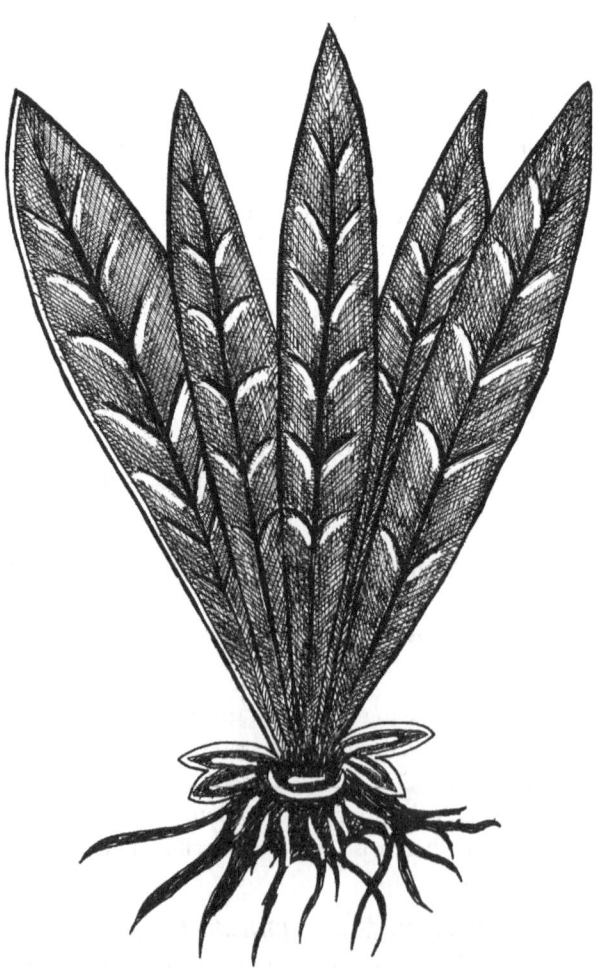

Polypody

85. Polypody (*Polypodium vulgare* L.), *radiola*, *Eforfearn*
This plant, which is called *radiolum* and another name, polypody, is like a fern, and it grows in stony places and on ruins. It has two rows of beautiful spots on each leaf, and they shine like gold.

(85:1) For headache, take the plant we call *radiolum* and clean it very well. Simmer it in vinegar and smear the head with it. It will relieve the headache.

86. Asparagus (*Asparagus officinalis* L.), *herba sparagiagrestis*, *Wuduceruille*[116]

(86:1) For pain or swelling of the bladder, take the roots of the plant called *sparagiagrestis* and another name, asparagus; simmer it down in water by three-fourths, then drink it for seven days on an empty stomach. They should bathe for many days, but they should not get into nor drink cold water. The person will feel healthy in a wonderful way.

(86:2) For toothache, take the juice of this same plant that we call *sparagi*, give it to drink and some to hold in their mouth.

(86:3) For sore veins, take the roots of this same plant pounded with wine and give them to drink. It helps.

(86:4) If an evil person enchants another out of spite, take the dried roots of this same plant, give them to eat with well water. Sprinkle the person with the water. They will be freed from the enchantment.

87. Savine (*Juniperus sabina* L.), *sabine*, *Sauine*

(87:1) For the king's disease,[117] which is called *aurignem* in Latin and means painful joints and foot swelling in our language, take this plant, which is called *sabinam*, and by another name like it, savine, give it to drink with honey. It will relieve the pain. It does the same thing mixed with wine.

(87:2) For headache, take the same plant, savine, well pounded in vinegar and mixed with oil. Rub it on the head and the temples. It will help remarkably.

(87:3) For carbuncles, take the savine plant mixed with honey and smear it on the sore.

88. Small Snapdragon (*Antirrhinum orontium* L.), *canis caput*, *Hundes Heafod*[118]

(88:1) For soreness and swelling of the eyes, take the roots of the plant called *canis caput* in Latin and in our language, snapdragon, simmer them in water, and then bathe the eyes with the water. It will quickly soothe the pain.

89. Blackberry or Bramble (*Rubus fruticosus* L.), *erusti*, *Bremel*

(89:1) For earache, take the plant called *erusti* and another name, blackberry, when soft, and pound it. Then take the juice, lukewarm, and drip it into the ear. It lessens the pain and effectively heals.

(89:2) For a woman's periods, take the berries of this same plant when they are soft—take three times seven of them—and simmer them down in water by two-thirds.[119] Give this to drink on an empty stomach for three days, but make a new drink each day.

(89:3) For heart pain, take the leaves of this plant pounded by themselves. Lay them on the left nipple. The pain will go away.

(89:4) For fresh wounds, take the flowers of this same plant and lay them on the wounds. It will heal the wounds without any delay or danger.

(89:5) For pain in the joints, take some of this same plant and simmer it down in wine by two-thirds. Bathe the joints with this wine, and all the illness in the joints will be relieved.

(89:6) For snakebite, take the leaves of the same plant that we call *erusti*, freshly pounded, and lay them on the bite.

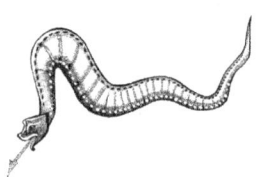

90. **Yarrow (*Achillea millefolium* L.), *millefolium*, Gearwe**

(90:1) About the plant called *millefolium* and in our language yarrow, it is said that Lord Achilles discovered it, and that with this same plant he cured those who were hit by an iron weapon and were wounded. It is also said some men named it *achylleos* because of this, and also that he cured a man named Thelephon with this plant.

(90:2) For toothache, take the roots of this same plant we call *millefolium*. Give them to eat on an empty stomach.

(90:3) For wounds that have been caused by something made of iron, take the same plant pounded in grease and smear it on the wounds. It will cleanse and heal the wounds.

(90:4) For swellings, take the same plant *millefolium* pounded in butter. Smear it on the swelling.

(90:5) If someone has difficulty passing water, take the juice of this same plant with vinegar and give it to drink. It cures wonderfully.

(90:6) If a wound has cooled, take the same plant, *millefolium*, pound it small, and mix it with butter. Put this on the wound; it will quickly recover feeling and warm up.

(90:7) If someone's head breaks out in rashes, or strange swellings appear on the face, take the roots of this same plant and fasten them around the neck. This will benefit them greatly.

(90:8) For the same condition, take the same plant, powder it, put it on the sores, and soon they will become slightly inflamed.[120]

(90:9) If someone's veins have hardened or their digestion is difficult, take the juice of this same plant; mix wine, water, and honey together with the juice. Give this to drink warm and they will quickly improve.

(90:10) Again for intestinal and abdominal pain, take the same plant and dry it, then make it into a fine powder. Put five spoonfuls of the powder into three[121] of good wine. Give them this to drink. This will benefit any internal condition they may have.

(90:11) If they develop hiccoughs or heartburn after taking that, take the roots of this same plant and pound them well. Put them in good beer and give this to drink lukewarm. I expect that it will truly benefit them, both for hiccoughs or for any other painful internal condition.

(90:12) For headache, take the same plant, make a poultice with it, and lay it on the head. It will quickly take the pain away.

(90:13) For bites of the kind of snake called "spalangius," take twigs and leaves of the same plant, simmer them in wine, pound them up fine, and apply this to a bite if it is scabbing over too quickly. Then take the plant and honey, mix them together, apply this to the bite, and it will quickly become slightly inflamed and heal.

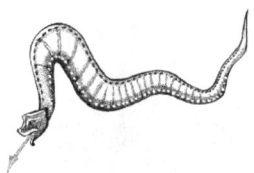

(90:14) To prevent snakebites: if anyone wears this plant and carries it with them on their way, they will be shielded from every kind of snake.

(90:15) For bite of a mad dog, take the same plant and grind it with wheat seeds. Put them on the bite, and this will quickly heal it.

(90:16) Again, for snakebite, if the wound is swollen, take twigs of this same plant, simmer them in water, grind them very small, and lay them soaking wet on the wound. If the wound is open, take the same plant dry, pound it very small, mix it with honey, and treat the wound with it. It will quickly heal.

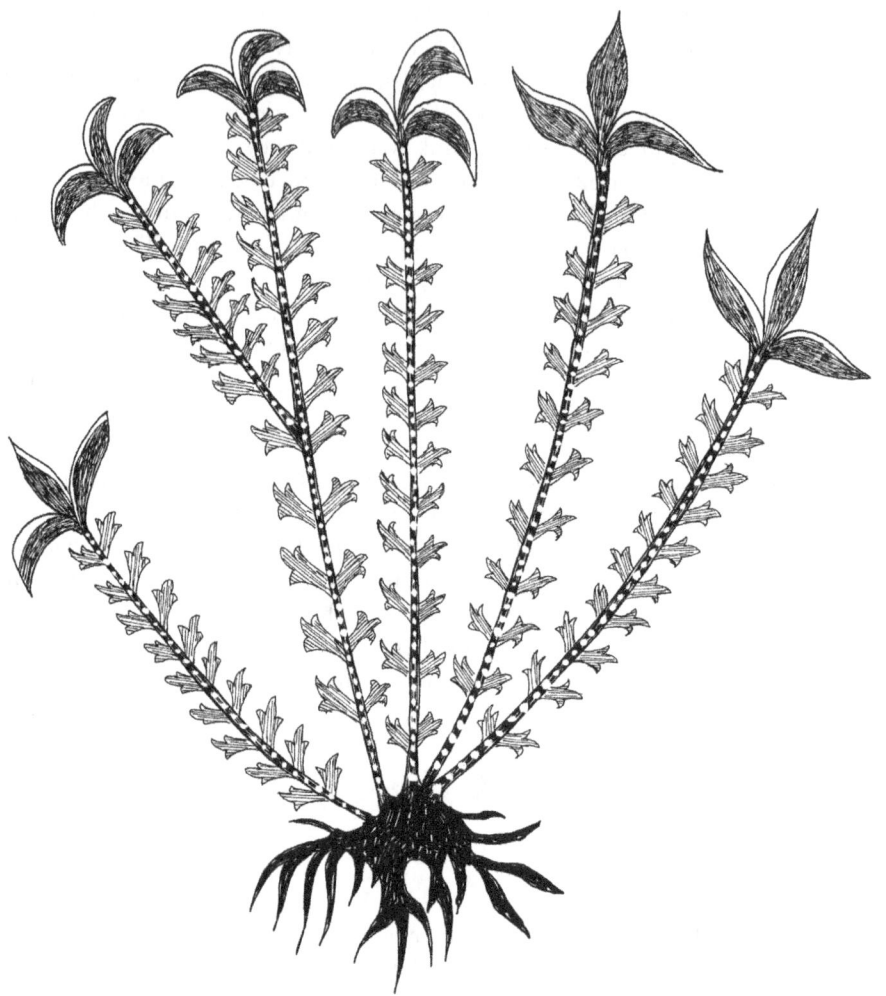

Rue

91. Rue (*Ruta graveolens L.*), *rute, Rude*

(91:1)   For nosebleed, take the plant that is called *rutam* and another name, rue, and put it in the nostrils often. It controls the nosebleed in a wonderful manner.

(91:2)   For swellings, take the same plant, *rutam*, give it to eat fresh a little at a time or to take in a drink.

(91:3)   For stomachache, take the seeds of this same plant, sulphur, and vinegar. Give this to eat on an empty stomach.

(91:4)   For pain and swelling of the eyes, take the same plant, *rutan*, pounded well, and lay it on the sore eyes. Also the pounded roots smeared on will cure the pain very well.

(91:5)   For the illness that is called *litargum*, and in our language forgetful-ness, take the same plant, *rutam*, soaked in vinegar. Sprinkle it on the face.

(91:6)   For dimness of the eyes, take the leaves of this same plant, give them to eat on an empty stomach, and give them to drink in wine.

(91:7)   For headache, take the same plant and give it to drink in wine. Pound that same plant and press out the juice into vinegar. Smear it on the head. The plant also helps heal carbuncles.

92. Horsemint (*Mentha longifolia* or *silvestris* L.), *mentastrus* (*Horsminte or Minte*)

(92:1)   For earache, take the juice of the plant called *mentastrum* and another name … mixed with strong wine. Put this into the ear. In case worms are growing there, they should be destroyed using this.

(92:2)   For a very bad skin condition,[122] take the leaves of this same plant and give them to eat. The person will certainly be healed.

93. Dwarf Elder or Danewort (*Sambucus ebulus* L.), *ebulus*, *Wealwyrt or Ellenwyrt*

(93:1)   For bladder stones, take the plant called *ebulum* and another name, dwarf elder, and some call danewort, and pound it with its leaves when it is tender. Give this to drink in wine. It will clear up the condition.

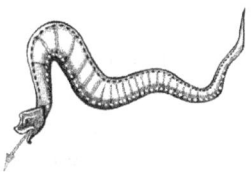

(93:2)   For snakebite, take the same plant we call *ebulum*, and before you cut it up, hold it in your hands and say this three times, nine times: *Omnes malas bestias canto*, that is in our language, I enchant and overcome all evil beasts.[123] Cut it up into three parts with a sharp knife, and while you are doing this, think of the person you want to heal using it. When you turn to the job, do not look around and about—be focused. Take the plant and pound it, then lay it on the bite. They will recover quickly.

(93:3)   For dropsy, take the pounded roots of this same plant, wring out enough from it so that you have four cups and add half a jug of wine. Give to drink once a day, and it will greatly help the dropsy.

Also, within half a year, it will clear out all the fluids caused by dropsy.

94. Pennyroyal (*Mentha pulegium* L.), *pollegium*, *dweorgedwosle*[124]

This plant, called *pollegium* and another name, pennyroyal, is good in many kinds of remedies although many people do not know it, because this plant has two varieties, masculine and feminine. The masculine one has white flowers, and the feminine red or brown; both are beneficial, wonderful, and have wondrous powers; they bloom with the brightest color just about when other plants are withering and fading.

(94:1) For abdominal pain, take the *pollegium* plant and cumin, pound them together with water and place this on the navel. The person will heal quickly.

(94:2) Again, for stomachache, take the same plant, *pollegium*, pound it, and wash it with water. Give it to drink in vinegar. It will relieve the upset stomach very well.

(94:3) For itching of the private parts, take the same plant, simmer in gently boiling water, and then let it cool until one can drink it. Drink it, and it will relieve the itching.

(94:4) Again, for abdominal pain: this plant relieves it well when eaten, and when fixed to the navel so that it cannot fall off. It will quickly alleviate the pain.

(94:5) For fever that comes every third day, take branches of this same plant, enfold them in wool, and fumigate the patient with it before the fever is due to strike. If this plant is fastened around the head, their headache will be relieved.

(94:6) If a stillborn child is inside a woman, take three springs of this plant, so fresh that they have a strong smell, pound them in aged wine, and give this to drink.

(94:7) For anyone suffering from nausea aboard ship, take the same plant, *pollegium*, and wormwood. Pound them together with oil and vinegar and rub them often with it.

(94:8) For bladder pain and for the stones that develop there, take the same plant, *pollegium*, pounded well and two cups of wine. Mix them together and give this to drink. The bladder will quickly become much better, and within a few days, it will heal up the condition, and the stones that developed will be sent out.

(94:9) If anyone suffers pain around the heart or chest, they should eat of this same plant, *pollegium*, and drink of it on an empty stomach.

(94:10) If someone suffers a cramp, take the same plant and two cups of vinegar, and drink this on an empty stomach.

(94:11) For swelling of the stomach and abdomen, take this same plant, *pollegium*, give it to eat by itself or pounded and simmered in wine or water. The condition will be relieved quickly.

(94:12) For pain of the spleen, take the same plant, *pollegium*, and simmer it in vinegar. Give it to drink warm.

(94:13) For aching loins and sore thighs, take equal amounts of this same plant, *pollegium*, and pepper and mix them together. When you are bathing, apply this where it hurts most.

95.   Catmint/Nepeta (*Mentha solvestris*), *nepitamon*, Nepte

This plant is called *nepitamon* or another name, catmint, and the Greeks call it *menthe orinon*.

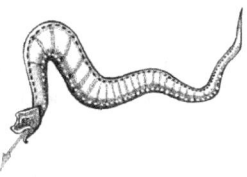

(95:1)   For snakebite, take the plant we call *nepitamon*, pound it in wine, wring out the juice, and give it to drink in wine. Then take the pounded leaves of the same plant and lay them on the wound.

96.   Hog's Fennel or Sulphurwort (*Peucedanum officinale* L.), *peucedana*, *Cammoc*

The plant is called *peucedana* and another name, hog's fennel.

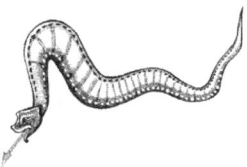

This plant, which we call *peucedanum*, can make snakes flee by its smell.

(96:1)   For snakebite, take the same plant, *peucedanum*, *betonican*, deer's grease or marrow, and vinegar. Mix this together and smear it on the wound; it will heal.

(96:2)   For the condition the Greeks call *frenesis*, which is witlessness of the mind in our language, that is, when the head becomes very hot, take the same plant, *peucedanum*, pound it in vinegar, and sprinkle the head with this. It heals very well.

97.   Elecampane (*Inula helenium* L.), *hinnula campana*, *Sperewyrt*

(97:1)   For bladder pain, take this plant called *hinnula campana* and another name, elecampane, wild celery seed, asparagus, and fennel root, pound them together, and give this to drink lukewarm. It heals with certainty.

(97:2)   For toothache and loose teeth, take the same plant and give it to eat on an empty stomach. It firms up the teeth.

(97:3)   For worms [*rengwyrmas*] around the navel, take the same plant, *hinnula*, pound it in wine, and lay it on the abdomen.

98.   Ribwort Plantain (*Plantago lanceolata* L.), Narrow-Leaved Plantain or Ribwort, *cynoglossa*, *Ribbe*[125]

The plant is called *cynoglossam* and another name, ribwort, and some also call it *linguam canis*.

(98:1)   For snakebite, the plant we call *cynoglossam* heals effectively when pounded and taken in wine.

(98:2)   For a fever that comes every fourth day, take this same plant, *cynoglossam*, the one with four leaves, pound it, and give it to drink in water. It will bring them relief.

(98:3)   If the ears don't work right, and if a person can't hear well, take the same plant, *cynoglossam*, pounded and warmed in oil. Drip it into the ear, and it will help in a wonderful manner.

99. Saxifrage (*Saxifraga granulata* L.), *saxifraga*, Sundcorn

The plant called *saxifragam* and another name, saxifrage, grows on hills and in rocky places.

(99:1)   For stones in the bladder, take the plant we call *saxifragam*, pound it in wine, and give in warm water to anyone suffering and feverish. It is so effective, that those who tried it said that it breaks up the stones on that same day, sends them out, and leads to health.

100. Ivy (*Glechoma hederacea* L.), *hedera nigra*, Eorþifig[126]

(100:1)   For stones in the bladder, take seven to eleven shoots of the plant called *hederan nigran* and another name, ivy, crushed in water. Give this to drink. It will collect the stones in the bladder in a wondrous way and will destroy them and send them out when passing water.

(100:2)   For headache, take the same plant, *hederam* and rose juice soaked in wine. Rub this on the temples and the face, and the pain will lessen.

(100:3)   For pain in the spleen, on the first attack, take three shoots of this same plant, on the next, five; at the third attack, take seven; at the fourth time, nine; at the fifth, eleven; at the sixth, thirteen; the seventh time, fifteen; at the eighth, seventeen; at the ninth, nineteen; and at the tenth, twenty-one. Give to drink daily in wine, but if there is fever present, give it in warm water. Great improvement and strength will result.

(100:4)   For the bite of a poisonous critter called *spalangiones*,[127] take the juice of the roots of the same plant we call *hederan* and give it to drink.

(100:5)   To treat wounds, take the same plant, simmer it in wine, and lay it on the wounds.

(100:6)   If the nostrils smell bad, take the juice of this same plant, clarified, and pour it into the nostrils.

(100:7)   If the ears do not work well and if someone does not hear well, take the juice of this same plant, very clean, in wine, and drip this into the ears. They will be healed.

(100:8)   So that the head will not ache because of the heat of the sun, take tender leaves of this plant, pound them in vinegar, and smear this on the face. It also prevents any other pain that bothers the head.

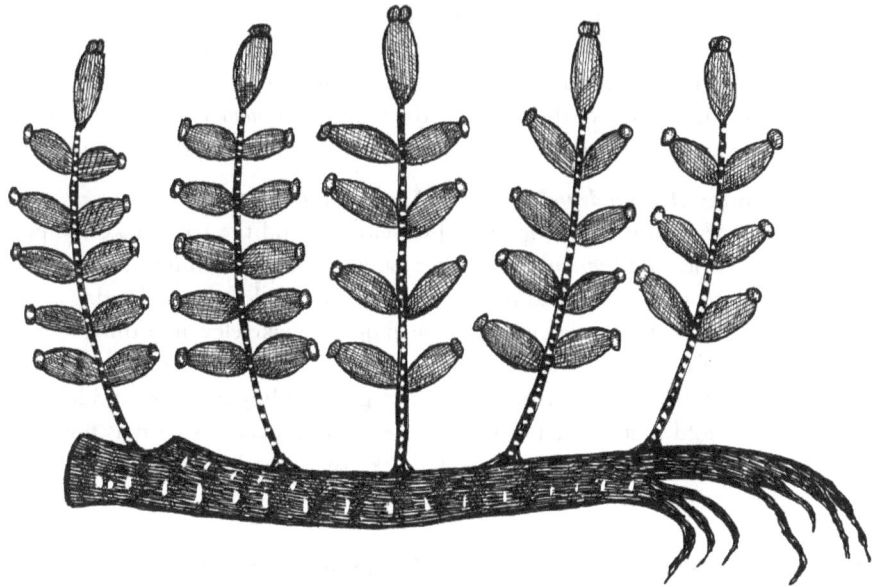

Wild Thyme

101. Wild Thyme (*Thymus serpyllum* L.), *serpillus*, *Organe*

(101:1) For headache, take the juice of the plant called *serpillum* and another name, wild thyme, oil, and burned salt made into a fine powder. Mix everything together, smear the head with this, and it will be healed.

(101:2) Again, for headache, take the same plant, *serpillum*, simmered. Pound it in vinegar and smear it on the temples and the face.

(101:3) If someone is burned, take the same plant, *serpillum*, one stalk of vervain, one ounce of silver shavings, and three ounces of roses. Pound all of these in a mortar, add wax to this, and half a pound of bear and deer grease. Simmer this together, purify it, and smear it on the burns.

102. Wormwood (*Artemisia absinthium* L.), *absinthius*, *Wermod*

This plant, called *absinthium* and another name, wormwood, grows in cultivated soil, on hills, and in rocky places.

(102:1) For removing bruises and other sores from the body, take the plant *absinthium*, simmer it in water, put it in a cloth, and put it on the sore. If the flesh is tender, simmer it in honey and lay it on the sore.

(102:2) If worms [OE *rengwyrmas*] are harming the area around the navel, take equal amounts of the same plant, *absinthium*, horehound, and lupine. Simmer them in sweetened water or in wine. Put it on the navel two or three times, and it will kill the worms.

103. Sage (*Salvia officinalis* L.), *salfia*, *Saluie*

(103:1) For itching of the private parts,[128] take the plant called *saluian*, simmer it in water, and smear this water on the private parts.

(103:2) For itching of the rear, take the same plant, *salfian*, simmer it in water, and bathe the rear with this water. It relieves the itch very well.

104. Coriander (*Coriandrum sativum* L.), *coliandra*, *Celendre*

(104:1) If worms [OE *rengwyrmas*] develop around the navel, take the plant called *coliandrum* and another name, coriander; simmer it down in oil by two-thirds, and put it on the sores and also on the head.

(104:2) So that a woman may give birth quickly, take eleven or thirteen seeds of this same *coliandran* plant, bind them with a thread to a clean linen cloth. Take a person who is a virgin,[129] a boy or a girl, and let them hold it at the left thigh near her private parts. As soon as the entire process of birth is completed, take the remedy away immediately, so that some of the intestines do not follow.

105. Wild Purslane (*Portulaca oleracea* L.), *porclaca*, no OE word

(105:1) For excessive flowing of semen,[130] the plant called *porclaca* and another name … helps effectively, either eaten by itself or with different drinks.

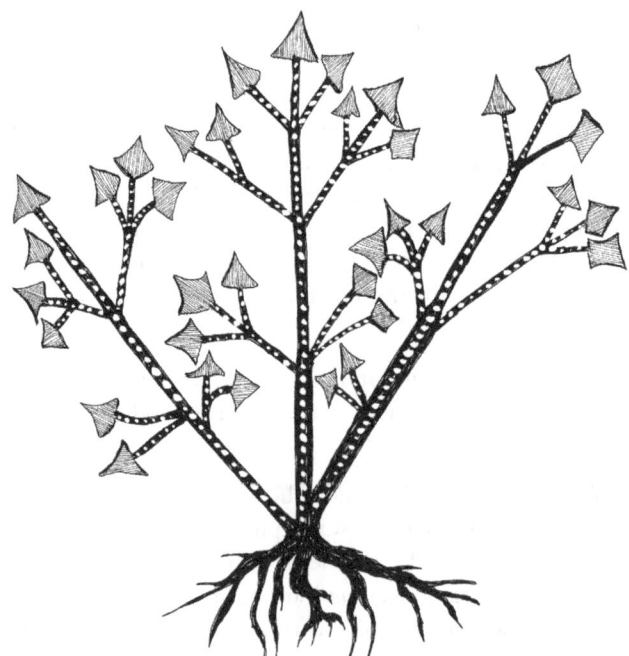

Chervil

106. Chervil (*Anthriscus cerefolium* L.), *cerefolia*, *Cerfille*

(106:1) For stomachache, take three fresh sprouts from the plant called *cerefolium* and another name, chervil, and pennyroyal. Grind them well in a wooden mortar together with one spoonful refined honey and fresh poppy.[131] Simmer them together and give this to eat. It will quickly strengthen the stomach.

107. Brook or Water Mint (*Mentha acquatica or hirsuta* L.), *sisimbrius*, *Brocminte*

(107:1) For bladder pain and for inability to pass water, take the juice of this plant called *sisimbrium* and another name, brook mint. Give this to the suffering person to drink in warm water if feverish, or if not, give it in wine. You will cure them wondrously.

108. Alexanders or Horse Parsley (*Smyrnium olusatrum* L.), *olisatrum*, no OE name

(108:1) Again, for bladder pain and inability to pass water, take the plant we call *olisatrum* and another name …, pound it into simmered wine and give it to drink. It greatly improves the ability to pass water.

109. Lily (*Lilium* spp. L.), *erinion*, *Lilie*

The plant called *erinion* and another name, lilium.

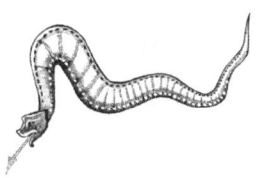

(109:1) For snakebite, take the plant we call lily and *bulbum*, the plant that is also called by another name, narcissus,[132] pound them together, and give this to drink. Then take the plant *bulbum* pounded, lay it on the bite, and it will heal.

(109:2) For swellings, take pounded lily leaves and lay them on the swelling. It will certainly cure it and reduce the swelling.

110. Caper-Spurge (*Euphorbia lathyris*), *titlmallos calatites*, no OE name

This plant called *titymallos calatites* and another name, caper spurge, grows in wet places and on the shore.

(110:1) For abdominal pain, take a shoot of the plant *titymalli*, pound it into wine so that there are two cups of wine, add to it two spoonfuls of the juice of this plant, and give this to drink on an empty stomach. It will heal a person.

(110:2) For warts, take the milky sap from this plant and the juice of celery-leaved crowfoot and put it on the warts. On the third day, it will heal up the warts.

(110:3) For bad skin conditions,[133] take the flowers of this same plant simmered in resin and apply it.

111. Sow-Thistle (*Sonchus oleraceus* L.), *carduum silfaticum*, *Wuduþistel*

This plant, called *carduum silfaticum* and another name, sow-thistle, grows in meadows and along roadways.

(111:1) For stomachache, take the upper part of the flower head of the plant we call *carduum silfaticum* when it is soft and fresh, and give this to eat in sweetened vinegar. It will soothe the soreness.

(111:2) So that you do not fear encountering any evil,[134] pick this same plant, *carduum silfaticum*, at daybreak when the sun first comes up—let it be when the moon is in Capricorn—and keep it with you. As long as you bear it on you, no evil will come to you.

112. Lupin (*Lupinus* L.), *lupinus montanus*, no OE word[135]

This plant, which is called *lupinum montanum* and another name …, grows along hedges and in sandy places.

(112:1) For worms [OE *wyrmas*] that irritate around the navel, take the *lupinum montanum* plant, pounded, and give it to drink in one cup of vinegar. Without delay, it will drive out the worms.

(112:2) If the same thing bothers children, take the same plant, *lupinum*, and wormwood, pound them together and put this on the navel.

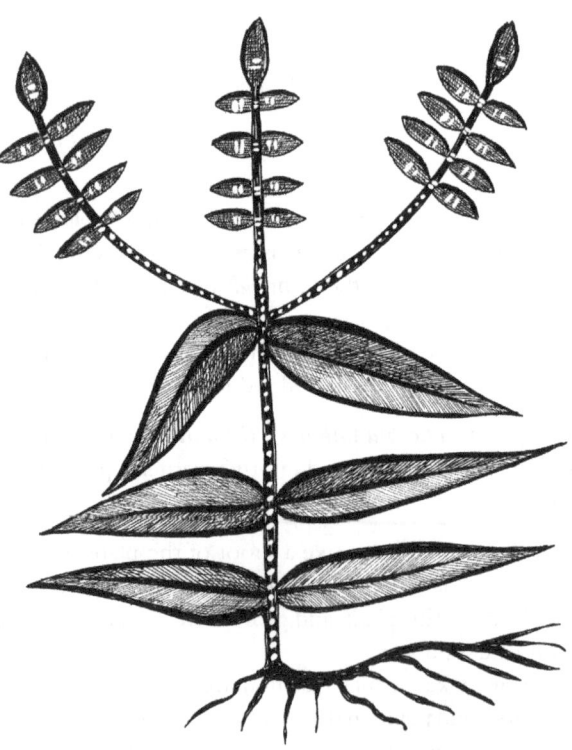

Spurge Laurel

113. Spurge Laurel or Spurge Flax (*Daphne laureola* L. or *gnidium* L.), *lactyrida*, *Giðcorn*

This plant, which is called *lactyridem* and another name, spurge laurel, grows in cultivated and sandy soils.

(113:1) For stopped up intestines, take the seeds of this plant (they are the berries) well washed. Give this to drink in warm water. It will soon move the bowels.

114. Lettuce (*Chondrilla juncea* L.), *lactuca leporina*, no OE word[136]

This plant, which is called *lactucam leporinam* and another similar name, *lactucam*, grows in cultivated and in sandy soils. About this plant, it is said that the hare, when it is tired in the summer from the intense heat, heals itself with this same plant Because of this, it is named *lactuca leporinam*.[137]

(114:1) For feverishness, take the *lactucam leporinam* plant and lay it under a person's pillow without their knowing it. They will be cured.

115. Squirting Cucumber (*Ecballium elaterium* Rich.), *cucumeris siluatica*, *Hwerhwette*[138]

This plant, called *cucumerem siluaticum* and another name, squirting cucumber, grows near the sea and in hot places.

(115:1) For sore joints and for foot conditions, take the root of this plant that we call *cucumerem silfaticum*, simmer it down in oil by two-thirds, and smear it on.

(115:2) If a child is not born right,[139] take the roots of this same plant simmered down by two-thirds and wash the child with it. Also, if anyone eats the fruit of this plant on an empty stomach, he will be endangered; for that reason, everyone should restrain from eating it on an empty stomach.

116. Hemp (*Cannabis sativa* L.), *cannane silfatica*, *Henep*

This plant, called *cannane silfatica* and another name, hemp, grows in rough places, along roads, and hedges.

(116:1) For sore breasts, take the plant *cannauem siluaticam* pounded in lard, lay it on the breasts, and it will diminish the swelling. If any inflammation is present, it will clear it up.

(116:2) For frostbite, take the fruit of this same plant pounded with nettle seeds and soaked in vinegar, and put it on the sore.

117. Wild Rue (*Ruta montana*), *ruta montana*, *Rude*[140]

This plant, called *rutam montanam* and another name, wild rue, grows on hills and uncultivated places.

(117:1)　For dim eyesight and for bad scars, take the leaves of the plant we call *rutam montanam* simmered in aged wine. Put this in a glass vessel, and then smear it on.

(117:2)　For a sore chest,[141] take the same plant, *rutam siluaticam*, and pound it in a wooden vessel. Then take as much as you can pick up with three fingers, put it into a pot, and add to it one cup of wine and two of water. Give this to drink and let the person rest for a while; they will be better quickly.

(117:3)　For liver pain, take a handful of this same plant, a jug and a half of water, and the same amount of honey. Simmer this together and give it to drink for three days, more if they need it. You will heal them.

(117:4)　If someone cannot pass water, take nine stalks of this same *rute siluatice* and three cups of water; pound them, then add half a jug of vinegar. Simmer them together and then give this to drink continually for nine days. They will be cured.

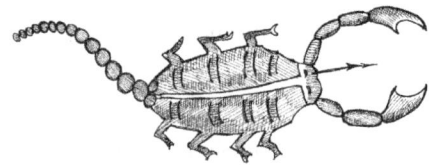

(117:5)　For bite of the snake called *scorpius*, take the seeds of the plant called *rute siluatice*, pound them in wine, and give it to drink. It will alleviate the pain.

118.　Tormentil (*Potentilla heptaphylla* L. or *Potentilla recta* L.), septifolium, Seofenleafe

This plant, which is called *eptafilon* and another name, *septifolium*, and also some call tormentil, grows in gardens and in sandy soil.

(118:1)　For foot disease, take the *septifolium* plant pounded and mixed with saffron. Smear the juice on the feet. In three days, it will take away the pain.

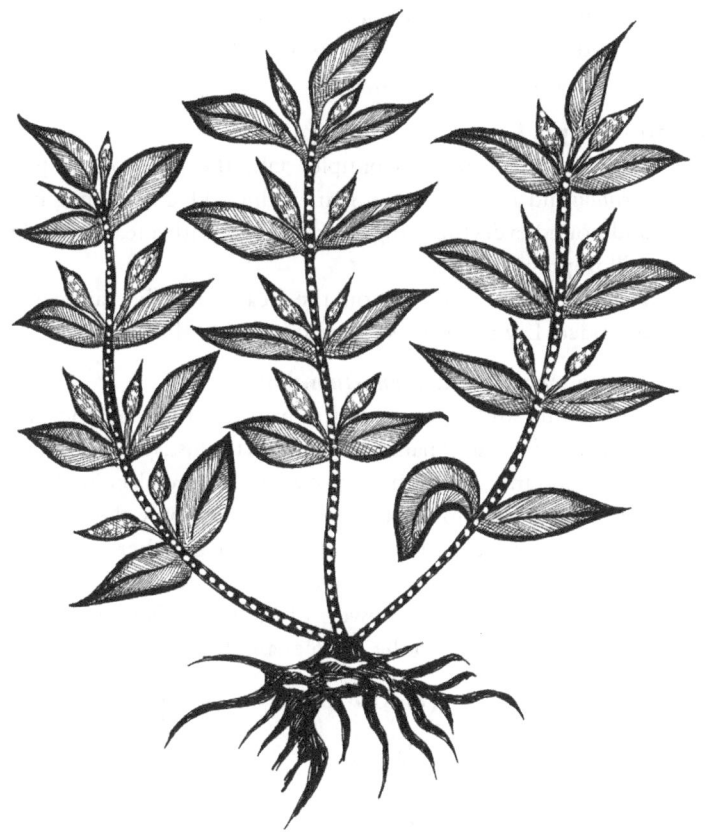

Basil

119. Basil or Wild Basil (*Ocimum basilicum* or *Calaminthe vulgare* L.), *ocimus*, Mistel

(119:1)   For headache, take the plant called *ocimum* and another name, basil, pound it with rose or myrtle juice or with vinegar and lay it on the face.

(119:2)   For eye pain and swelling, pound this same plant in good wine and smear this on the eyes. You will heal them.

(119:3)   For kidney pain, do the same thing and give it to drink with the skin of apples that are named *malum granatum*.[142]

120. Wild Celery (*Apium graveolens* L.), *apium*, Merce

(120:1)   For eye pain and swelling, take the plant called *apium* or wild celery pounded well with bread; lay it on the eyes.

121. Ivy (*Hedera chrysocarpa* Walsh), *hedera*, Ifig[143]

This plant, called *hedera crysocantes* and another name, ivy, is called *crysocantes* because it bears seeds that are like gold.

(121:1) For dropsy, take 20 seeds of this plant, crush them into a jug of wine. Give three cups of this wine to drink for seven days; the illness will be sent away by passing water.

122. Mint (*Mentha* spp. L.), *menta, Minte*

(122:1) For skin infections and pimples, take the juice of the plant called *mentam* and another similar name, mint; add to it sulphur and vinegar, and pound everything together. Apply it with a feather, and the sores will improve quickly.

(122:2) If bad sores or cuts are on the head, take the same plant, mint, pounded. Lay it on the sores, and it will heal them.

123. Dill (*Anethum graveolens* L.), *annetum, Dile*

(123:1) For itching and soreness of the private parts, take the plant called *anetum* and another name, dill; burn it to dust, then take the dust and honey and mix it together. First wash the sore place with water, then bathe it with warm myrtle juice, and then apply the remedy to it.

(123:2) If a similar condition troubles a woman, give her the same remedy using the plants we just talked about from her midwife.

(123:3) For headache, take the flowers of the same plant and simmer them with oil. Apply this to the temples and fasten it to the head.

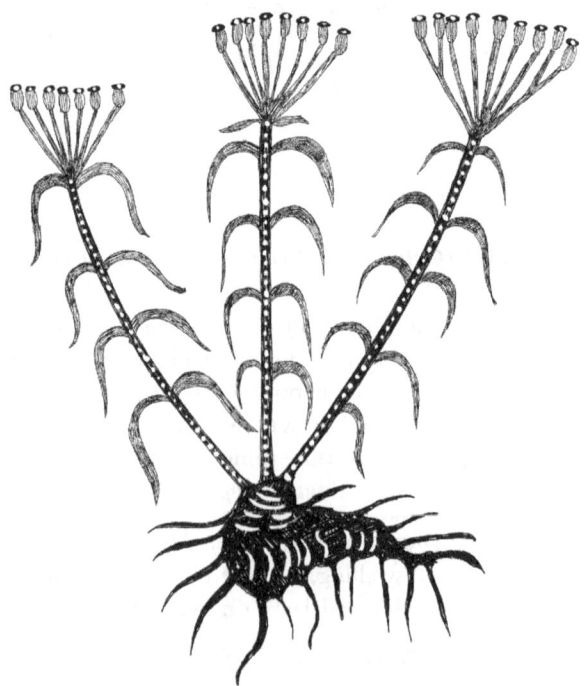

Wild Marjoram

124. Wild Marjoram or Sweet Marjoram (*Origanum vulgare* or *majorana* L.), *organum*, *Organe*

(124:1) This plant, called *origanum* and another similar name, marjoram, has a hot, strong nature and it breaks up coughs, subdues bad blood and foot disease,[144] and helps with shortness of breath and liver disease.

(124:2) For coughs, take the same plant, marjoram, and give it to eat. You will be surprised at its effects.

125. Houseleek (*Sempervivum arboreum* L.), *semperuiuus*, *Sinfulle*

(125:1) For accumulations of diseased fluids in the body, take the plant called *sempervivum* and another name, houseleek; lard, bread, and coriander. Pound them together as you would make a poultice and lay this on the affected area.

126. Fennel (*Foeniculum vulgare*), *feniculus*, *Finul*

(126:1) For coughing and shortness of breath, take the roots of the plant called *fenuculum* and another name, fennel, pound it in wine, and drink it on an empty stomach for nine days.

(126:2) For bladder pain, take a handful of the same plant that we call *fenuculum* when fresh, and fresh roots of wild celery and of asparagus, and put them in a new earthenware pot with one jug of water. Simmer down by three fourths. Let them drink this on an empty stomach for seven days or more, and let them take a bath, however not a cold one, nor should they drink cold water. The bladder pain will be relieved without delay.

127. Rue (*Ruta chalepensis* L.), *erifion*, *Liðwort*[145]

This plant, called *erifion* and by another name, rue, was originally grown in Gaul, that is in the land of the Franks, on a mountain called Soractis. It looks like wild celery, has red flowers like garden cress, and it has seven roots and the same number of stems. It propagates itself in uncultivated places, but not moist ones. It blooms at all times and has seeds like beans.

(127:1) For lung diseases, take the *erifion* plant, pounded as for making a poultice. Lay this on the sore spot, and it will heal it. Then take the juice of this same plant, give it to drink, and you will be surprised at the power of this plant.

128. Comfrey (*Symphytum officinale* L.), *sinfitus albus*, *Halswyrt*

(128:1) For a woman's periods, take the plant called *sinfitum album* and another name, comfrey, dry it, and pound it into fine powder. Give it to drink in wine, and it will soon get the periods under control.

129. Parsley (*Petroselinum hortense* Huff.), *petrosilinum*, *Petersilie*

The plant is called *triannem* or *petroselinum*, and some also call it a similar name, parsley.

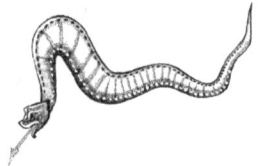

(129:1) For snakebite, take four grams of the *petroselini* plant made into very fine powder and give this to drink in wine. Then take the pounded plant and lay it on the wound.

(129:2) For nerve pain, take the same plant, *petroselinum*, pounded, lay it on the painful place, and it will quickly heal the nerve pain.

130. Cabbage or Colewort (*Brassica oleracea* L. or *napus* L.), *brassica*, *Caul or Cawel*

(130:1) For any swelling, take the shoots of the plant called *brassicam siluaticam* and another name, cabbage, pound and mix them with aged lard, and make this as you would make a poultice. Put this onto a thick linen cloth and lay it on the sore.

(130:2) For a pain in the side, take the same plant, *brassicam siluaticam*, and apply where it is sore, mixed as we just told you.

(130:3) For foot disease, take the same plant, *brassicam*, mixed the same way we said earlier. The longer the preparation stands, the more effective and healing it will be.

131. Sweet Basil (*Ocimum basilicum* L.), *basilisca*, *Nædderwyrt*

(131:1) This plant, called *basilisca* and another name, basil, grows where there is a snake that has the same name, *basiliscus*.[146] Actually, there is not one kind of basil, but three. One is *olocryseis*, that is, as said in our language, that it shines like gold. Another kind is *stillatus*, which is "spotted" in our language; it looks as though it has golden head. The third kind is *sanguineus*, that is blood-red, and also looks as if its head were golden. The basil plant comes in all these types.

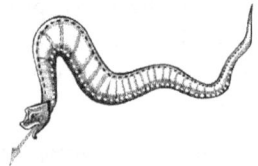

If anyone has this plant with them, none of the following kinds of snakes can harm them. The first snake, *olocryssuss*, is named *eriseos*, and whatever it sees it blows on and sets on fire. The second, *stillatus*, is called *crysocefalus asterites*; whatever it sees dries up and disappears. The third kind is named *hematites* or *crysocefalus*. Whatever it sees or touches it destroys so that nothing is left but the bones. The basil plant has all of their strength, and if anyone has the plant with them, they will be strong against all kinds of snakes.

This plant is like rue: it has red milky juice like greater celandine, and it has purple flowers. Anyone who wants to pick it should purify themselves and mark around it with gold and silver, with deer horn and ivory, with bear's tooth and bull's horn, and lay around it fruit sweetened with honey.

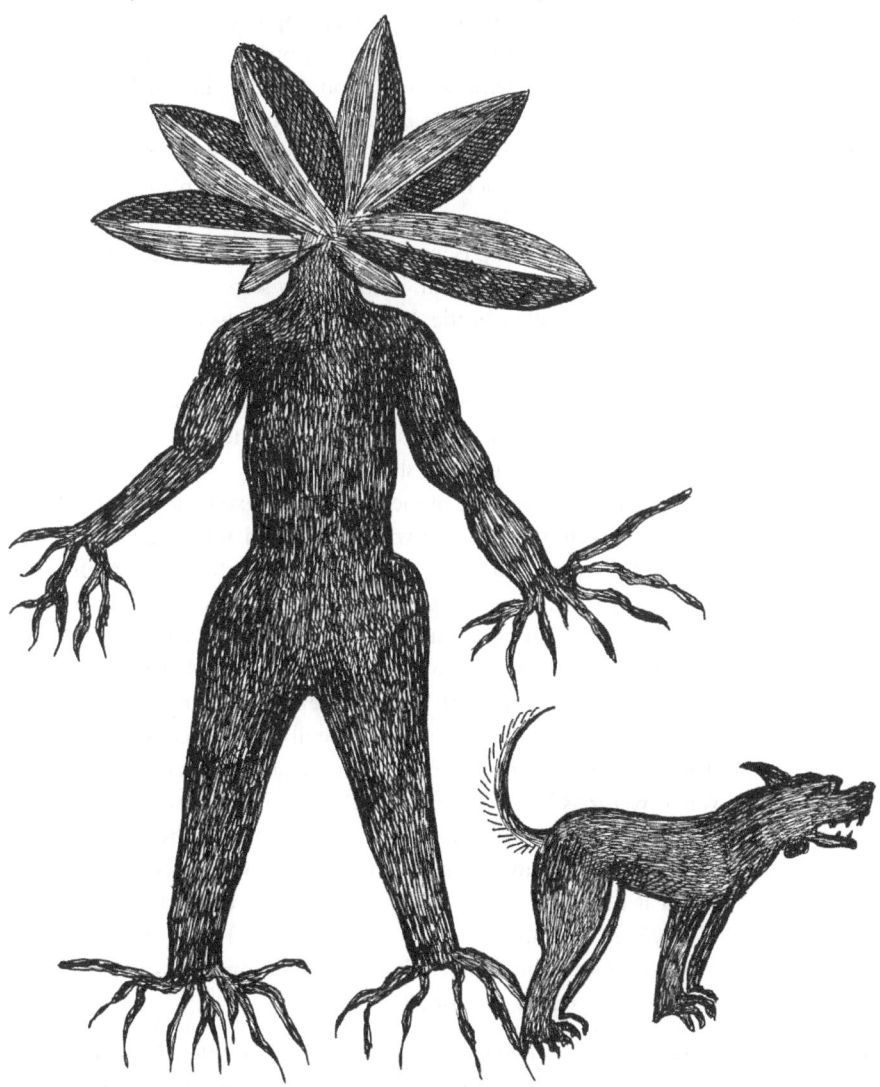

Mandrake

132. Mandrake (*Mandragora officinarum or autminalis*), mandragora, no OE word

This plant called *mandragoram* is large and glorious to see, and it is beneficial.[147] You must gather it in this manner: when you approach the plant, and you will recognize it because it shines at night like a lantern, when you first see its head, mark around it quickly with an iron tool lest it flee from you. Its power is so great and powerful that it wants to flee quickly when an impure person approaches it. Because of this, you must mark around it with an iron tool, and then you must dig around it, being careful not to touch it with the iron; however, you can dig the earth strenuously with an ivory staff. When you see its hands and feet, fasten them. Take the other end and fasten it around a dog's neck (make sure the dog is hungry). Throw some meat in front of him so that he cannot reach it unless he snatches the plant up with him. About this plant, it is said that it has such great powers, whatever pulls it up will quickly be deceived in the same way. Because of this, as soon as you see that it has been pulled up, and you have power over it, immediately seize it, twist it, and wring the juice from its leaves into a glass bottle. If you need to help people with it, then help them as follows.

(132:1) For headache and for sleeplessness, take the juice and smear it on the face, and use the plant in the same way to relieve headache. You will be surprised at how quickly sleep will come.

(132:2) For earache, take the juice of the same plant mixed with oil of spikenard and pour it into the ears. You will be surprised at how quickly it heals.

(132:3) For foot disease, even if it is severe, take from the right and from the left hand [of the plant], of each three pennies' weight and powder it. Give it to drink in wine for seven days, and the person will be cured; not just that the swelling will go down, but it will also relieve nerve spasms and cure pain, both in a wonderful manner.

(132:4) For lunacy, that is for possession by devils, take three pennies' weight from the body of this same plant, *mandragore*, and give it to drink in warm water as best the person is able. Quickly they will be healed.

(132:5) Again, for nerve spasms, take one ounce by weight from the body of this plant and pound it into a fine powder. Mix it with oil and then smear it on whomever has the aforementioned condition.

(132:6) If anyone sees any grievous evil in their home, take the plant *mandragoram* to the center of the house—however much they have of it—and it will drive out all evil.

133. Rose Campion (*Agrostemma coronaria*), lichanis stephanice, Læcewyrt[148]

(133:1) This plant, which is called *lichanis stefanice* and another name, rose campion, has long, luxuriant, purple leaves, its stem has bushy shoots, and it has yellow flowers on the upper part of the stem. The seeds of this plant given in wine help greatly against all kinds of snakes and scorpion stings. Some say about its strength, that if a person lays it on a scorpion, it will bring the scorpion powerlessness and disease.

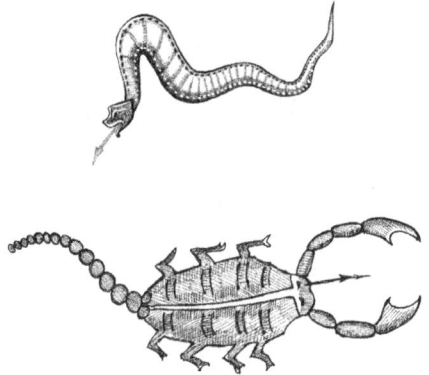

134. Burdock (*Arctium lappa* L.), *action,* no OE word

This plant, called *action* and another name, …, has leaves like a gourd, but larger and firmer, and it has at its roots a large stalk that is more than two yards long. It has a seed like a thistle on the upper part of the stem, but it is smaller and red in color.

(134:1) If a person coughs up blood and phlegm together, take four pennies' weight of the seeds of this plant and nuts from the cones of pine trees, and pound them together so that you make something like an apple. Give this to the patient to eat; it will heal them.

(134:2) For pain in the joints, take the same plant, pounded and made into a poultice. Smear it on the soreness, and it will improve it. It also cures old wounds in the same manner.

135. Southernwood (*Artemisia abrotanum* L.), *abrotanus, Supernewuda*

There are two kinds of this plant, which is called *abrotanum* and another name, southernwood. This one is the kind that has large branches and very small leaves, looking as though they were really hairs. It has very small flowers and seeds, has a good strong smell, and is bitter to the taste.

(135:1) For shortness of breath, bone pain, and difficulty passing water, the seeds of this plant help when pounded and drunk in water.

(135:2) For pain in the side, take the same plant and *betonican,* pound them together, and give to drink.

(135:3) For poison and for snakebite, take the same plant, *abrotanum,* and give it to drink in wine. It helps very much. Also, pound it into oil and smear it on the body. It also helps cure fever chills. Moreover, the seeds of this plant, scattered about or set on fire, effectively put [snakes] to flight.[149]

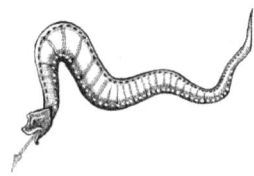

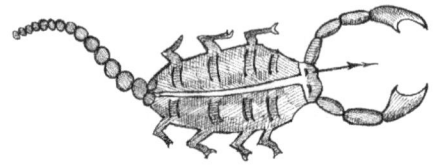

(135:4) For bite of snakes we call *spalangiones* and *scorpiones*, this plant is effective.

(135:5) For eye pain, take the same plant, *abrotanum*, simmered with the plant called *melacidoniam* and another name, *codoniam* [quince], and mixed with bread as you would make a poultice. Apply this to the soreness, and the pain will be soothed.

This plant is, as we said before, of two kinds: one is female, the other male. All have the same effects on the conditions we just listed.

136. Water Parsnip (*Sium latifolium* L.), *sion*, *Laber*

This plant, which is called *sion* and another name, water parsnip, grows in watery places.

(136:1) For bladder stones, take the plant and give to eat simmered or raw. It will send out the stones when passing water.

(136:2) Also, this same plant helps greatly with very loose stools and unsettled intestines.

137. Heliotrope (*Heliotropium europaeum* L. or *H. Supinum* L.), *eliotropus*, *Sigilhweorfa*[150]

This plant, called *eliotropus* and another name, heliotrope, grows in rich, cultivated soil,[151] has rough, broad leaves that are very much like wild basil and it has round seeds in three colors.

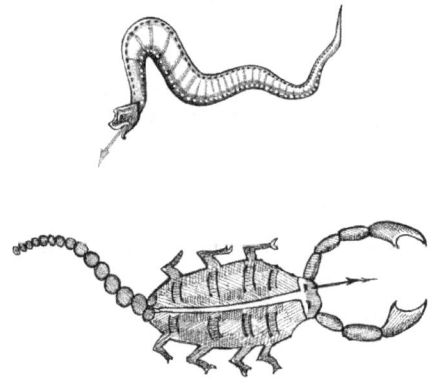

(137:1) For all kinds of snake and scorpion bites, take the roots of the *eliotropos* plant, give this to drink in wine, and put it pounded on the wound. It will help a great deal.

(137:2)   If worms around the navel irritate the intestines, take this same plant, and hyssop, salt, and watercress, and pound them together. Give this to drink in water, and it will kill the worms.

(137:3)   For warts, take the same plant and salt and pound them together. Put this on the warts, and it will take them away. For this reason, it is also called *uerrucaria* [wart plant].

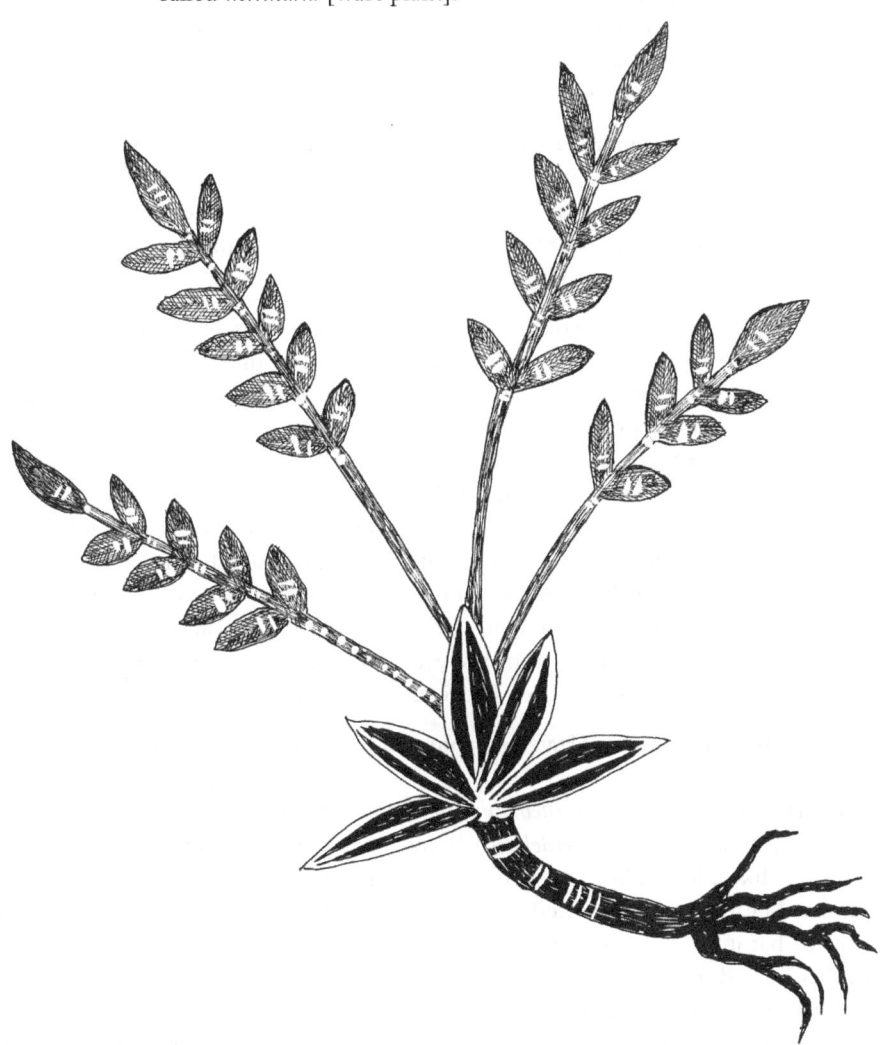

Field Marigold

138. Field Marigold (*Calendula arvensis* L.), speritis, no OE name[152]
This plant, which is called *spreritis* and another name, …, has small, luxuriant leaves, and its root sends out many branches that are laid near to the ground. It has yellow flowers, and if you crush it between your fingers, it has a smell like myrrh.

(138:1) For fever chills, take the *spreritis* plant and simmer it in oil. At the time the fever begins its onset, smear it on the person.

(138:2) For the bite of a mad dog, take the same plant, pound it into a powder, then take a spoonful and give it to drink in warm water, and the person will recover.

(138:3) For pain of the spleen, take a good handful of this same plant and a jug of milk. Simmer them together and give to drink half in the morning and half in the evening as long as the person needs it. The spleen will be healed.

139. Stonecrop (*Sedum album or acre* L.), *ayzos minor*, no OE word

This plant, which is called *ayzos minor* and another name, …, grows along roadways and in rocky places, on hills, and on old burial grounds. From one root, it sends out many small shoots, and they are full of many small, long, pointed, sharp, succulent leaves full of juice. The root of this plant is useless.

(139:1) For skin infections, eye pain, and conditions of the feet, take this plant without the roots, and pound it with fine flour in the way you would make a poultice. Apply this to these conditions and it will heal them.

(139:2) For headache, take the juice of this same plant and juice of roses. Mix them together and smear this on the head. The pain will be soothed.

(139:3) For bite of worms we call *spalangiones*, take the same plant, *aizos*, pounded in wine and give it to drink. It heals effectively.

(139:4) For very loose stools and unsettled intestines and for worms that harm the intestines, this same plant helps very much.

(139:5) For any condition of the eyes, take the juice of this same plant and smear it on the eyes. It effectively heals the condition.

140. White Hellebore (*Veratrum album* L.), *elleborus albus*, *tunsingwyrt* or *wedeberge*

This plant, which is called *elleborum album* and another name, white hellbore (*tunsingwyrt*, and some call *wedeberge*) [white hellebore],[153] grows on hills, and it has leaves like a leek. The roots and the entire plant should be picked about midsummer because it is well suited to making remedies. To be recognized about this plant is that it has a small root, which is not so straight that it is not bent a little; it is brittle and fragile when it is dried, and when it is broken, it smells as though it sent out smoke, and it is slightly bitter to the taste. The larger roots are long, hard, and very bitter to the taste, and they have the violent and dangerous power that they often choke a person quickly. As we said before, one should dry this root and cut it into lengths like peas. Ten pennies' weight of this root will make many remedies for many conditions; however, it should never be given by itself because of its strength, but mixed with some other food in the amount commensurate with the illness, that is, if the condition is very serious, give it to drink in beer or dark gruel.[154]

(140:1) For someone with very loose stools, give this to eat in pea juice or with the plant called *oriza*[155] with flour; however, all these should be first simmered in light beer and softened.

(140:2) Indeed, this plant heals up all old, grievous, and incurable conditions, so that a person will be healed even though they thought their health was to be despaired of.

141. Ox-Eye Daisy or Marguerite (*Chrysanthemum segetum*), *buoptalmon*, no OE word[156]

(141:1) This plant, which is called *butoptalmon* and another name, ..., has tender stems and leaves like fennel, and it has yellow flowers that look like eyes, from which it got its name. It grew originally in the city of Meonia. The pounded leaves of this plant made into a poultice heal up any bad boils and calluses.

(141:2) For damage to the body coming from an overabundance of bile, take the juice of this plant and give it to drink. It will restore the natural color, and the person will look as though coming from a hot bath.

142. Gorse (*Ulex europaeus* L.), *tribulus*, Gorst[157]

This plant, which is called *tribulus*, and another name, gorse, has two varieties: one grows in gardens and the other out in the fields.

(142:1) If the body is very hot, take this plant *tribulum* pounded, and lay it on.

(142:2) For bad taste and putrefaction in the mouth and throat, take the *tribulum* plant simmered and mixed with honey. It will heal the mouth and throat.

(142:3) For bladder stones, take the pounded fresh seeds of the same plant and give them to drink. It helps effectively.

(142:4) For snakebite, take five pennies' weight of the pounded fresh seeds of this plant and give them to drink. In addition, take the plant with its seeds and pound it and lay it on the bite. It will drive out the poison.

(142:5) The seeds of this plant taken in wine help against a poisonous drink.

(142:6) For fleas, take the same plant simmered with its seeds and sprinkle it about the house. It kills the fleas.

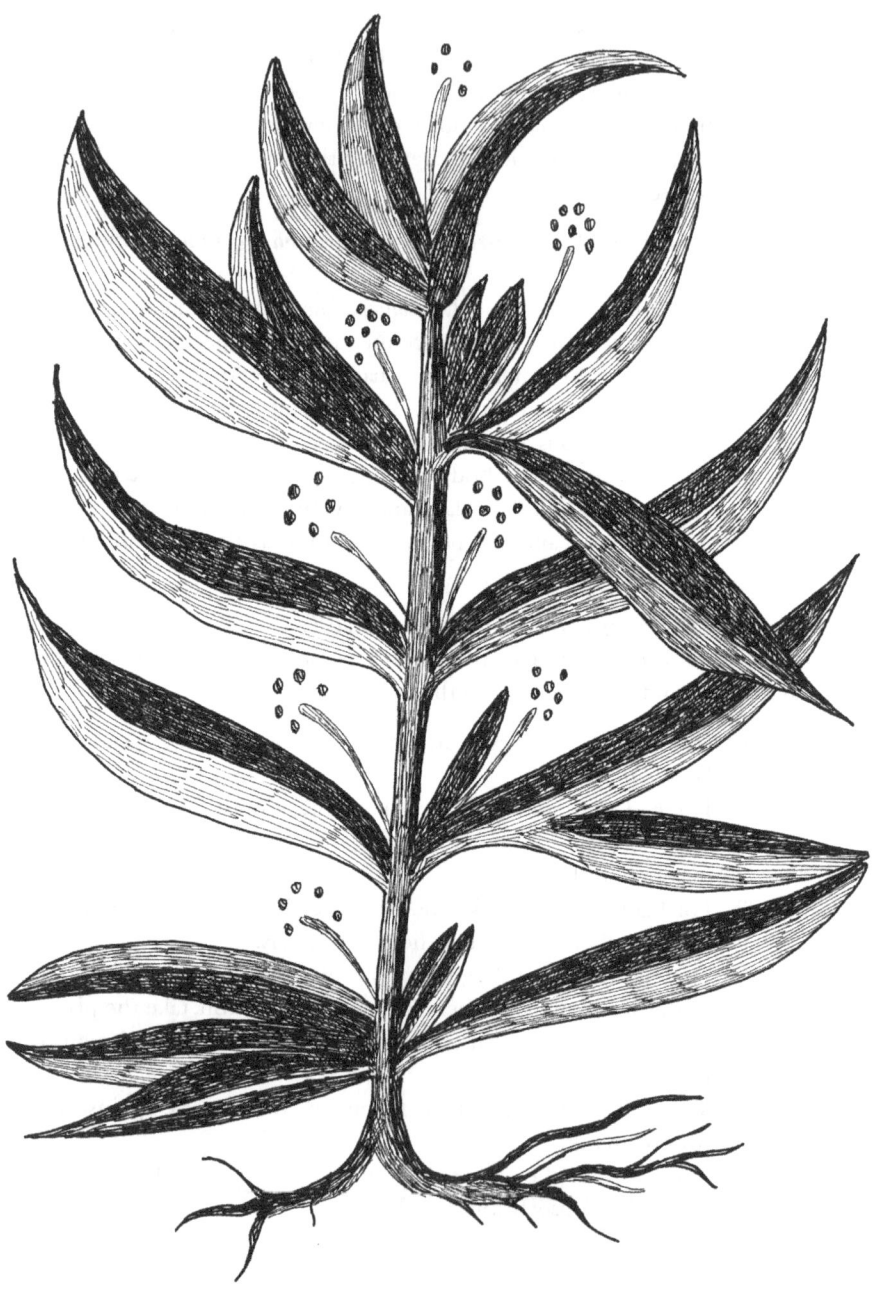

Fleabane

143. Fleabane or Spikenard (*Conyza squarrosa* or *Inula pulicaria* L.), *conize*, no OE word

(143:1)   This plant, which is called *conize* and another name, …, has two varieties: one is large, the other small. The smaller one has small, slight leaves that smell good. The other has large, succulent leaves with an unpleasant smell, and its roots are not used. However, the stem of this plant, including the leaves, if set on fire and scattered about chases away snakes. Also, when it is pounded and made into a poultice, it heals up snakebites. It also kills gnats, mosquitoes, and fleas and cures all their bites. It helps in passing water if there is difficulty doing so, and it cures jaundice and helps epilepsy when given in vinegar.

(143:2)   This plant, *conize*, simmered in water and laid under a seated woman, purifies the womb.[158]

(143:3)   If a woman has difficulty giving birth, take the juice of this same plant soaked in wool, and put it into her private parts; it will quickly induce birth.[159]

(143:4)   For fever chills, take the same plant and simmer in oil. Take the oil and smear it on the body. The fever will disappear.

(143:5)   For headache, take the smaller of the plants and make it into a poultice. Lay this on the soreness, and it will be relieved.

144. Thorn–Apple (*Datura stramonium* L.), *trycnos manicos*, *Foxes Glofa*[160]

(144:1)   For skin conditions, take the leaf of the plant called *trycnos manicos* and another name, thorn–apple, and make it into a poultice. Smear it on the sores, and they will heal.

(144:2)   For a pimply body, which the Greeks call *erpinam*, take the same plant, which we call *trycnos manicos*, and fine flour, and make it into a poultice. Apply this to the sores, and they will heal.

(144:3)   For headache, for stomach burn, and for hard swellings, take the same plant pounded in wine and smear it on the sore places. They will be healed.

(144:4)   For earache, take the juice of the same plant with juice of roses and drip it into the ear.

145. Licorice (*Glycyrrhiza glabra* L.), *glycyrida*, no OE word

(145:1)   For a dry fever, take the plant called *glycyridam* and another name, …, and boil it gently in warm water. Give it to drink, and it helps effectively.

(145:2)   This same plant also heals pain in the chest, liver, bladder, and kidneys when taken with warm wine. It also relieves the thirst of thirsty people.

(145:3)   For conditions of the mouth, the roots of this plant eaten or drunk help and heal the conditions. It also clears up wounds that are washed with it. The root does the same things, although not as effectively.

146. Soapwort (*Saponaria officinalis* L.), *strutium*, no OE word

(146:1)   If a person cannot pass water, take the roots of the plant we call *strutium* and another name, …, and give to eat. It will stimulate passing water.

(146:2)   For liver disease, shortness of breath, and for heavy coughing, take one spoonful of this plant, pounded into a powder; give it to drink in light beer, and it will help. It also heals up any kind of intestinal disturbance and chases out the condition.

(146:3)   For bladder stones, take the roots of this same plant *strutium* and of *lubasticam* [lovage], and of the plant called *capparis* [capers], pound them together and give this to drink in light beer. It soothes the bladder and sends out the stones. It also soothes pain in the spleen.

(146:4)   For a bad skin condition, take the same plant, flour, and vinegar. Pound them together and apply them to the irritation. It will heal.[161]

(146:5)   This same plant simmered in wine with barley flour clears up all callouses and boils.

147. Orpine (*Sedum telephium* L.), *aizon*, no OE word

(147:1)   This plant is called *aizon* and another name, …, looks like it is always alive. It has a stem more than a yard long that is the thickness of a finger. It is full of juice and has succulent leaves that are the length of a finger. It grows on hills and sometimes is planted inside a wall.[162] Pounded with flour, this plant helps many bodily conditions, such as erupting sores, a festering body, and pain, heat, and burning of the eyes. It helps all these conditions.

(147:2)   For headache, take the juice of the same *aizon* plant mixed with juice of roses. Apply this to the head, and it relieves the pain.

(147:3)   For a bite from a snake is called *spalangionem*, take the same plant *aizon* and give it to drink in hot wine.

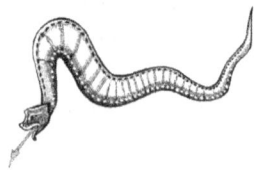

(147:4)   Do the same thing for very loose stools, for intestinal worms, and for a bad chill. It will help.

148. Elder (*Sambucus nigra*), *samsuchon*, *Ellen*[163]

(148:1)   For dropsy, take the plant called *samsuchon* and another name, elder, and give it to drink simmered; it slows the onset of dropsy. It also helps with the inability to pass water and to move the bowels.

(148:2)   For carbuncles and for other skin eruptions, take the dried leaves of the same *samsuchon* plant pounded and mixed with honey. Apply this to the sore. It will burst and then heal.

(148:3) For a scorpion's sting, take the same plant, salt, and vinegar; pound them together and make them into a plaster. Apply this to the sting, and it will clear up.

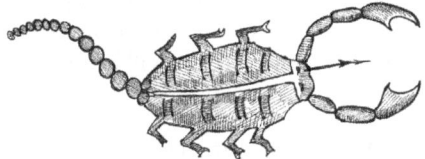

(148:4) For extremely hot and swollen eyes, take the same plant mixed with flour and made into a poultice. Smear it on the eyes, and the discomfort will be relieved.

149. French Lavender (*Lavandula stoechas* L.), *stecas*, no OE name

This plant, which is called *stecas* and another name, …, has many seeds; they are small and slight, and the plant is like rosemary, except that it has somewhat larger and stiffer leaves.

(149:1) Take this plant simmered and give it to drink. It helps chest pain.

(149:2) It is also usual for people to add this to many good drinks.

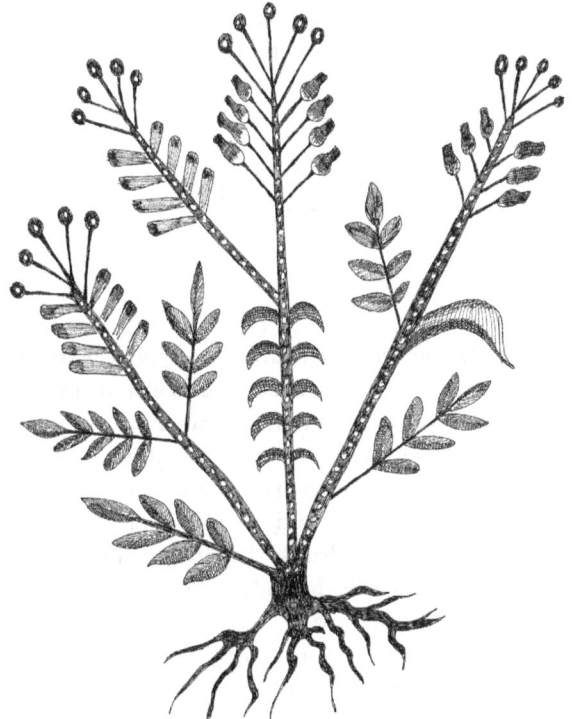

Shepherd's Purse

150. Shepherd's Purse (*Capsella bursa-pastoris* L.), *thyaspis*, no OE name

This plant, which is called *thyaspis* and another name, …, has small divided leaves one finger in length that bend toward the earth. It has a long thin stem with purple flowers on the upper part, and its seeds are generated along the entire stem. All of this plant is strong and bitter. If the juice of this plant is pressed out and a cupful is drunk, all the bitter taste that comes from bile will be sent out by natural movement of the bowels and by vomiting.

(150:1)   This same plant cleans the intestines of harmful congestions and it also stimulates a woman's periods.[164]

151. Wood-Sage or Sage-Leaved Germander (*Teucrium scorodonia* L.), *polios*, no OE word

This plant, which is called *polios* and another name, *omnimorbia*, and also some call … grows on hills. It sends out many shoots from one root, and on its upper part, it has seeds like flower heads. It has an unpleasant smell and tastes a little sweet.

(151:1)   For snakebite, take the juice of the plant *polios* simmered in water and give it to drink. It will heal the bite.

(151:2)   For dropsy, do the same; it relieves the abdomen.

(151:3)   For pain of the spleen, take the same plant *polios*, simmer it in vinegar, and give to drink. It effectively relieves the pain in the spleen. This same plant strewn or burned in the house chases away snakes. It also heals fresh wounds.

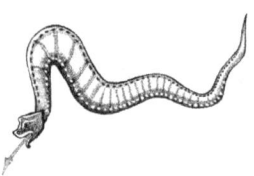

152. St. John's Wort (*Hypericum perforatum* L.), *ypericon*, no OE word

(152:1)   This plant, which is called *hypericon* and another name, *corion*, because it looks like cumin, has leaves like rue, and many branches grow from one stalk and they are red. It has flowers like a wall-flower, and round somewhat long berries, like barley, in which is the seed, which is dark and smells like tar.[165] It grows in cultivated places. Pounded and drunk, this plant stimulates passing water and it brings on monthly periods very well if laid under her private parts.[166]

(152.2)   For fever that returns every fourth day, take the same plant, pounded, and give it to drink in wine.

(152.3)   For swelling and pain of the leg shanks, take the seed of this same plant and give it to drink in wine. Within 40 days, the person will be healed.

153. Globe Thistle (*Echinops sphaerocephalus* L.), *acantaleuce*, no OE word

This plant, which is called *acantaleuce* and another name, …, grows in stony places and on hills. It has leaves like wild teasel, but they are softer, whiter, and also bushier, and it has a stem more than two yards long and as wide as a finger or a little more.

(153:1) If someone coughs up blood and also for stomach ache, take the same plant *acantaleuce* and pound it into powder. Give a spoonful to drink in water, and it will help.

(153:2) To stimulate passing water, take the same plant pounded when it is juicy, and give it to drink. It will make passing water happen.[167]

(153:3) For bad bruises, take the same plant, make it into a poultice, and lay it on the sore; it will clear it up. A decoction of this same plant relieves toothache if it is held warm in the mouth.

(153:4) For cramps, take pounded seeds of this plant and give it to drink in water, and it will soothe them. The same drink also prevents snakebites.

(153:5) Also, if the plant is worn about the neck, it chases snakes away.

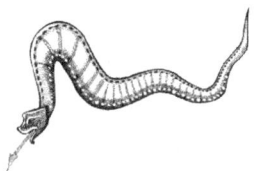

154. Scotch Thistle (Onoropordon *acanthium* L.) (*Acanthus mollis* L.), *acanton*, *Beowyrt*[168]

This plant, which is called *acanton* and another name, Scotch thistle, grows in pleasant and wet places and sometimes stony ones.

(154:1) To stimulate the bowels and the passing of water, take the dried roots of this same plant pounded into powder. Give this to drink in warm water.

(154:2) For lung disease and for any intestinal ailments, this same plant eaten or drunk just as we said earlier helps a great deal.

155. Cumin or Caraway (*Cuminum cyminum* L.; *Carum carvi* L.), *quimminon*, *Cymen*

(155:1) For stomachache, take the seeds of the plant that is called *quimminon* and another name, cumin, simmered in oil and mixed with bran, then simmered together. Make it into a poultice and put it on the abdomen.

(155:2) For shortness of breath, take the same plant, *quimminon*, water, and vinegar and mix them together. Give this to drink; it helps effectively. Also, if drunk in wine, it heals up snakebite.

(155:3) If the abdomen is swollen and hot, take the same plant pounded with grapes or with flour made from beans and make it into a poultice. It will heal the swelling.

(155:4) It also stops nosebleed when mixed with vinegar.

156. Carline Thistle (*Carlina acaulis* L.), *camelleon alba*, *Wulfes Tæsl*

This plant, which is called *camelleon alba* and another name, carline thistle, has rough and thorny leaves, and has in its middle a round and thorny flower head; its flowers are brown, and it has white seeds and white roots with a strong smell.

(156:1) If worms in the intestines bother the area around the navel, take the juice from the roots or powder them and give to drink in water in which marjoram or pennyroyal was simmered. It sends out the worms plentifully.

(156:2) Five pennies' weight of the root of this same plant taken in wine relieves dropsy, and it has the same effect for difficulty in passing water when simmered and then drunk.

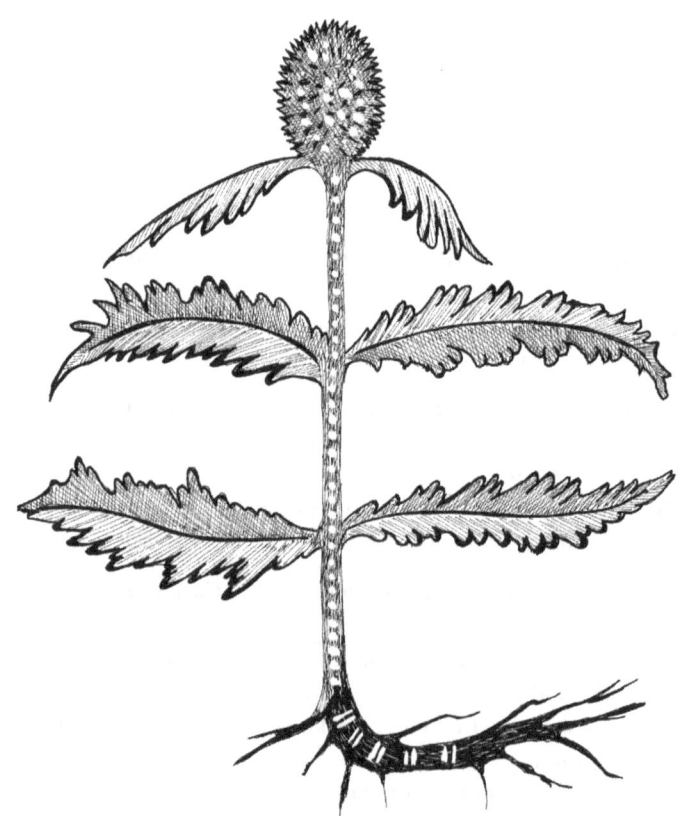

Spotted Golden Thistle

157. Spotted Golden Thistle or Cardoon (*Scolymus maculatus* or *S. hispanicus* L.), *scolymbus*, no OE word[169]

(157:1)   This plant, called *scolimbos* and another name, …, simmered in wine and drunk removes foul smell from armpits and the rest of the body.

(157:2)   This same plant cures passing foul-smelling water and provides healing food for people.

158. Iris (*Iris illyrica, I.* spp. L. *or germanica* L.), *Iris illyrica*, no OE word

This plant, called *iris illyricam* and another name, …, is named for the diversity of its blossoms, and because its colors are thought to resemble a rainbow in the sky, called *iris* in Latin, and because it grows best and strongest in the country of *Illyrico.*[170] It has leaves like the iris the Greeks call *xifian*, and it has strong roots with a strong odor. It should be folded up in a linen cloth and hung in the shade so that it can thoroughly dry, because its nature is hot and sedative.

(158:1)   For deep coughs that a person cannot clear away because they are thick and soft, take ten pennies' weight of the finely pounded and powdered root of this plant and give it to drink in light beer on an empty stomach: four cups for three days or until they are better. In the same way, the powder of this same plant taken in light beer induces sleep and soothes intestinal discomfort.

(158:2)   In the same way, the powder of this same plant heals snakebites. The same quantity of the powder of this plant, as we said before, mixed with vinegar and drunk benefits a man[171] whose semen spontaneously ejects—the disease the Greeks call gonorrhea. Indeed, if the same quantity is mixed with wine, it will stimulate a woman's periods even though they have been gone for some time.

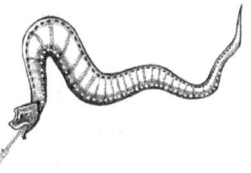

(158:3)   For hard boils and painful swellings, take the whole root of this plant dried thoroughly and then soaked. Pound it then to soften it and make it into a poultice. Put it on the sores, and they will leave.

(158:4)   It also helps a headache when mixed with vinegar and juice of roses.

159. Sea–Onion, Squill (*Urginea maritima* L.) *(?)*; *eleborum album*, no OE name[172]

(159:1)   For liver diseases, take the plant *eleborum album* and another name, ..., dried and pounded into powder. Give it to drink in warm water, six spoonfuls of the powder. It will heal the liver. The same thing helps against all poisons when taken in wine.

160. Larkspur (*Delphinium ajacis* L.), *delfinion*, no OE word

(160:1)   For fever that comes on a person every fourth day, take the juice of the plant called *delfinion* and another name, ..., carefully gathered and pounded and mixed with pepper. There should be an odd number of peppercorns, that is, on the first day, 31, and the next day, 17, and the third day, 13. If you give this before the fever's onset, the person will quickly find relief.

161. Viper's Bugloss (*Echium plantagineum* or *vulgare* L.), *aecios*, no OE word

This plant, called *æcios* and another name, ..., has seeds that look like a snake's head and long stiff leaves, and it sends out many stems. It has thin, somewhat thorny leaves, and brown flowers between the leaves. Between the flowers, it has, as we said before, seeds that look like a snake's head. Its root is small and dark.

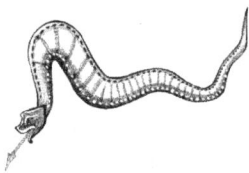

(161:1)   For snakebite, take the root of this same *aecios* plant and give it to drink in wine. It helps both before and after the bite. The same drink also relieves pain in the loins, and the dried plant stimulates breast milk. Truly, there is power in the plant, in its root, and its seeds.

162. Moneywort (*Lysimachia nummularia* L.), *centimorbia*, no OE word

(162:1)   This plant, which is named *centimorbia* and another name, ..., grows in cultivated places, in stony places, on hills, and in pleasant places. From one piece of turf it sends out many shoots. It has small, round, divided leaves, and it has the power to heal. If a horse is injured on the back or on the shoulder and the wound is open, take this plant, thoroughly dried and pounded into powder, sprinkle it onto the wound and the plant will heal it. You will be amazed by its effectiveness.

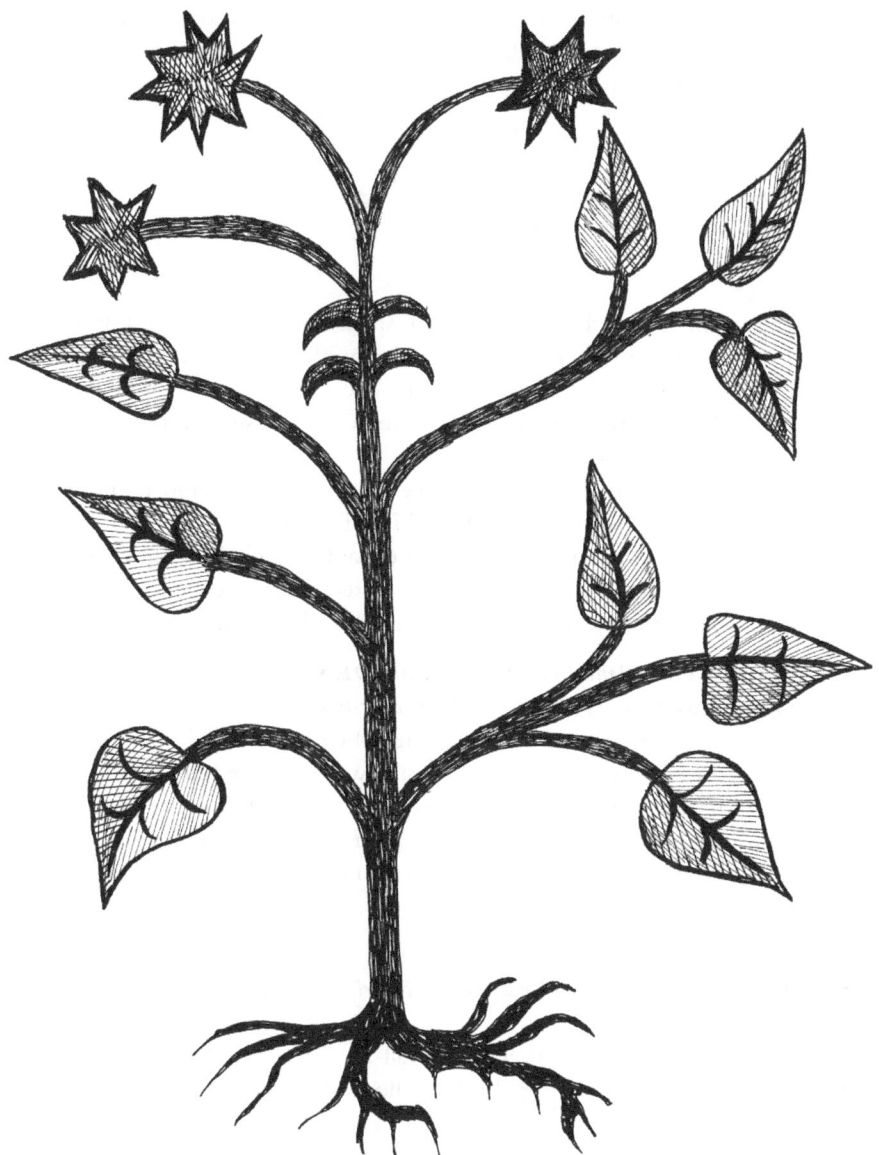

Water Germander

163. Water Germander or Barrenwort (*Epimedium alpinum* L. or *Teucrium scordium* L., scordias?) no OE word[173]

This plant, called *scordias* and another name, …, smells like a leek and because of this is called *scordios*. This plant grows on the moors and it has round leaves that are bitter to the taste. It has a four-edged stem and reddish-yellow flowers.

(163:1) To stimulate passing water, take the fresh, pounded *scordios* plant in wine or the dried plant simmered in wine. Give this to drink, and it stimulates passing water.

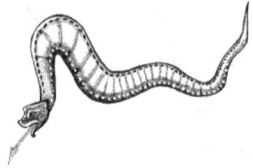

(163:2) The same thing helps with snakebite, all types of poison, and stomachache, and as we said before, with having trouble passing water.

(163:3) For formation of phlegm in the chest,[174] take ten pennies' weight of the same plant mixed with honey. Give one spoonful to eat, and the chest will be purged.

(163:4) For conditions of the feet, take the same plant pounded into vinegar or water. Give it to drink, and it will help.

(163:5) For fresh wounds, take the same plant, pounded, and smear it on the wounds. It will heal them. Also, mixed with honey, it purges and heals old wounds, and powdered, it inhibits skin from growing.

164. Bishop's Weed (*Ammi maius*), **ami, no OE word**

(164:1) This plant, called *ami* and another name, *miluium*, and some call …, has good seeds for medications when given in wine. It helps move the bowels, with difficulty passing water, and for bites of wild animals. It also brings on women's periods. For blemishes on the body, the seed of this same plant pounded in honey clears up the blemishes.

(164:2) For paleness and discoloration of the body, the same: that is, that you apply the same thing to the body, or give to drink, and it will take the discoloration away.

165. Wall-Flower or Daisy (*Cheiranthus cheiri* L., *Bellis perrinis* L.) (?), *uiola, Banwyrt*[175]

This plant, called *uiolam* and another name, wall-flower, comes in three varieties: one is dark purple, one white, and the third is yellow. The yellow one, however, is best to use in remedies.

(165:1) For pain and inflammation of the womb, pound the same plant and put it under the woman; it will help. In the same way, it also starts her periods.

(165:2) For various problems with a person's rear, called *ragadas*, primarily for a discharge of blood, take the pounded leaves of this same plant and make them into a poultice. It heals all these disorders.

(165:3) The leaves of this same plant pounded and mixed with honey heal canker sores of the teeth, from which the teeth often fall out.

(165:4) To stimulate a woman's periods, take ten pennies' weight of the seeds of this plant, either pounded and drunk in wine, or mixed with honey and put on her private parts. It brings about her periods and carries out the child from the womb.

(165:5) For pain of the spleen, take the roots of this same plant pounded in vinegar. Lay it on the spleen and it will be of benefit.

166. Sweet Violet *(Viola odorata L.)*, *uiola purpurea*, no OE word

(166:1) For fresh wounds and also for old ones, take the leaves of the plant called *uiola purpurea* and another name, …, and lard in equal quantities. Apply this to the wounds, and it will effectively heal them. It also reduces swellings and callouses.

(166:2) For a stomach that feels hard, take the flowers of this same plant mixed with honey and soaked in very good wine. The stomach hardness will be soothed.

167. Unidentified

This plant, called *zamalentition* and by another name, …, grows in stony places and on hills.

(167:1) For all wounds, take the *zamaltentition* plant powdered thoroughly in unsalted lard, and smear it on the wounds. All will be healed.

(167:2) For ulcerous wounds, take the dried plant pounded into a fine powder. Apply this to the wounds, and it will purge the pain from the wounds.

168. Alkanet *(Anchusa tinctoria L.)*, *ancusa*, no OE name

This plant, called *ancusa* and another name, …, grows in cultivated places and on smooth ones. You should pick it in the month people call *Martius*. There are two varieties of this plant: one the Africans call *barbatum*. The other is very good for medications, and it was originally grown in the country people call Persia. It has sharp, thorny leaves without stalks.

(168:1) For a bad burn, take the roots of the *ancusa* plant soaked in oil and then mixed with wax like you would make a plaster or poultice. Apply this to the burn, and it will heal it up in a wonderful manner.

169. Fleawort or Fleaseed *(Plantago psyllium L.)*, *psillios*, *Coliandre*[176]

This plant is called *psillos* because it has seeds like flea and for this reason, it is also called *pulicarem* in Latin and some people call it, …. It has small, hairy leaves, and its stem is bushy with branches. It is by nature dry and weak, and it grows in cultivated places.

(169:1) For hard boils and other swellings filled with diseased matter, take a pint of the pounded seed from this plant and two cups of water, and mix them together. Give this to drink. Take some of the same seeds, make them into a plaster, lay them on the sore, and it will be healed.

(169:2)   For a headache, do the same soaked with rose juice and water.

170. Dog Rose, Eglantine *(Rosa canina or rubiginosa L.)*, no OE word[177]

This plant, called *cynosbatus* and another name, …, when picked from its stem is harsh on the throat and disagreeable as food. But nevertheless, it purifies the chest and all things that are either sour or bitter even though it harms the stomach. Nevertheless, it greatly benefits the spleen. If the flowers of this plant are drunk, they affect a person in such a way that the bowels and passing water will discharge the illness. And it also purifies blood flow.

(170:1)   Again, for pain of the spleen, take the well-cleaned bark from the root of this plant and lay it on the spleen. It will be of use to it and beneficial. The person who undergoes this treatment should lie facing up lest they feel impatient about the strength of this treatment.

171. Peony *(Paeonia L.)*, *aglaofotis*, no OE name[178]

This plant, called *aglaofotis* and another name, …, shines at night like a lamp and it helps with many conditions.

(171:1)   For fever that comes on a person every third and every fourth day, take the juice of this same plant, *aglaofotis*, mixed with oil of roses. Smear it on the sick person; undoubtedly you will help them.

(171:2)   If anyone suffers rough seas while rowing, take the same plant and set it on fire to make incense; the rough waves will be restrained.

(171:3)   For cramps and tremors, take the same plant for someone to have with them. If they have it, every evil will fear them.

172. Caper *(Capparis spinosa L.)*, *Capparis*, *Wudubend*

(172:1)   For pain of the spleen, take the root of the plant called *capparis* and another name, caper; pound it into powder and make it into a poultice. Lay this on the spleen, and it will dry it up. But yet, fasten the person, lest they shake the medication off them because of the pain. After three hours, lead them to the bath, bathe them well, and they will be much better.

173. Eryngo *(Eryngium supp.)*, *eringius*, no OE word

This plant, called *eringius* and another name, …, has soft leaves when it first grows and they are sweet to the taste and one eats them just like other plants. Thereafter they are sharp and thorny. It has white or green stalks, on the upper part grow sharp, thorny prickles. It has a long root whose outer part is black, and it has a good smell. This plant grows in fields and in rough places.

(173:1)   To stimulate passing water, take the plant we call *eringius* pounded and give it to drink in wine. Not only will it stimulate passing water, but also women's periods and bowel movements, and it reduces swellings. In addition, it helps with liver diseases and snakebites.

(173:2)   The same eaten with the seeds of the plant called *olisatrum* [Alexanders or horse parsley] also benefits many abdominal conditions.

(173:3)   For swelling of the breasts, take the same plant made into a poultice, and lay it on the breasts. It will dispel all the diseased matter from the breasts.

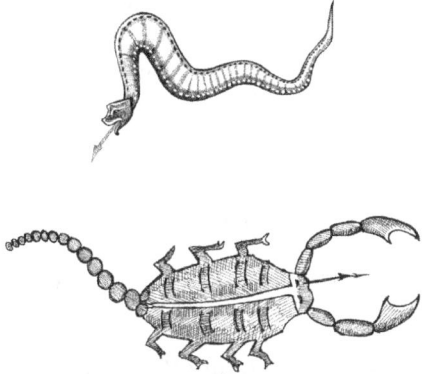

(173:4)   For sting of a scorpion and for all bites from snakes and mad dogs, take the same plant and make it into a plaster. Lay it on the wound (the wound is first to be opened up with something made of iron). After it is laid on, make sure the sick person does not perceive the smell. Prepared the same way, this same plant greatly benefits skin conditions, and it also relieves foot disease if one puts it on at the onset.

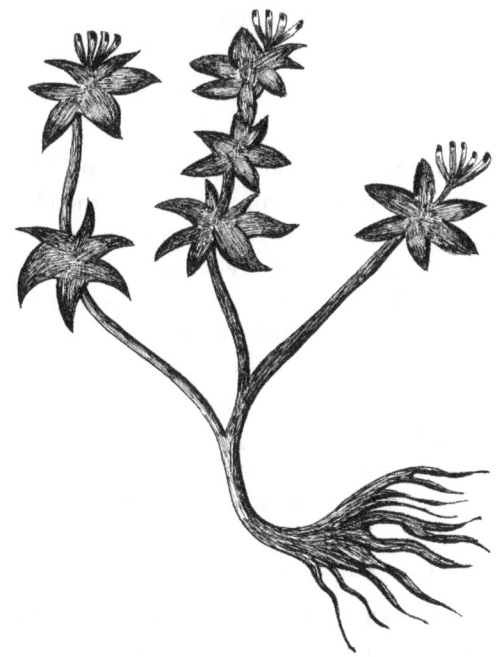

Cleavers

174. Cleavers (Clivers) (*Galium aparine* L.), *philantropos*, Clate

This plant is called *philantropos*—in our language, that is "loving people"—because it quickly adheres to a person and it has seeds like a human navel. It is also called another name, cleavers (clivers). It sends out many branches that are long and four-sided, and its leaves are stiff. It has big stems and white flowers and seeds that are hard, round, and hollow in the middle, and, as we said before, they look like a human navel.[179]

(174:1) For bites from snakes and for the worms that people call *spalangiones*, take the juice of this plant mixed in wine. Give it to drink, and it will be of benefit.

(174:2) For earache, take the juice of this same plant, drip it into the ear, and it will relieve the pain.

175. Yarrow (*Achillea* spp.), *achillea*, no OE word[180]

The plant called *achillea* and another name, ..., grows in cultivated soil and near water; it has yellow and white flowers.

(175:1) For fresh wounds, take pounded flower heads of this plant and lay them on the wound. They will take away the pain, will heal the wounds, and stop the bleeding.

(175:2) If women are troubled by fluid flowing from their private parts, take the same plant, soaked, and lay it beneath the woman, who is seated. Its smell will control all her fluid.[181]

(175:3) Also this same plant drunk in water greatly relieves very loose stools. This plant is called *achillea* because it is said that Lord Achilles often used it to treat wounds.

176. Castor-Oil Plant (*Ricinus communis* L.), *ricinus*, no OE word

(176:1) To turn away hail and storms: if you have the plant called *ricinum*[182] and another name, ..., in your possession or you hang its seeds in your house or have it or its seeds some place, it will turn back a hail storm. If you hang it or its seeds aboard a ship, it is surprising how it calms all storms. You must pick this plant while saying this: *Herba ricinum, precor uti adsis meis incantationibus et auertas grandines, fulgora, et omnes tempestates, per nomen omnipotentis Dei qui te iussit nasci.* That is in our language: *Ricinum* plant, I ask that you be present while I sing, and that you turn away the hail and lightning flashes and every storm, through the name of almighty God, who caused you to be made.

Also, you must be pure when you pick the plant.

177. Black Horehound (*Ballota nigra* L.), *polloten*, no OE name

This plant, called *polloten* and another name, *porrum nigrum*, and also some call ... has thorny, dark, rough stems and broader leaves than a leek but darker. They have a strong smell, and its power is sharp.

(177:1) For dog bite, take the leaves of this plant pounded with salt. Lay this on the wounds, and it will heal them in a wonderful manner.

(177:2) Again, for wounds, take the leaves of this plant pounded with honey and lay them on the wounds. It will heal every wound.

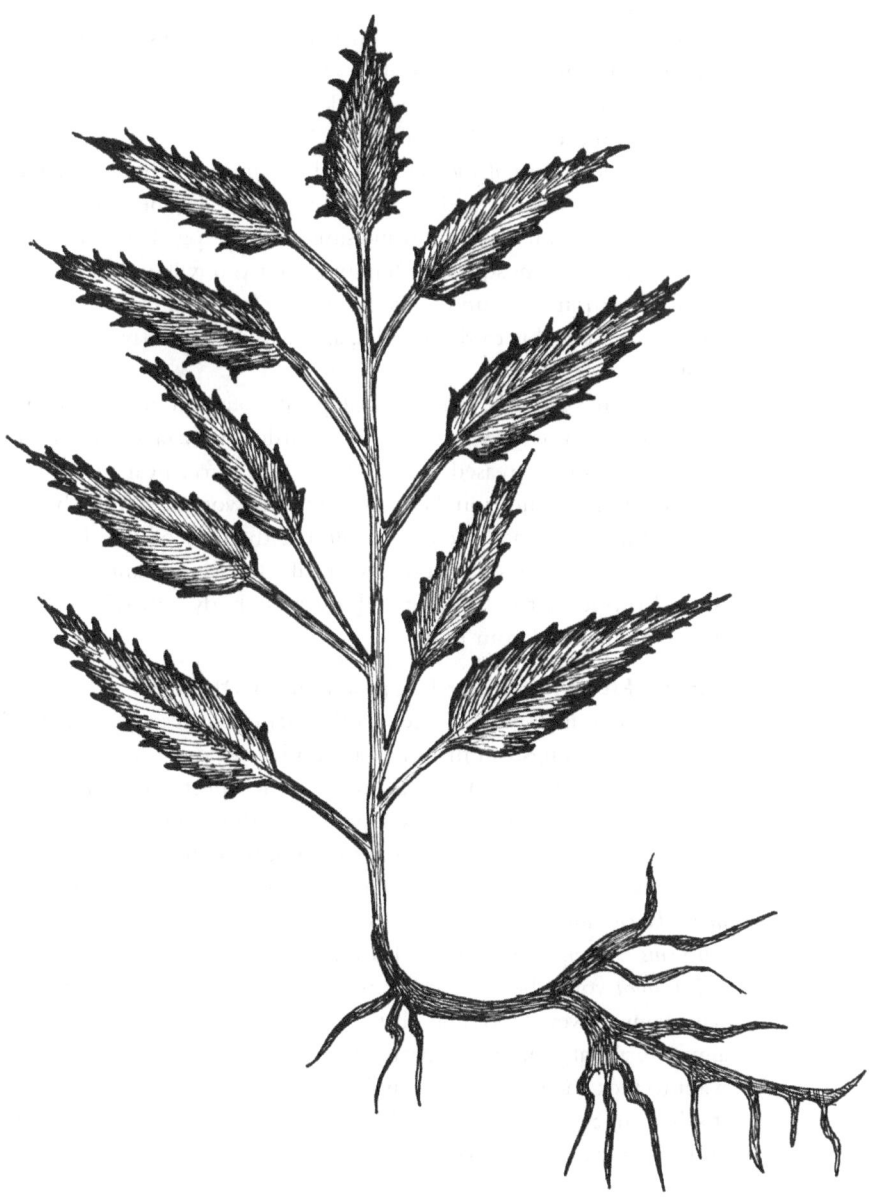

Nettle

178. Nettle (*Urtica dioica* L.), *urtica*, *Netele*

(178:1) For wounds that are frozen, take the juice of this same plant, called *urticam* and another name, nettle, mixed with the sediment in oil with a little salt added, and put it on the wound. Within three days, it will be healed.

(178:2) For swellings, do the same thing, that is, put it on the swelling in the same manner, and it will be healed.

(178:3) If any part of the body has been struck, take the same plant, pounded, and lay it on the wound. It will be healed.

(178:4) For pain in the loins, if they are injured because something happened to them or because of a chill or anything else, take the juice of this plant and oil in equal quantities and simmer them together. Put this on where it hurts the most, and within three days, you will heal the person.

(178:5) For foul, putrefied wounds, take the same plant pounded and add a little salt. Fasten this to the wound, and within three days, it will be healthy.

(178:6) For a woman's periods, take the same plant, pounded thoroughly in a mortar so that it is very soft. Add to it a little honey, take some moist wool that has been teased well, and then use it to smear the private parts with the medication. Then give it to the woman, so that she can lay it under her. That same day, it will stop the flow of blood.[183]

(178:7) So that the cold does not bother you, take the same plant soaked in oil and rub it on the hands and all over the body. You will not feel the cold on any of your body.

179. Greater Periwinkle (*Vinca major* L.), *priapisci*, no OE word

(179:1) This plant, called *priapisci* and another name, *uicaperuica*, is helpful against many things, but first of all against being possessed by demons, then against snakes, wild animals, poison, any threat, envy, and terror, and so that you have blessings. If you have the plant with you, you will be happy and always satisfied. You must pick the plant saying the following: *Te precor uicaperuica multis utilitatibus habenda ut uenias ad me hilaris florens cum tuis uirtutibus, ut ea mihi prestes, ut tutus et felix sim semper a uenenis et ab iracundia inlesus.* That is then in our language: I pray you, *uica peruica* you who have many uses, that you come to me happily with your powers blooming, that you ensure I will be protected and always fortunate and not be harmed by poison or by anger. When you want to pick the plant, you should be free of any stain. You must pick it when the moon is 9 nights old, and 11 nights, 13 nights, 30 nights, and when it is 1 night old.

180. Common Gromwell (*Lithospermum officinale* L.), *lithospermon*, *Sunnancorn*

This plant, called *lithospermon* and another name, …, grows in Italy, originally in Crete, and it has larger leaves than rue and straight. At its top, it has white, round stones, like pearls, the size of peas, and they are as hard as pearls, and also bunched together. They are hollow inside and the seeds are inside.

(180:1)   For bladder stones and for difficulty passing water, take five pennies' weight of these stones and give them to drink in wine. It will break up the stones and promote passing water.

181. Stavesacre (*Dephinium stafisagria* L.), *stauisagria*, no OE word

The plant called *stauisagria* and another name …, has leaves like a grapevine and a straight stem, and it has triangular green pods with seeds the size of peas that are sour and dark, they are white inside and bitter to the taste.

(181:1)   For general bodily discomfort,[184] take 15 kernels of the seeds of this plant pounded in light beer. Give it to drink, and it purges the body through vomit. After the person has drunk the drink, they should walk around and get the circulation going before they vomit. When the person begins to vomit, they should often drink light beer, lest the power of the plant burn the throat and choke them.

(181:2)   For scaly skin and scabs, take the seeds of this same plant and roses and pound them together. Smear it on the dry places, and they will heal.

(181:3)   For toothache and sore gums, take seeds of this same plant and simmer them in vinegar. Have them hold some of the vinegar in their mouth for quite a while. It will cure the toothache, sore gums, and all putrefaction in the mouth.

182. Eryngo (*Eryngium* supp. L.), *gorgonion*, no OE word[185]

(182:1)   This plant, called *gorgonion* and another name, …, grows in shady places and wet ones. About this plant it is said that its root looks like the head of a snake people call gorgon, and that its branches, so it is also said, have the eyes, nose, and color of snakes.

(182:2)   Also its root makes any person look like itself, whether the color of gold or of silver. If you want to pick the plant with its root, be careful that the sun does not shine on it, lest its color and strength be changed by the sun's brightness. Cut it only with a curved and very hard iron tool; and whoever intends to cut it must turn away from it because it is not permitted that anyone see its entire root. Whoever has this root with them will ward off all evil footsteps leading toward them; indeed, because of it, the evil one will either turn away or yield to them.

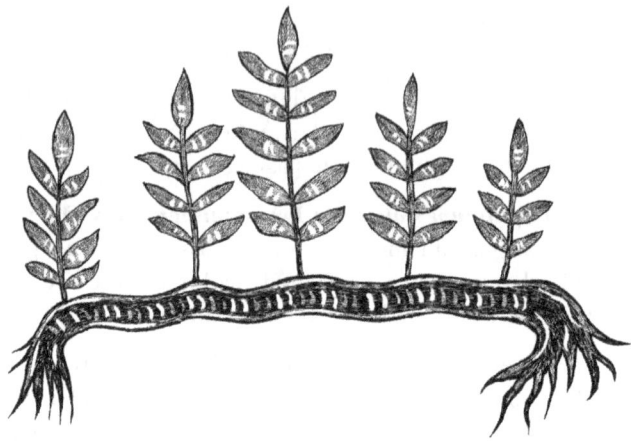

Melilot

183. Melilot (*Melilotus officinalis* L.), *milotis*, no OE word

(183:1) This plant, called *milotis* and another name, ..., grows in cultivated places and wet ones. You should pick this plant when the moon is on the wane in the month of August. Take the root of this plant, fasten it to a weaving thread, and hang it around your neck. During that year, you will not have dim eyes, or if it has already happened to you, it will quickly disappear, and you will be healthy. This remedy is tested.

(183:2) For muscle spasms, take the juice of this same plant, rub it on, and the condition will abate. Also, it is said about this plant that it flowers twice a year.

184. Tassel Hyacinth (*Muscari comosum* Mill.), *bulbus*, no OE word[186]

This plant, called *bulbus* and another name, ..., has two varieties: one is red and helps stomach pain, while the other is more bitter to the taste, is called *scillodes*, and is also more beneficial for the stomach. Both are powerful, and when eaten as food, they strengthen the body.

(184:1) For swellings and foot disease and for any injury, take this plant pounded by itself or mixed with honey. Put it on the soreness as needed.

(184:2a,b) For dropsy, take this same plant, as we said before, pounded, and lay it on the abdomen. Mixed with honey, it also heals up dog bites. If it is mixed with pepper and applied, it stops a person from sweating. It also lessens stomach pain.

(184:3) For open sores that generate themselves, take the root of this plant pounded with oil, wheat flour, and soap, the same as you would make a poultice, and lay it on the wounds. It also cures the condition the Greeks call *hostopyturas*, that is, a flaky scalp, and also one called *achoras*, or scabies, which very often makes the hair fall out. In addition, it clears the face of pimples when pounded with vinegar or honey.

(184:4) Also, taken with vinegar, it heals internal swelling and ruptures.

About this plant, it is said to be begotten by dragon's blood on mountaintops in thick groves.

185. Bitter Cucumber (*Citrullus colocynthis*), colocynthisagria, no OE word[187]

This plant, called *colocynthisagria*, that is *curcurbita agrestis*, which is also called *frigillam*, just like other gourds expands its branches over the ground. It has divided leaves like a cucumber and round and bitter fruit, which should be picked at the time just when its green gives way to yellow.

(185:1) To move the bowels, take two pennies' weight of the tender inside of the fruit without the seeds pounded in light beer. Give this to drink. It will move the bowels.

Notes

Betony (1)

1 *on clænum dunlandum.* C=clean downlands. DOE=*dun*=hill. *clænsian*=to cleanse, purify.

2 *gefriþedum* = sheltered. C=shady.

3 *nihtgengum* = evil night spirit. C=monstrous nocturnal visitors.

4 *molde, -an* = dust, earth, etc. C=mold

5 *gewyrc to duste.* C = reduce it to dust.

6 *scearfian* = scrape, shred. C = scrape, but shred would make more sense here before the plant (possibly dried) was made into a powder.

7 This is a departure from the Latin text, and also from Dioscorides, in which the pounded betony is put on the broken skull to heal the fractured bones. Might this Old English version of the remedy be instead for migraine headache, when the head indeed feels '*tobroken*'?

8 *seoð on wætere to þriddan dæle.* C = boil it down to the third part. Modern usage is to reduce liquid by so much, usually by simmering (not boiling) a long time.

9 *wring þæt wos* (*wos* is juice) C=wring the wash.

10 *Wiþ sidan sare.* C = for sore of side.

11 *twega* = two. C = three to agree with the Latin original!

12 *Gif mannes innoð* [literally insides] *to fæst sy. innoð* = intestines, abdomen, sometimes womb. *Fæstnyss* is blockage. C = If a man's inwards be too fast.
The chapter on betony was originally a longer stand-alone Latin work; the chapters following are from the Latin Herbarius of Pseudo-Apuleius.

Plantain (2)

13 *genime wegbræden seaw ðære wyrte, gedo þæt hio blacu sy.* C= take the juice of waybread the wort and contrive that it be lukewarm. Culpepper advises clarifying the juice of the greater plantain plant before giving it to drink. DOE gives "pale" as the meaning of *blacu*; close to the idea that (clarified) plant sap is intended here.

14 *fordwineð.* C = dwindle.

15 *do on sumes cynnes ealo* (C says it is *cald* (cold), not *ealo* (ale) in MS V) C=put it on cold of some kind.

16 C=if a man be overgrown in wamb.

17 C=always one cup for a discharge.

18 *licoma sy ahearded*. C=a man's body be hardened. It is unlikely the whole body would be hard; instead, this remedy would soften a hard lump somewhere on the body, a use Culpepper lists for plantain.

19 *to clame*. C = work it to clam (a clammy substance).

20 *wunda hatunge*. C=heats of wounds.

21 *tyddernysse* = weakness C=every days tenderness of a man inwardly. A custom in Germany used to be to take a small shot of some kind of schnapps mid-morning to overcome "the dead time." Perhaps this was a long-standing custom.

Cinquefoil (3)

22 *bewrit þriwa* ... C = scratch it thrice with the least finger and the thumb. DeV = mark round (for the verb). The action is intended to loosen the soil around the plant, since the next instruction is to pull the plant up.

23 *cymeð him to bote*. C=that will come to him for a boot (remedy).

24 *cwepað cræftige men*. C=aver crafty men.

25 *cancer ablendan*. C=blind a cancer, or prevent its discharging.

26 *Ðu scealt ... gewyrcean þa wyrt*. C = thou shalt work up the wort.

Vervain (4)

27 Grieve notes that vervain must be picked before flowering and dried promptly, and, with regard to the remedy just before this one, she notes that since ancient times, the vervain plant has been crushed and worn about the neck for certain conditions. Culpepper says vervain flowers at Midsummer, which agrees well with the advice about when to gather this plant for medicinal use.

28 C=For a head sore ... it will make to wane the sore of the head.

29 C= wheaten corns hole.

30 C=if the scratch is blind.

Henbane (5)

31 C=swart in hue. Two varieties of henbane are used medicinally; *Hyoscyamus niger* and *Hyoscyamus albus*, i.e., black and white henbane. In its description of the plant, the *Herbarium* seems to specify that it is talking about white henbane, not black. Yet most authorities on herbals identify it as the black variety. Both have similar medicinal properties. I leave the final decision to herbalists and botanists, but flag the issue here.

32 C=For lungs addle (disease) ... with high wondering he will be healed.

Snakeweed (6)

33 Literally snakeplant (*nædre wort*) in Old English; also called adderwort and viperina in modern English.

34 C= it healeth wondrously the rent.

"Bee Plant" (7)

35 In the first edition, I followed several authorities in calling this plant "sweet flag," but newer studies are calling that identification into question. As a consequence, here I use a literal translation of the Old English name; i.e., bee plant. DOEPN identifies this plant as *Melissa officinalis* L. because of the reference to its preventing bees from swarming ("wegen der Verwendung gegen das Abschwärmen der Bienen"). Dioscorides III, 18, and Grieve also say that Melissa is said to delight bees. How the reference to bees originally got into the uses for this plant is not known; it is in the Latin version as well. *Acorus*, or *Akoron* in Dioscorides I, 2 is *Iris pseudacorus* or yellow flag, a cousin to sweet flag. In

a 2022 private communication, M.A. D'Aronco said she is leaning toward yellow iris. The illustration in Cotton Vitellius C. iii would support identifying this plant as sweet flag; its major feature, according to Grieve, is a large rhizome that grows sideways, not down, from which numerous roots grow. Grieve also mentions its sword-shaped leaves. The sideways-growing rhizome, the roots, and sword-shaped leaves are all shown in the manuscript illustration. A definitive identification may one day be made.

36 C=*ac hym gelicað*: it will like them well.

37 *blewð*: C=blows.

Lion's Foot or Lady's Mantle (8)

38 DeV explains in a note that the Latin original, *defixus* (tied up in a knot by witchcraft), has such a meaning; and he translated the Old English here, *sy cis*, as 'to be under a spell'. However, C=be choice (fastidious or nauseated when eating), which is the meaning given in BT and the DOE. The remedy as written suggests something more than simple nausea when eating; the healer is "unbinding" the patient from some kind of unspecified condition. (*Aristolochia* is birthwort.)

39 *Curanderas* frequently prescribe remedies for *mal de ojo*, conditions caused by being looked at by someone with an evil eye. Several other ailments are caused by being put (or putting oneself) under a spell of some kind. The conditions are said to be easily recognized if one is trained to diagnose them. Birthwort (20) is twice prescribed in the *Herbarium* as a smudge stick to provide healing smoke.

Celery-Leaved Crowfoot (9)

40 C=clofthing or cloffing; C has the correct botanical identification but an unusual English translation. The plant is a type of buttercup.

41 *hwæt horwes on bið*. C=anything of foulness.

Buttercup (10)

42 C=clove wort. BT has "buttercup," and this is a type of buttercup.

43 *ða sweartan dolh*. C=the swart scars.

Mugwort (11)

44 Literally, this says to turn away the eyes of an evil person, but I believe it is another reference the *mal de ojo* (evil eye). C=evil eyes of evil men. He also adds here "he, the man of the house" to explain who in the house would have the plant; the Old English says literally "in the house where one has it (the plant) inside."

Mugwort/Tansy (12)

45 No painting appears for this plant in the Cotton manuscript, although in the contents list, *herba artemisia tagantes* (chapter 12) is listed as another kind of mugwort. Cockayne's numbering of the mugworts reflects the Latin original(s), which had three separate chapters for the *artemisias*, a very large family of bitter plants. Dioscorides, too, lists three *artemisias* in a row as III, 127, 128, and 129, but they do not correspond exactly to the OE. That three *artemisias* occur together is noteworthy, and the identification may have changed over the centuries to match where the compiler lived. D'A says that André identifies this plant as *Tanacetum vulgare L.* or tansy. Bierbaumer, C, and De V=*Artemesia dracunculus* (tarragon).

Roman Wormwood (13)

46 *Artemesia pontica* is roman wormwood; *artemesia leptefilos* is southernwood (III, 128 in Dioscorides); not listed by this name in Grieve who calls southernwood *artemesia abrotanum*). D'A says that André identifies this plant as *Artemisia campestris* L. Because of the number of *artemesias* in any locale, a practitioner would have to learn which one was meant from someone who knew them well.

47 One of the figures on the title page (19r) is Chiron the centaur.

Dock (14)

48 Rumex is a genus that includes about 200 types of docks and sorrels. Exactly which species is meant here is uncertain. "Cabbage leaf" is described in chapter 130, where C and DeV identify it as *Brassica napus* or rape (also colewort), a type of mustard. D'A identifies it as *Brassica oleracea*, cabbage, citing Maggiulli, *Nomenclatura delle piante*, p. 173. C uses cabbage leaf here.

Dragonwort (15)

49 C, DeV, and D'A identify this plant as *Dracunculus vulgaris* or *Arum dracunculus L.* and the plant in chapter 6, *nædre wyrt*, as *Polygonum bistorta*. Hunt identifies both as "bistort" (*Polygonum bistorta*). Grieve says that the *Arum* family is enormous and that the roots are used for many purposes; her description of how arums grow is very close to the drawing in the Cotton ms.

50 C puts the plant name in Greek here; however, the OE version has the Latin name.

51 Groves of trees have been holy places from the most ancient times in many cultures; see Sir James G. Frazer, *The Golden Bough* (New York: The Macmillan Company, 1940).

52 Clearly a step is missing in the instructions—that of applying the medicine.

Orchis (16)

53 C gives a Greek name here that is not in the original. C calls this plant ravens leek, but notes that it is in the Orchis (orchid) family.

54 *earfoðliche wundela*. C=difficult wounds.

Gentian (17)

55 C=Field Wort (*Erythraea pulcella* Sw.), Bierbaumer has Autumn Gentian (*Gentiana amarella* L.), all in the same family of plants. D'A and DeV agree on *Gentiana lutea* L.

56 *heo framað to eallum drenceom*. C=is beneficial for all drinks (antidotes). Grieve explains at length how gentian root was used in many kinds of tonics.

Sowbread (18)

57 C has *Cyclamen hederaefolium*, which Grieve says is very close to the species that Bierbaumer and DeV prefer. Grieve notes that the roots are a favorite food of swine, hence the name.

58 *wiþ þæt ðæt mannes fex fealle*. literally: if the hair of a person falls out. DeV says in a note that the translator confused *deplere* with *depilare*. The Latin original DeV uses has *Ad caput deplendum*. But the meaning is not appreciably different in either case.

59 *heortece*. C=heartache, which is different from heartburn—pain in the heart—in modern English.

Knotgrass (19)

60 C= Untrodden to Pieces, a literal translation of the OE name of this plant.

61 *butan smice gewyl*. C=boil it without smoke. The meaning may not be without smoke from the fire, but without the plume of vapor a liquid makes when it is boiling fast.

62 *titta sár wifa*. C=for sore of titties of women.

63 The custom of speaking to plants before picking them (with the allied caution of not picking too many of the same plant in any one locality to save the species) is a basic tenet for many who collect medicinal plants in the wild.

Birthwort (20)

64 *swylce deofulseocnyssa*. The hallucinations often associated with high fevers and similar conditions could be described in such a way. C= devil sickness or demoniacal possession.

65 Grieve's description of the various *Aristolochias* bears out the need for caution in using the correct amount of this plant; too much of it will cause terrible pain in the abdomen and bowels.

66 *ahwæned*. C=vexed. However, BT shows the Latin as *vexare, contristare, molestare*; all connote being upset or afraid more than angry. The Latin cited by DeV is *contristus*.

Meadow Saffron (22)

67 Perhaps dung heaps or privies are meant here, known sources of rich soil.

Ashwagandha (23)

68 *This is a change from the first edition*, where no modern English plant name is supplied. C, DeV, Bierbaumer=lily of the valley. D'A, citing Maggiulli and André, identifies the plant as *herba apollinaris* (*Withania somnifera*). Hunt suggested *apollinaris* might have been a name used for lily of the valley, foxglove, mandrake, and black nightshade. The plant *Withania somnifera* is used in Ayurvedic medicine and called ashwagandha. It has become popular and is now packaged and sold in most commercial pharmacies under that name; poison gooseberry, the only English name found, is seldom listed as a medicinal plant. The DOEPN gives its identification as ashwagandha.

69 Apollo is another figure named on the title page (19r).

Chamomile (24)

70 As an example of C's style: For sore of eyes, let a man take ere the upgoing of the sun, the wort which is called Χαμαίμηλον. C supplies the Greek letters for the name although they are not in the manuscript and he has "ooze" for "juice."

71 Picking plants before the sun is hot and is also customary so that few volatile oils and saps are dissipated by the heat.

Wall Germander (25)

72 DeV notes here that *Heort* is probably from *heorot*, hart, because deer are said to like to eat it and lists other possible identifications for it.

Wild Teasel (26)

73 This is a method used to determine dosage based largely on the patient's body weight and physical condition.

Madder (29)

74 DeV, Bierbaumer=wayfaring-tree (*Viburnum lantana* L.), which Grieve says is never used for medicinal purposes. DeV says in his note to this entry that the plant is difficult to identify. C identifies it as *Sambucus ebulus*.

Water Dock (30)

75 C identifies this plant as *Cochlearia anglica* and calls it "bright-coloured hydele." DeV says this may well be the plant Pliny and Dioscorides claim cured the Roman soldiers of scurvy when they were in the Rhine country.

76 *syle drincan be þære mihte þe hwa mæge þurch hit self.* C=give it to drink by the might, which each one may (according to a man's strength), through itself without danger ....

Prickly Lettuce (31)

77 Why the plant is collected without smoke is not known.

Asphodel (33)

78 Identifying both this plant and the plant in chapter 53 as "asphodel" should be considered placeholder names until their true identity can be established. See discussion in DOEPN under OE *wudurofe* and also English "asphodel." For many reasons, asphodel and sweet woodruff became intertwined in manuscripts. I follow D'A's identifications in both chapters, but with reservations.

79 **Centaury (35 and 36)**

C, DeV, Bierbaumer=Yellow Centaury. Tobyn, Denham and Whitelegg list numerous references to both kinds of century in the index to their book; Grieve discusses several types of centaury plants, grouping them under *Erythraea centarium*, as does Hunt.

80 Chiron is shown on the title page (19r).

81 *gyf hwa þonne on þas frecnysse befealle.* C= if anyone then fall into this mischief. Centaury was widely used for fever, according to Grieve. The Latin original in DeV does not say why this is prescribed, but simply gives the remedy.

82 C translates the OE as spasm of sinews, but BT and DeV also translate *sinu (seonu)* as nerve, sinew, or tendon.

Beet (37)

83 C, DeV= beet (with doubts) *Here, my initial identification of this plant as burdock has been corrected to beet,* in line with D'A and others. Hunt says *personacia* is a name given to large-leaved plants including burdock, beet, and water-lily. Latin *personata/personatia* means burdock.

84 *wið niwe wunda þa þe þone wætan gewyrceaþ.* C= for new wounds which work up the wet or humor.

Mallow (41)

85 *7 þæt sy binnan þrim dagum gewylled, swa we ær cwædon, to healfan dæle.* C=let that be boiled within three days, as we said before, to a half part.

Alkanet (42)

86 C, DeV, Bierbaumer=Bugloss or Hound's Tongue (*Cynoglossum officinale* L.) All of them question its identification. In the list of synonyms, "glofwyrt" appears to be an error here (as DeV claims) because it is the vernacular name given earlier for Ashwaganda (23).

Sea-Onion (43)

87 No translation or explanation is given for the Greek term, which means chilblains.

"Wild Gladiolus" (47)

88 This plant name should be considered a place-holder for a future definitive identification. Opinions are varied. C, DeV= unbranched burr-reed (*Sparganium emersum*). The DOEPN updates Bierbaumer in identifying this as *Gladiolus italicus*, agreeing with André 1985. M.A. D'Aronco thinks it may be sword-grass (private communication 2022). It appears to be a wild grassy type plant, of which there are many kinds.

True Maidenhair (48)

89 C, DeV, Bierbaumer=*Callitriche verna* L., water starwort.

Garlic (49)

90 D'A=this is said to be the plant Mercury gave Ulysses to escape from Circe; thought to be a kind of garlic with a yellow flower (citing Grieve, André, and Maggiulli for the identification). DeV identifies it as butterwort (*Pinguicula vulgaris* L.) and Cockayne as houseleek (*Sempervivum tectorum*).

Heliotrope (50)

91 DeV and Bierbaumer say this is cat's ear (*Hypochoeris glabra* L.). Both reject C's identification of the plant as *Achillea tomentosa*.

Common Maidenhair (52)

92 C, DeV=Yellow clover (*Trifolium procumbens* L.)

93 *on ealdum husstedum.* C=in old house-steads (tofts).

Asphodel (53)

94 See note to chapter 33, asphodel, above. Certainly, the uses given for the plant in this chapter are similar to those often found for sweet woodruff, the identification Bierbaumer and the DOEPN give for this plant.

Dropwort (55)

95 C, DeV=dropwort, but *Oenanthe pimpinellifolia.*

Throatwort (56)

96 C, Bierbaumer=narcissus but *Campanula trachelium* L.

Spleenwort (57)

97 Many suggestions have been made about the identification of this plant. D'A gives the meaning listed in the heading. C = either of the *Scrofularias* mentioned. DeV and Bierbaumer = *Asplenium ceterach* L. or *Phyllitis scolopendrium* L. See full discussion with numerous references in DOEPN under OE *brunwyrt.*

98 *uppan þas wyrte gewearp.* C=scraped intestines with this plant.
Butcher's Broom (59)

99 *wiþ dropan.* C=the wrist drop. DOE, DeV=gout.
Aster or Chickweed (61)

100 A good case could be made for identifying this plant either as aster, following D'A based on André, or as chickweed (*Stellaria media*) following C and DeV. About aster, D'A= chickweed does not grow on stony ground; however, Grieve says chickweed grows virtually everywhere and also notes that chickweed flowers open about 9 a.m. and are said to remain open for 12 hours, thus, in the night. The final word is not in on the identity of this plant.
Croton (65)

101 *This is a change from the first edition* in supplying a modern English name for the plant and identifying it as *Croton tiglium*, an emetic fitting the remedy here. It replaces the identification of an unnamed plant as *Croton tinctoria* L., which has no medicinal uses.
Peony (66)

102 *Maligranati* is pomegranate, though whether it would have been known in England at the time is not certain and may be why it is left in Latin. Cockle, the DOE identification, is a weed growing in grain fields that does indeed produce seeds.

103 Although in modern English, insanity has largely replaced lunacy (from the French word for moon), lunacy captures the medieval concept of what caused it. The moon was believed to cause "lunacy," and the Old English word for it is "month-sickness," months being measured in moons.
Vervain/Gypsywort (67)

104 DOEPN, D'A list both plants as possibilities; DOE=vervain. DeV=columbine (*Aquilegia vulgaris* L.). C= vervain.
Bryony (68)

105 DOEPN, DOE, list both bryony and hops as possibilities. C=*Hummulus lupus* or hops.
White Water Lily (69)

106 *heo þæs innoðes unryne gewrið.* C=it restrains ill running of the inward.
Thistle (70)

107 Tentative identification. D'A identifies it as a type of thistle with soft spines. However, DOEPN, C, DOE, DeV, and Bierbaumer= clover (*Trifolium pratense* L.). Both clover and thistle are used medicinally; however, only the aerial parts of clover are traditionally used; roots of thistle (and other parts) are used. The manuscript illustration does not look like clover or thistle.
Woad (71)

108 C and DeV call attention to the fact that whoever made the translation did not put the English name for woad here, but apparently by mistake copied the Latin for the next line, which reads, "for snakebite," which is the meaning of the Latin phrase. But DeV also points out the interesting fact that the same mistake occurs in MSS B and H.
Great Mullein (73)

109 D'A and DeV consider the OE text here to be mistaken in giving the OE name for this plant as *feldwyrt*. Both supply mullein as the correct identification. The Cotton MS illustration looks much like mullein. *Feldwyrt* is identified and translated as yellow gentian in DOEPN and DOE and is the name of the plant in chapter 17.
Herba Heraclea (74)

110 C gives no name and deems its illustration "fantastic." DeV= *Centaurea calcitrapa* L., star thistle, based on a gloss in MS Bodley 130, which C had earlier rejected because of the image in the Cotton MS. The present identification is based on D'A, which is based on André's identification: ironwort. *Sideritis* is believed to heal wounds caused by anything iron.

111 **Black Nightshade (76)**
C, DeV=*Atropa belladonna*; D'A=*Solanum nigrum* as well as their reading. Both plants belong to the Solanacea family.

112 DOE, DOEPN=*cypressus* means a type of cypress tree, galingale, or henna, and cyprus was also a medical name for privet.
Couch Grass (79)

113 D'A, based on André and his explanation that the "grass that has three branches" mentioned in the Latin description and shown clearly in the manuscript illustration is couch-grass, not quitch, *Agropyrum repens* L., suggested by C and DeV, and preferred in DOE. DOEPN = couch grass.
Iris (80)

114 *breost*, which can be chest or breasts. C=breasts. The Latin *praecordia* would favor chest.
Rosemary (81)

115 The Old English term, *wyrtbett*—plant bed or garden plot—supports the idea that many of these plants were grown in special beds, as discussed in chapter 3.
Asparagus (86)

116 DeV =wild chervil (*Anthriscus silvestris*); D'A, DOEPN=wild asparagus. Chervil has no medicinal properties; asparagus has many.
Savine (87)

117 *wiþ þa cynelican adle*. Literally, "king's disease" which DeV and the DOE note was a condition that the king could cure, here, jaundice, particularly jaundice associated with gout. C uses the Latin, *ad morbum regium*, in his translation. See Marc Bloch, *The Royal Touch: Sacred Monarchy and Scrofula in England and France*, trans. J.E. Anderson (London: Routledge & Kegan Paul, 1973).
Snapdragon (88)

118 Both the Latin and OE names literally mean "dog's head." DOEPN has a lengthy entry about its meaning.
Blackberry or Bramble (89)

119 In case numerology is involved in the directions, the instructions are translated as given.
Yarrow (90)

120 Slight inflammation is a sign a sore is beginning to heal.

121 The Old English has simply "three of wine," which could be an erroneous omission of cups or another specified amount, or indicate an assumption that the reader would know the proper ratio of this herb to liquid.
Horsemint (92)

122 DeV includes a lengthy note about the possible skin conditions meant by *hreofl/hreofla*. The DOE includes leprosy among them, which DeV does not.
Dwarf Elder or Danewort (93)

123 For many who collect plants, especially in the wild, speaking to a plant when it is cut explaining why one is gathering it is not at all unusual.
Pennyroyal (94)

124 The Old English word for this plant, *dweorgedwosle*, has *dweorge*, dwarf, as its first element. In his notes DV suggests that the plant name relates to the role dwarfs were thought to play in affecting health. The DOEPN, on the other hand, explains that here the word simply connotes the dwarf, or smaller, type of a plant and traces that use etymologically. This plant occurs throughout the OE medical texts; whether one sees a connection to dwarfs or to an ancient diminutive form of the name could be important to many studies, especially where magic is alleged to be involved.

Ribwort/ Plantain (98)

125 *This is a change from the first edition*, where its preferred identification is listed as 'hounds tongue' (*Cynoglossum officinale*). It was based on André and D'A. Since then the DOEPN has appeared with a persuasive discussion of its identification as ribwort plantain, under the OE name *ribbe*. Ribwort plantain has a wide variety of medicinal uses. The Cotton manuscript page on which its illustration occurs is badly damaged, so it cannot be of much help.

Ivy (100)

126 The first edition gives *Hedera helix* L. (common ivy) as the botanical name for this plant, in accordance with D'A. There is no doubt the plant is ivy. However, Bierbaumer and DeV=*Glechoma hederaceum*, ground-ivy. Opinion of philologists is mixed about which of the two kinds of ivy is correct, ground or common ivy. Medical herbalists would be good arbiters. The information in Grieve supports ground ivy; i.e., its long history of many medicinal uses contrasted with that of common ivy. DOEPN now lists both kinds as possibilities. Another issue is whether berries or tender branches (OE *croppas*) are to be used.

127 DeV has a note about what kind of venomous insect or serpent this may have been, pointing out that the Latin name *spalangiones* is often used both for snake and spider. Many venomous bites could have been treated pretty much the same. C=tarantula.

Sage (103))

128 *gescapa*. C=shapes (or the verenda).

Coriander (104)

129 *nime ðonne an man þe sy mægðhades man, cnapa oþþe mægden*: literally, "take then a person who is a virginal person, boy or girl." It is the virginal person who holds the cloth; however, the OE wording is not too clear about who is meant.

Wild Purslane (105)

130 *wiþ swiðlichne flewsan þæs sædes*; literally, for excessive flowing of seed. C=for violent gonorrhœa. Neither DeV nor BT have a note about the condition meant here.

Chervil (106)

131 *ameredes hiniges 7 grene popig*. C= spoilt honey and a green poppy. *Grene* is used to mean fresh many times in this work.

Lily (109)

132 C and DeV note that the translator made a mistake here and translated the Latin *lilii bulbum* (bulb of the lily) as two different plants.

133 **Caper Spurge (110)**
   hreofl. C=leprosy. As noted several times, the term applies to a wide variety of skin rashes and irritations and might have included leprosy.

Sow Thistle (111)

134 *wiþ þæt ðu nane yfele gean cymas ðe ne ondræde*. C=In order that thou may dread no ill gaincomers.

Lupin (112)

135 C, DeV, Bierbaumer=*Lupinus albus*.

Lettuce (114)

136 Bierbaumer, DeV=*Lactuca virosa* L.

137 The Latin means literally hare's lettuce.

Squirting Cucumber (115)

138 According to D'A, this cucumber is a wild species that grows near the sea in warm places. Bierbaumer, DeV=cucumber (*Cucumis sativus* L.).

139 *Gif cild misboren sy*, literally, if a child is "mis-born," which could be born prematurely or misshapen.

140 **Rue (117)**
Note that the name for the type of rue shifts from *montana* to *siluatica* within this chapter, and as usual, the OE name is not used. For a lengthy discussion of rue's long use as a medicinal plant, see chapter 27 in Tobyn, Denham, and Whitelegg.

141 Although the Latin differentiates between women's breasts (*mamilla*) and the chest/ breast as seat of the heart (*praecordia*), the OE does not. The remedy seems to be more for chest pain than for sore breasts (take the drink and rest). In either case, the drink is supposed to soothe the person. *Wiþ ðære breostan sare.* C=sore of the breasts.
Basil (119)

142 C says this is a pomegranate. *Mālum* is apple in Latin.
Ivy (121)

143 See notes to chapter 100 above, on another species of ivy.
Marjoram (124)

144 The condition I translate as foot disease or condition is Old English *dropa* (m.), translated in many dictionaries as gout; a retroactive diagnosis I avoid. The DOE lists its primary meaning as "drop, drops," as in a drop of rain, water, or medicine. Many fewer examples are listed there for *dropa* in the medical texts than in other types, and DOE supplies meanings in medical contexts as varied as gout, rheum, and cholera. In this instance, the conditions for which the plant is said to be beneficial are quite dissimilar (*dropa*, liver disease, and shortness of breath). More work is needed on such terms to ascertain the meanings they could actually have in a medical setting.

145 **Rue (127)**
DeV gives goat's rue, *Galega officinalis*, for this plant. See note above at rue (107).
Basil (131)

146 The OE name for the plant, *nædderwyrt*, literally is "snake plant."
Mandrake (132)

147 The root of a mandrake plant is large and somewhat shaped like a human being. Many legends have grown up around it; a recent mention is in the Harry Potter series. See Anne Van Arsdall, "Exploring what was understood by 'mandragora' in Anglo-Saxon England," and Van Arsdall, H. Klug, and P. Blanz, "The Mandrake Plant and Its Legend: A New Perspective," both *Old Names-New Growth: Proceedings of the Second Anglo-Saxon Plant Name Survey Conference*, eds. Peter Bierbaumer and Helmut Klug. Frankfurt am Main: Peter Lang, 2009.
Beginning with chapter 133, the Herbarium of Pseudo-Apuleius is no longer the source, but another work, which in the early-medieval world was attributed to Dioscorides, titled Liber medicinae ex herbis feminis. See DeV, lv-lx, for a discussion of sources; also J.M. Riddle, "Pseudo-Dioscorides' Ex herbis feminis and Early Medieval Medical Botany," Journal of the History of Biology 14 (1981) 43–81 for the history of this work and its long association with the Herbarium.
Campion (133)

148 DOEPN – *Plantago lanceolata* (ribwort plantain, native to England) or *Silene coronaria* L (rose campion, foreign).
Southernwood (135)

149 The OE text does not tell us what is put to flight. C supplied the word snake, which is in the Latin version.
Heliotrope (137)

150 Various authorities say it is impossible distinguish the herb described here from the one in chapter 64, also heliotrope. C, DeV = marigold. DOEPN = various possibilities.

151 *on fættum landum 7 on beganum.* C=on fat lands and on cultivated ones.

Field Marigold (138)

152 C and DeV give scarlet pimpernel (*Anagallis arvensis*).

White Hellebore (140)

153 Two Old English names are given for this plant, mirrored in the translation because it is unusual in this work. The plant appears to have been highly valued for remedies.

154 *on blacan briwe*. C=black brewis. BT= a thick broth made of meal. DOE, DeV=pottage. Gruel seems to capture what it might have been; something between a broth and a soup/pottage.

155 *oriza*. C=rice. This word is not in BT or DeV. It is the Latin word for rice: the OE uses the Latin name as written but as a plant name.

Ox-Eye Daisy or Marguerite (141)

156 DeV and D'A list several other possibilities for this plant, all of them in the Crysanthemum family, and DeV discusses possible mistranslations that may be in the original OE translation.

Gorse (142)

157 *This is a change from the first edition*, because of more recent access to additional resources. C, DeV, DOE, DOEPN=gorse, which <u>has</u> known medicinal uses.

Fleabane/Spikenard (143)

158 C translates the plant's use into Latin.

159 C gives this entire entry in Latin, and translates the OE *cennan* as *parere*, to give birth. The Latin original has *abortionem praegnantibus facit*.

Thorn-Apple (144)

160 DOE notes that the OE name *foxes glofa* was used for a number of plants, none of them foxglove (*Digitalis purpurea*). DOEPN = either thorn-apple (*Datura stramonium*) or foxglove. DeV and D'A discuss the origin of the name and the plants it may connote. A distinctive aspect of the *Datura* family is the seed pod, which is round and covered with thorns.

Soapwort (146)

161 C again translates the condition *hreofl* as leprosy; see notes at 91 and 110 above.

Orpine (147)

162 Illustrations of early-medieval gardens often show many small raised garden plots in which individual kinds of plants are grown. These plots are enclosed by a large garden wall.

Elder (148)

163 *This is a change from the first edition*, where, following André, the plant is identified as sweet marjoram. C, DeV, DOEPN, DOE =elder (*Sambucus nigra* L.); in addition, the illustration in the Cotton MS looks more like the leaves of an elder bush than of marjoram.

Shepherd's Purse (150)

164 C translates into Greek the phrase about stimulating women's periods.

St. John's Wort (152)

165 *7 þæt sweart 7 on swæce swylce tyrwe*. C=swart and in smack as tar.

166 C writes the word for menses in Greek and calls the genitals "naturalia."

Globe Thistle (153)

167 The translation of this passage is a particularly good example of Cockayne's style: For stirring of the mie or urine, take this same wort, so oozy, pounded, give to drink; it forth leadeth the mie.

Scotch Thistle (154)

168 D'A and DeV give this identification. DOE and DOEPN give many possibilities as to which plant it might be. C= *Cnicus erioforus*, a wooly leaved thistle.

Spotted Golden Thistle (157)

169 *This is a change from the first edition,* based on a more careful reading of André and additional research. Golden thistle is a plant in the Bible DeV= artichoke (*Scolymus cardunculus* L.)

Iris (158)

170 *This is a slight change from the first edition,* in that the species of iris is not specified. *Iris illyrica* has been used medicinally since antiquity, but so have many other species of iris. German or bearded iris, the identification in the first edition, is also called orris root, and also well known for its medicinal properties. Illyria was a Roman province in the Balkan peninsula.

171 At this point, C translates the rest of the passage into Latin, with the words for gonorrhea and menses given in Greek.

Sea-Onion, Squill (159)

172 Identification of this plant is quite uncertain. In notes, DeV and D'A say that no such plant or remedy are found in any edition of *De herbis femininis,* the assumed source of this chapter. It cannot be satisfactorily identified through the DOEPN.

Water Germander, Barrenwort (163)

173 Identification of this plant is problematic, because the plant names mentioned have few attested medicinal uses. See same or similar plant at chapter 72. *Scordo* means garlic in Greek. Identifications from C, DeV, D'A.

174 *Wið þæs gerynnincge þæs worsmes ym ðs breost.* C=For the running of ratten about the breasts. Chest is intended in the original, not breasts; the Latin original in DeV is fragmentary, but MS O lists this remedy *Ad pectus.*

Wall-Flower (165)

175 Identified variously as daisy, century, comfrey, violet, wild pansy in André, DeV, D'A, DOE, DOEPN, or as André notes at p. 330, *uiola* " designates very numerous and very different plants," (my translation of André).

Fleawort (169)

176 D'A notes that the plant illustrated in the MS is coriander, as its caption indicates, but that the remedies describe uses for *psyllium;* however, the confusion began centuries before. All the Latin versions and all the extant mss of *De herbis femininis* make the same mistake. C translates it as coriander, and notes the confusion over what it is.

Dog Rose (170)

177 *This is a change from the first edition,* where the plant is identified as sweet-briar, one of several possibilities found at the time. DeV notes about the last statement in the chapter, that the OE translator missed the meaning of the Latin, which reads "lest, being unable to endure the potency of the medicine, he should scatter the remedy."

Peony (171)

178 C says it is *Peonia officinalis* L.; peony. DeV notes that this chapter is not found in any of the Latin texts he consulted, and identifies it as sunflower (*Helianthus annuus* L.)

Cleavers (Clivers) (174)

179 C seems to have skipped over some of the OE. He has "… it is stiff in leaves, and it hath a great stalk, and in the middle is hollow, as we before said, in the manner in which a mans navel is."

Yarrow (175)

180 DeV has sneezewort (*Achillea ptarmica* L.).

181 C translates the whole entry into Latin. His Latin translation and the supposed Latin original as given in DeV do not read the same. The Latin is talking about heavy menstruation, whereas the OE does not say this is specifically menstrual (*monaðlic*) flux; from the OE, it could be merely a discharge.

Castor-Oil (176)

182 Not found in any Latin text, according to DeV; André lists it in Pliny and Dioscorides. C adds in italics after the name of the plant, "and which is not a native of England."

Nettle (178)

183 C translates the whole section into Latin.

Stavesacre (181)

184 For yfelan wætan means literally, for evil waters, i.e., bodily fluids. C=evil humors. Whether *wætan* means humor here and the extent to which humoralism was widely known at the time this work was translated is not yet fully known.

Eryngo (182)

185 *This is a change from the first edition*, where the plant was not named. C, DeV, D'A, Bierbaumer=Field eryngo or sea holly. Other possible species are *E. maritinum*, *E. campestre* L.

186 **Tassel Hyacinth (184)**

DeV = Onion (*Allium cepa* L.)

Bitter Cucumber (185)

187 DeV= Cucumis colocynthis. This is the only chapter in the Cotton MS that does not begin with a plant illustration.

REFERENCES AND ONLINE RESOURCES

Works by (T) Oswald Cockayne (other than on Greek philology)

————*The Civil History of the Jews from Joshua to Hadrian; with a Preliminary Chapter on the Mosaic History.* London: John W. Parker, West Strand, 1845. Often reprinted.

————*Short Stories Founded on European History. England, First Series.* London: Society for Promoting Christian Knowledge, 1846. Often reprinted.

————*Outlines of the History of France.* London: Society for Promoting Christian Knowledge, 1846.

————*Short Stories from European History. France.* London: Society for Promoting Christian Knowledge, 1849. Often reprinted.

————*Outlines of the History of Ireland.* London: Society for Promoting Christian Knowledge, 1851.

————*The Life of Marshal Turenne.* London: Longman's Travellers' Library, 1853.

————*Narratiunculae Anglice Conscriptae: De Pergamenis Exscribebat Notis Illustrabat Eruditis Copiam.* Soho Square [London]: Iohannem R. Smith, 1861.

————*Spoon and Sparrow, Σ ΠΕΝΔΕΙΝ AND ΨΑΡ, Fundere and Passer; or, English Roots in the Greek, Latin, and Hebrew: Being a Consideration of the Affinities of the Old English, Anglo-Saxon, or Teutonic Portion of Our Tongue to the Latin and Greek; with a Few Pages on the Relation of the Hebrew to the European Languages.* London: Parker, Son, and Bourn, 1861.

————ed. *Leechdoms, Wortcunning, and Starcraft of Early England: Being a Collection of Documents for the Most Part Never before Printed, Illustrating the History of Science in This Country before the Norman Conquest.* 3 vols. London: Her Majesty's Stationery Office, Rolls Series, Vol. 35, 1864–66. Revised by Charles Singer, London: The Holland Press, 1961.

————ed. *Leechdoms, Wortcunning, and Starcraft of Early England: Being a Collection of Documents for the Most Part Never before Printed, Illustrating the History of Science in This Country before the Norman Conquest.* 3 vols. London: Her Majesty's Stationery Office, Rolls Series, Vol. 35, 1864–66. Reprint. London: Kraus Reprint Ltd., 1965.

————*The Shrine: a Collection of Occasional Papers on Dry Subjects.* London: Williams and Northgate, 1864–70. Some published as individual pamphlets.

————*Seinte Marherete: The Meiden ant Martyr.* London: EETS, Trübner & Co., 1866.

————*Hali Meidenhad, An Alliterative Homily of the Thirteenth Century.* London: EETS, Trübner & Co., 1866.

————Mr. Cockayne's Narrative. Privately printed 1869. Held in Archives of King's College School.

————and Edmund Brock, eds. *þe Liflade of St. Juliana: From Two Old English Manuscripts of 1230 A.D.* London: Trübner and Co., 1872.

————"The Death of King Oswald," in *Notes and Queries.* No. 281, May 17, 1873, 397–8.

References

Aarsleff, Hans. *The Study of Language in England, 1780–1860.* Princeton: Princeton University Press, 1967.

Ackerknecht, Erwin H. *A Short History of Medicine.* New York: Ronald Press, 1955.

Amherst, Alicia M. Tyssen. "A Fifteenth Century Treatise on Gardening. By 'MAYSTER ION GARDENER.'" *Archaeologia* 1894.

André, Jacques. *Lexique des termes de botanique en latin.* Paris: Klincksieck, 1956.

Anonymous reviewer. "Anglo-Saxon Leechdoms: Medicine and Astronomy in the Dark Ages." *Dublin University Magazine* Vol. 69 (May 1867).

Arthur, Ciaran. *'Charms', Liturgies, and Secret Rites in Early-Medieval England.* Anglo-Saxon Studies 32. Woodbridge: Boydell Press, 2018.

Banham, Debby. "Dun, Oxa and Pliny the Great Physician: Attribution and Authority in Old English Medical Texts." *Social History of Medicine* Vol. 24, No. 1 (2011): 57–73.

Bankert, Dabney A. *Joseph Bosworth and the Making of His Old English Dictionary, 1820–1921.* University of Toronto: Pontifical Institute of Medieval Studies, Publications of the Dictionary of Old English, 2022.

Baring-Gould, Sabine. *Early Reminiscences: 1834–1864.* New York: E.P. Dutton & Co., 1922.

Bartrip, Peter. "Secret Remedies, Medical Ethics, and the Finances of the British Medical Journal." In *The Codification of Medical Morality: Historical and Philosophical Studies of the Formalization of Western Medical Morality in the Eighteenth and Nineteenth Centuries,* ed. Robert Baker, Vol. 2. Dordrecht: Kluwer Academic Publishers, 1995.

Bately, Janet M. "Old English Prose before and during the Reign of Alfred." *Anglo-Saxon England* Vol. 17 (1988): 93–138.

Beccaria, Augusto. *I Codici di Medicina del Periodo Presalernitano (Secoli Ix, X e XI).* Roma: Edisioni de Storia e Letteratura, 1956.

Bierbaumer, Peter. *Der botanische Wortschatz des Altenglishen.* Vols. 3 Frankfurt/M: Peter Lang, 1975.

Biller, Peter and Joseph Ziegler, eds. *Religion and Medicine in the Middle Ages.* Woodbridge: York Medieval Press, 2001.

Bloomfield, Josephine Helm. "Diminished by Kindness: Frederick Klaeber's Rewriting of Wealhtheow." *Journal of English and Germanic Philology* Vol. 93 (April 1994): 183–203.

Bonser, Wilfrid. *The Medical Background of Anglo-Saxon England: A Study in History, Psychology, and Folklore.* London: The Wellcome Historical Medical Library, 1963.

Bosworth, Rev. Joseph. *The Origin of the Germanic and Scandinavian Languages and Nations: with a Sketch of their Literature, and Short Chronological Specimens of the Anglo-Saxon, Friesic, Flemish, Dutch, the German from the Meso-Goths to the Present Time, the Icelandic, Danish, Norwegian, and Swedish: Tracing the Progress of these Languages and their Connection with the Anglo-Saxon and the Present English.* London: Longman, Rees, Orme, Brown, and Green, 1836.

Brewer, Charlotte. "Walter William Skeat." In *Medieval Scholarship: Biographical Studies on the Formation of a Discipline,* ed. Helen Damico. New York: Garland Press, 1998.

Brice-Yisma, Hananja and Frances Watlkins, eds. *Herbal Exchanges: In Celebration of the National Institute of Medical Herbalists 1864–2014*. London: Strathmore Publishing, 2014.

Brown, Peter. *The World of Late Antiquity*. London: Harcourt Brace Jovanovich, 1971.

Brown, Peter. *The Rise of Western Christendom: Triumph and Diversity, A.D. 200–1000*. Chichester: Wiley-Blackwell, 2013.

Burridge, Claire. "Healing Body and Soul in Medieval Europe: Medical Remedies with Christian Elements." *Studies in Church History* Vol. 58 (June 2022): 46–67. Open access at https://doi.org/10.1017/stc.2022.3

Bynum, W.F. *Science and the Practice of Medicine in the Nineteenth Century*. Cambridge: Cambridge University Press, 1994.

Cameron, M.L. "The Sources of Medical Knowledge in Anglo-Saxon England." *Anglo-Saxon England* Vol. 11 (1983): 135–15.

Cameron, M.L. "Anglo-Saxon Medicine and Magic." *Anglo-Saxon England* Vol. 17 (1988): 191–215.

Cameron, M.L. *Anglo-Saxon Medicine*. Cambridge: University of Cambridge, 1993.

Chance, Jane, ed. *Women Medievalists and the Academy*. Madison: University of Wisconsin Press, 2005.

Chavez, Thomas E. *An Illustrated History of New Mexico*. Albuquerque: University of New Mexico Press, 2004.

Collins, Minta. *Medieval Herbals: The Illustrative Traditions*. Toronto: British Library and University of Toronto Press, 2000.

Copeland, Rita. *Rhetoric, Hermeneutics, and Translation in the Middle Ages: Academic Traditions and Vernacular Texts*. Cambridge: Cambridge University Press, 1991.

Crosby, Jr. and W. Alfred. *The Columbian Exchange: Biological and Cultural Consequences of 1492*. Westport, CT: Greenwood Publishing Co., 1972.

Crossgrove, William. "The Vernacularization of Science, Medicine, and Technology in Late Medieval Europe: Broadening Our Perspectives." *Early Science and Medicine* Vol. 5, No. 1 (2000): 47–63.

Culpepper, Nicholas. *Culpepper's Herbal*, ed. David Potterton. New York: Sterling Publishing, 1983.

D'Aronco, M.A. "The Botanical Lexicon of the Old English Herbarium." *Anglo-Saxon England* Vol. 17 (1988): 15–33.

D'Aronco, M.A. "The Old English Pharmacopoeia: A Proposed Dating for the Translation." *AVISTA Forum Journal* Vol. 13, No. 2 (2003): 9–18.

D'Aronco, M.A. "How English Is 'Anglo-Saxon' Medicine? The Latin Sources for Anglo-Saxon Medical Texts." In *Britannia Latina: Latin in the Culture of Great Britain from the Middle Ages to the Twentieth Century*, ed. Charles Burnett and Nicholas Mann. London: The Warburg Institute/Turin: Nino Aragano, 2005.

D'Aronco, M.A. "The Benedictine Rule and the Care of the Sick: the Plan of St Gall and Anglo-Saxon England." In *The Medieval Hospital and Medical Practice, AVISTA Studies in the History of Medieval Technology, Science, and Art*, ed. Barbara Bowers. Aldershot: Ashgate, 2007.

D'Aronco, M.A. and M.L. Cameron. *The Old English Illustrated Pharmacopoeia*. Copenhagen: Rosenkilde and Bagger, 1998.

Dachez, Roger. *Histoire de la médecine: De l'Antiquité à nos jours*. Paris: Éditions Tallandier, 2021.

De Vriend, Hubert Jan. *The Old English Herbarium and Medicina de Quadrupedibus*. Early English Text Society. O.S. 286. New York: Oxford University Press, 1984.

Deegan, Marilyn and Donald G. Scragg, eds. *Medicine in Early Medieval England*. Manchester: University of Manchester, 1989.

Dioscorides. *De Materia Medica*, trans. Lily Y. Beck, third rev. edition Hildesheim; New York: Olms-Weidmann, 2017.

Doyle, Conan T. "Anglo-Saxon Medicine and Disease: A Semantic Approach." 2 Vols. Ph.D. dissertation, Corpus Christi College, Cambridge, 2011. Vol. 2, "Appendix: Bald's Leechbook" 2017, available open access: https://doi.org/10.17863/CAM.14430

Duffin, Jacalyn. *History of Medicine: A Scandalously Short Introduction.* Third edition. Toronto: University of Toronto Press, 2021.

Duke, James A. *Handbook of Medicinal Herbs.* Boca Raton: CRC Press, 2002.

Everett, Nicholas. *The Alphabet of Galen: Pharmacy from Antiquity to the Middle Ages.* Toronto: University of Toronto Press, 2012.

Flechner, Roy and Maire NiMhaonaigh, eds. *The Introduction of Christianity into the Early-Medieval Insular World: Converting the Isles I.* Turnhout: Brepols, 2016.

Francia, Susan and Anne Stobart, eds. *Critical Approaches to the History of Herbal Medicine: From Classical Antiquity to the Early Modern Period.* London: Bloomsbury, 2014.

Getz, Faye. *Medicine in the English Middle Ages.* Princeton: Princeton University Press, 1998.

Glaze, Florence Eliza. "The Perforated Wall: The Ownership and Circulation of Medical Books in Medieval Europe, ca. 800–120." Ph.D. dissertation, Department of History, Duke University, 2000.

Grape-Albers, Heide. *Spätantike Bilder aus der Welt des Arztes: Medizinische Bilderhandschriften der Spätantike und Ihre Mittelalterliche Überliferund.* Wiesbaden: Guido Pressler Verlag, 1977.

Grape-Albers, Heide. *Medicina Antiqua: Codex Vindobonensis 93.* London: Harvey Miller, 1999.

Grattan, J.H.G. and Charles Singer. *Anglo-Saxon Magic and Medicine.* London: Oxford University Press, 1952.

Grieve, M. *A Modern Herbal.* 1931; Reprint: New York: Dover Publications, 1971.

Griggs, Barbara. *Green Pharmacy: The History and Evolution of Western Herbal Medicine.* Rochester, VT: Healing Arts Press, 1997.

Gross, Arthur. "Wolframs Schlangenliste (*Parzifal* 481) und Pseudo-Apuleius." In *Licht der Natur: Medizin in Fachliteratur und Dichtung,* eds. J. Domes, W. Gerabek, B. Haage, C. Weißer und V. Zimmermann. Göppingen: Kümmerle Verlag, 1994.

Guyonvarc'h, Christian-J. *Magie, médecine et divination chez les Celtes.* Paris: Payot, 1997.

Hall, J.R. "William G. Medlicott (1816–83): An American Book Collector and His Collection." *Harvard Library Bulletin,* n.s., Vol. 1, No. 1 (Spring 1990): 13–46.

Hankins, Freda Richards. "Bald's Leechbook Reconsidered. " Ph.D. dissertation, University of North Carolina at Chapel Hill, 1991.

Hardman, Lizabeth. *The History of Medicine.* (juvenile audience) Detroit: Lucent Books, 2011.

Harrison, Freya and Erin Connelly. "Could Medieval Medicine Help the Fight Against Antimicrobial Resistance?" In *Making the Medieval Relevant,* eds. Carol Jones, Conor Kostick and Klaus Oschema. Berlin, Boston, MA: DeGruyter, 2019. Available online: https://doi.org/10.1515/9783110546316-005

Harvey, John H. "The First English Garden Book: Mayster Jon Gardener's Treatise and its Background." *Garden History* Vol. 13, No. 2 (1985): 83–101.

Hayden, Deborah. "Old English in the Irish Charms." *Speculum* Vol. 97, No. 2 (April 2022): 349–76.

Hilbelink, Aaltje Johanna Geertruida. *Cotton MS Vitellius C. iii of the Herbarium Apulei.* Amsterdam: NV Swets und Zeitlanger, 1930.

Holland, Bart K., ed., *Prospecting for Drugs in Ancient and Medieval European Texts: A Scientific Approach.* Amsterdam: Harwood Academic Publishers, 1996.

Hollis, Stephanie. "Scientific and Medical Writings." In *A Companion to Anglo-Saxon Literature,* eds. Phillip Pulsiano and Elaine Treharne. London: Blackwell Publishers, 2001.

Hollis, Stephanie and Michael Wright. *Old English Prose of Secular Learning.* Cambridge: D.S. Brewer, 1992.

Horden, Peregrine. "What's Wrong with Early Medieval Medicine." In *Cultures of Healing-Medieval and after: Collected Studies*. London: Routledge, Variorum Series, 2019.

Howald, Ernst and Henry E. Sigerist, *Antonii Musae de Herba Vettonica Liber, Pseudo-Apulei Herbarius, Anonymi de Taxone Liber, etc.* In *Corpus Medicorum Latinorum*, Vol. 4. Leipzig, 1927.

Hunt, Tony. *Plant Names of Medieval England*. Cambridge: D.S. Brewer, 1989.

Inglis, Brian. *A History of Medicine*. Cleveland, OH: World Publishing Co., 1965.

Jansen-Sieben, Ria ed., *Artes Mechanicae en Europe médiévale / en middeleeuws Europa*. Bruxelles: Archives et Bibliothèques de Belgique, 1989.

Jolly, Karen Louise. *Popular Religion in Late Saxon England: Elf Charms in Context*. Chapel Hill, NC: University of North Carolina Press, 1996.

Jones, Peter Murray. *Medieval Medicine in Illuminated Manuscripts*. London: British Library, 1998.

Keil, Gundolf. "Möglichkeiten und Grenzen frühmittelalterlicher Medizin." In *Das Lorscher Arzneibuch und die Frühmittelalterliche Medizin: Verhandlungen des Medizinhistorischen Symposiums im September 1989 in Lorsch*. eds. Keil Gundolf und Paul Schnitzer. Lorsch: Verlag Laurissa, 1991.

Keil, Gundolf und Paul Schnitzer, eds. *Das Lorscher Arzneibuch und die Frühmittelalterliche Medizin: Verhandlungen des Medizinhistorischen Symposiums im September 1989 in Lorsch*. Lorsch: Verlag Laurissa, 1991.

Kenneally, Daniel F. "Thomas Oswald Cockayne." Unpublished thesis. King's College, London, September 1999. Available at the archives of the college.

Kenneally, Daniel F. and Jane Roberts. "Oswald Cockayne." *Poetica* Vol. 86 (2016): 107–37.

Ker, Neil R. *Catalogue of Manuscripts Containing Anglo-Saxon*. Oxford: Clarendon Press, 1957.

Kesling, Emily. *Medical Texts in Anglo-Saxon Literary Culture*. Cambridge: D.S. Brewer, 2020.

Kett, J.F. "Provincial Medical Practice in England 1730–1815." *Journal of the History of Medicine and Allied Sciences* Vol. 19 No. 1 (Jan 1964): 17–29.

Keys, Thomas E. *The History of Surgical Anesthesia*. 1945; Reprint, New York: Dover Publications, 1963.

Knowles, David. *Great Historical Enterprises*. New York: Nelson, 1962.

Lapidge, Michael. "The School of Theodore and Hadrian." *Anglo-Saxon England* Vol. 15 (1986): 45–72.

Lesser, Zachary, ed. *The Book in Britain: A Historical Introduction*. Hoboken, NJ: John Wiley & Sons, 2019.

Leven, Karl-Heinz. *Geschichte der Medizin: von der Antike bis zur Gegenwart*. München: C.H. Beck, 2017.

Loudon, Irvine. *Medical Care and the General Practitioner 1750–1850*. Oxford: Clarendon Press, 1986.

Luft, Diana. *Medieval Welsh Medical Texts: Vol. 1, the Recipes*. Cardiff: University of Wales Press, 2020.

MacKinney, Loren. *Early Medieval Medicine*. Baltimore, MD: The Johns Hopkins Press, 1937.

MacMahon, M.K.C. "Henry Sweet." In *Medieval Scholarship: Biographical Studies on the Formation of a Discipline*, ed. Helen Damico. New York: Garland Press, 1998.

Mann, John. *Murder, Magic, and Medicine*. New York: Oxford University Press, 1992.

Maxwell, Herbert. "Odd Volumes – I." *Blackwood's Edinburgh Magazine* Vol. 163 (May 1898): 652–70.

McNeill, William H. *Plagues and Peoples*. New York: Doubleday, 1976.

Meaney, Audrey L. "Extra-Medical Elements in Anglo-Saxon Medicine." *Social History of Medicine* Vol. 24, No. 1 (2011): 41–56.

Miles, Frank and Graeme Cranch, *King's College School: The First 150 Years*. London: King's College School, 1979.

Millett, Bella. "The Saints' Lives of the Katherine Group and the Alliterative Tradition." *Journal of English and Germanic Philology* Vol. 87, No 1 (Jan 1988): 16–34.

Minnis, Alastair J. *Medieval Theory of Authorship*. Second edition. Philadelphia: University of Pennsylvania Press, 1984.

Momma, Haruko. "Old English as a Living Language: Henry Sweet and an English School of Philology," paper presented at the International Society of Anglo-Saxonists, Palermo, Italy, 1997.

Momma, Haruko. *From Philology to English Studies: Language and Culture in the Nineteenth Century*. Cambridge: Cambridge University Press, 2012.

Moore, Michael. *Los Remedios de la Gente: A compilation of Traditional New Mexican Herbal Medicines and Their Use*. Santa Fe, 1977.

Moreno Olalla, David. *Lelamour Herbal (MS Sloane 5, ff 13r-57r): An Annotated Critical Edition*. Pieterlen: Peter Lang Verlag, 2018.

Neuburger, Max. *History of Medicine*, trans. E. Playfair, Vol. II. London: Oxford University Press, 1915.

Nida, Eugene A. and William D. Reyburn. *Meaning Across Cultures*. Maryknoll, NY: Orbis Books, 1981.

Niedermann, Max, ed., *Marcellus Über Heilmittel*. Second edition, Vols. 2. Berlin: Akademie Verlag, 1968.

Niles, John and Maria A. D'Aronco, eds. *The Old English Herbal, Lacnunga, and Other Texts*. Dumbarton Oaks Medieval Library. Cambridge, MA: Harvard University Press, forthcoming in 2023.

Ogilvy, J.D.A. *Books Known to the English, 597–1066*. Cambridge, MA: Medieval Academy of America, 1967.

Olds, Barbara M. "The Anglo-Saxon Leechbook III: A Critical Edition and Translation." Ph.D. dissertation, University of Denver, 1984.

Olender, Maurice. *The Languages of Paradise: Race, Religion, and Philology in the Nineteenth Century*. Cambridge, MA: Harvard University Press, 2008.

Olsan, Lea. "Charms and Prayers in Medieval Theory and Practice." *Social History of Medicine* Vol. 16, No. 3 (Dec. 2003): 343–66.

Papper, E.M. *Romance, Poetry, and Surgical Sleep: Literature Influences Medicine*. Westport, CT: Greenwood Press, 1995.

Payne, Joseph Frank. *The Fitz-Patrick Lectures for 1903: English Medicine in the Anglo-Saxon Times*. London: Clarendon Press, 1904.

Pelteret, David A.E. *Slavery in Early Medieval England: From the Reign of Alfred until the Twelfth Century*. Woolbridge: The Boydell Press, 1995.

Peterson, M. Jeanne. *The Medical Profession of Mid-Victorian London*. Berkeley: University of California Press, 1978.

Pliny the Elder. *Natural History*, trans. H. Rackham, Vols. 10. London: Heinemann, 1938–62.

Porter, Roy. *The Greatest Benefit to Mankind: A Medical History of Humanity*. New York: W.W. Norton & Co., 1997.

Pulsiano, Phillip and Elaine Treharne, eds. A Companion to Anglo-Saxon Literature. London: Blackwell Publishers, 2001.

Riddle, John M. "The Textual Tradition of Dioscorides in the Latin West." In *Catalogus Translationum et Commentanorum*, ed. F. Edward Cranz, Vol. IV (1980): 1–143.

Riddle, John M. *Quid pro quo: Studies in the History of Drugs*. Brookfield, VT: Ashgate, 1992.

Riddle, John M. "Theory and Practice in Medieval Medicine." *Viator: Medieval and Renaissance Studies* Vol. V (1974): 157–84.

Riddle, John M. *History of the Middle Ages 300–1500*. Lanham: Rowman & Littlefield, 2008; rev. with Winston Black, 2015.

Rider, Catherine. "Medical Magic and the Church in Thirteenth Century England." *Social History of Medicine* Vol. 24, No. 1 (2011): 92–107.

Robinson, Victor. *Victory over Pain: A History of Anesthesia*. New York: Henry Schuman, 1946.

Rubin, Stanley. *Medieval English Medicine*. New York: Barnes and Noble, 1974.

Sanchez, Joseph P., Robert L. Spude, and Art Gomez. *New Mexico: A History*. Norman: University of Oklahoma Press, 2013.

Sauer, Hans. "Towards a Linguistic Description and Classification of the Old English Plant Names." In *Words, Texts and Manuscripts: Studies in Anglo-Saxon Culture Presented to Helmut Gneuss*, ed. Michael Korhammer et al. Cambridge: D.S. Brewer, 1992.

Sauer, Hans. "English Plant Names in the Thirteenth Century: The Trilingual Harley Vocabulary." In *Middle English Miscellany*, ed. Jacek Tisiak. Posnan: Motivex, 1996.

Sauer, Hans. "On the Analysis and Structure of Old and Middle English Plant Names." *The History of English* No.3 (1997): 133–61.

Scragg, Donald G. *Superstition and Popular Medicine in Anglo-Saxon England*. Manchester: University of Manchester, 1989.

Siegel, Rudolph E. *Galen's System of Physiology and Medicine*. Basel: S. Karger, 1968.

Sigerist, Henry E. *Studien und Texte zur frühmittelalterlichen Rezeptliteratur*. Leipzig: Verlag von J.A. Barth, 1923.

Singer, Charles. *From Magic to Science: Essays on the Scientific Twilight*. (1928); repr. New York: Dover Publications, 1958.

Singer, Charles. "The Herbal in Antiquity." *The Journal of Hellenic Studies* Vol. 47 (1927): 1–52.

Skeat, Rev. Walter W. *A Student's Pastime: Being a Select Series of Articles Reprinted from "Notes and Queries."* Oxford: Clarendon Press, 1896.

Stace, Clive A. *New Flora of the British Isles*. Fourth Edition. United Kingdom: C&M Floristics, 2019.

Stanley, E.G. *The Search for Anglo-Saxon Paganism*. Cambridge: D.S. Brewer, 1975.

Stannard, Jerry. "Marcellus of Bordeaux and the Beginnings of Medieval Materia Medica." *Pharmacy in History* Vol. 15, No. 2 (1973): 47–53.

Stannard, Jerry. "Botanical Data and Late Mediaeval 'Rezeptliteratur.'" In Gundolf Keil, *Fachprosa-Studien: Beiträge zur mittelalterlichen Wissenschafts- und Geistesgeschichte*. Berlin: E. Schmidt, 1982.

Stoll, Ulrich. "Das Lorscher Arzneibuch: Ein Überblick über Herkunft, Inhalt und Anspruch des ältesten Arzneibuchs deutscher Provenienz." In *Das Lorscher Arzneibuch und die Frühmittelalterliche Medizin: Verhandlungen des Medizinhistorischen Symposiums im September 1989 in Lorsch*, eds. Gundolf Keil und Paul Schnitzer. Lorsch: Verlag Laurissa, 1991.

Storms, Godfrid. *Anglo-Saxon Magic*. 1948; Reprint, The Hague: Martinus Nijhoff, 1974.

Stubbs, Stanley G.B. and Edward W. Bligh, *Sixty Centuries of Health and Physick*. London: Sampson Low, Marsten and Co., 1931.

Sweet, Henry. "The History of the TH in English" (1869). In *Collected Papers of Henry Sweet*, ed. Henry C. Wyld, Oxford: Clarendon Press, 1913. (First printed in the *Transactions of the Philological Society* 1868–69, 272–88.)

Sweet, Henry. Review of *Liflade of St Juliana*. *Academy III* Vol. 52 (15 July 1872): 278.

Sweet, Henry. *King Alfred's West Saxon Version of Gregory's Pastoral Care*, 1871; repr. London: Kegan Paul, Trench, Trübner & Co., Ltd., 1930.

Talbot, Charles H. *Medicine in Medieval England*. London: Oldbourne, 1967.

Thurston, C.B. *A Few Remarks in Defense of Dr. Bosworth and His Anglo-Saxon Dictionaries*. London: Macmillan and Co., 1864.

Tobyn, Graeme, Alison Denham, and Margaret Whitelegg. *The Western Herbal Tradition: 2000 Years of Medicinal Plant Knowledge*. Edinburgh: Elsivier, 2011.

Touwaide, Alain. "Quid Pro Quo: Revisiting the Practice of Substitution in Ancient Pharmacy." In *Herbs and Healers from the Ancient Mediterranean through the Medieval West*, eds. Anne Van Arsdall and Timothy Graham. Farnham: Ashgate, 2012.

Turner, Sharon. *The History of the Anglo-Saxons: Comprising the History of England from the Earliest Period to the Norman Conquest*. Fourth edition, Vols. 3, 1799–1805. Reprint, London: Longman, Hurst, Rees, Orme, and Brown, 1823.

Van Arsdall, Anne. "An Old World Herbal in the New World: the Badianus Manuscript." In *… un tuo serto di fiori in man recando; scritto in onore di M.A. D'Aronco*, ed. Patrizia Lendinara. Udine: Forum, 2007.

Van Arsdall, Anne. "Medical Training in Anglo-Saxon England: An Evaluation of the Evidence." In *Form and Content of Instruction in Anglo-Saxon England in the Light of Contemporary Manuscript Evidence*, eds. Patrizia Lendinara, Loridana Lazzari, and M.A. D'Aronco. Turnhout: Brepols, 2007.

Van Arsdall, Anne. "The Transmission of Knowledge in Early-Medieval Medical Texts: An Exploration." In *Between Text and Patient: The Medieval Enterprise in Medieval and Early Modern Europe*, eds. Florence L. Glaze and Brian K. Nance. Firenze: SISMEL, 2011.

Venuti, Lawrence. *The Scandals of Translation: Towards an Ethics of Difference*. London: Routledge, 1998.

Venuti, Lawrence. *Translation Changes Everything: Theory and Practice*. London: Routledge, 2013.

Voigts, Linda Ehrsam. "The Old English Herbal in Cotton MS Vitellius C III: Studies," Ph.D. dissertation, University of Missouri, 1973.

Voigts, Linda Ehrsam. "A New Look at the Manuscript Containing the Old English Translation of the *Herbarium Apulei*." *Manuscripta* Vol. 20 (1976): 40–59.

Voigts, Linda Ehrsam "The Significance of the Name Apuleius to the *Herbarium Apulei*." *Bulletin of the History of Medicine* Vol. 52 (1978): 214–27.

Voigts, Linda Ehrsam, and Robert P. Hudson. "A drynke þat men callen dwale to make a man to slepe whyle men kerven him: A Surgical Anesthetic from Late Medieval England." In *Health, Disease and Healing in Medieval Culture*, eds. Sheila Campbell, Bert Hall, and David Klausner. New York: St. Martin's Press, 1992.

Wallis, Faith and Robert Wisnovsky, eds. *Medieval Textual Cultures: Agents of Transmission, Translation and Transformation*. Berlin/Boston, MA: DeGruyter, 2016.

Ward-Perkins, Bryan. "Why did the Anglo-Saxons not Become More British?" *The English Historical Review* Vol. 115, No. 462 (June 2000): 513–33.

Ward-Perkins, Bryan. *The Fall of Rome and the End of Civilization*. Oxford: Oxford University Press, 2005.

Watkins, Frances. "Investigation of Antimicrobials From Native British Plants Used in 10th Century Anglo-Saxon Wound Healing Formulation" Ph.D. dissertation., University of East London, 2013.

White, Elizabeth, ed. *Keynsham and Saltford: Life and Work in Times Past 1539–1945*. Keynsham and Saltford Local Historical Society, 1990.

Online Resources (all verified current in December 2022)
American Herbalists Guild
   www.americanherbalistsguild.com
American Botanical Council and its journal, *Herbalgram*
   www.herbalgram.com
AVISTA: Association Villard de Honnecourt for the Interdisciplinary Study of Technology, Science, and Art, includes medicine as well.
   www.avista.org

Bosworth-Toller Anglo-Saxon Dictionary
   https://bosworthtoller.com/
British Society for the History of Science (BSHS)
   www.bshs.org.uk/
BSHS's *Viewpoint* has the pertinent:
   "Unity and Disunity in Academia," and "The Dark Age That Wasn't" www.bshs.org.uk/
      wp-content/uploads/Viewpoint116_ONLINE.pdf
British Library's British Newspaper Archive*s*:
   www.britishnewspaperarchive.co.uk/
CORE: UK Open access site for research papers and journals
   https://core.ac.uk
CROSSROADS:The Evolution of Early-Medieval Medicine in Global and Local Contexts
   www.earlymedievalmedicine.com/
Dictionary of Old English–University of Toronto
(letters a – i in 2022: available by subscription or through subscribing institutions)
   https://doe.artsci.utoronto.ca/
Dictionary of Old English Corpus–(nearly all words in Old English MSS)
   Use Google Search for "Dictionary of Old English Corpus" for ways to access
Dictionary of Old English Plant Names:
   http://oldenglish-plantnames.org/
Forschergruppe Klostermedizin (Research Group on Monastic Medicine)
   www.klostermedizin.de/
Herbal History Research Network:
   www.herbalhistory.org/home/
International Society for the Study of Early-Medieval England (ISSEME)
   www.isseme.org
Keynsham Historical Society Website:
   www.keysalthist.org.uk/
Merovingian World: Early-Medieval Northern Europe, including science and medicine
   https://merovingianworld.com/
National Institutes of Health (US): Center for Complementary and Integrative Health (formerly, Center for Complementary and Alternative Medicine)
   www.nccih.nih
National Institute of Medical Herbalists (UK)
   https://nimh.org.uk/
Society for Promoting Christian Knowledge (SPCK): www.lib.cam.ac.uk/collections/depa
   rtments/rare-books/collections/society-promoting-christian-knowledge-spck
Voigts-Kurtz/eTk and eVK2:Thorndike and Kibre (searchable databases for sources relating
   to medieval science and medicine)
   http://cctr1.umkc.edu/cgi-bin/medievalacademy

ALPHABETICAL INDEXES
OF PLANT NAMES

Behind each plant name is its chapter number in the translated *Herbarium*, located in Chapter 5. The Roman numerals are provided for cross-referencing with Cockayne, De Vriend, and D'Aronco and Cameron, and other editions using that style of numbering.

Name in modern English

Botanical name

Urginea maritima, 43 (XLIII)
Urginea maritima L., 159 (CLIX)
Urtica dioica L., 178 (CLXXVIII)

Veratrum album L., 140 (CXL)
Verbascum thapsus L., 73 (LXXIII)

Verbena officinalis, 67 (LXVII)
Verbena officinalis L., 4 (IV)
Vinca maior L., 179 (CLXXIX)
Viola odorata L., 166 (CLXVI)

Withania somnifera, 23 (XXIII)

Plant name found in medieval Latin manuscripts

abrotanus, 135 (CXXXV)
absinthius, 102 (CII)
acantaleuce, 153 (CLIII)
acanton, 154 (CLIV)
achillea, 175 (CLXXV)
action, 134 (CXXXIV)
aecios, 161 (CLXI)
aglaofotis, 171 (CLXXI)
agromonia, 32 (XXXII)
aizon, 147 (CXLVII)
ami, 164 (CLXIV)
ancusa, 168 (CLXVIII)
annetum, 123
apium, 120 (CXX)
apollinaris, 23 (XXIII)
aristolochia, 20 (XX)
arniglosa, 2 (II)
artemisia tagantes, 12 (XII)
artemisia, 11 (XI)
artemisia leptefilos, 13 (XIII)
Arum dracunculus, 15 (XV)
asterion, 61 (LXI)
astularegia, 33 (XXXIII)
ayzos minor, 139 (CXXXIX)
æliotropus, 50 (L)

basilisca, 131 (CXXXI)
batracion, 10 (X)
betonica, 1 (I)
brassica, 130 (CXXX)
brittanica, 30 (XXX)
bryonia, 68 (LXVIII)
buglossa, 42 (XLII)
bulbiscillitica, 43 (XLIII)
bulbus, 184 (CLXXXIV)
buoptalmon, 141 (CXLI)

caelidonia, 75 (LXXV)
camelleon, 156 (CLVI)
camemelon, 24 (XXIV)
canis caput, 88 (LXXXVIII)
cannane silfatica, 116 (CXVI)
Capparis, 172 (CLXXII)

carduum silfaticum, 111 (CXI)
centauria minor, 36 (XXXVI)
centauria maior, 35 (XXXV)
centimorbia, 162 (CLXII)
cerefolia, 106 (CVI)
chameælæ, 26 (XXVI)
chamedafne, 28 (XXVIII)
chamedris, 25 (XXV)
chamepithys, 27 (XXVII)
coliandra, 104 (CIV)
colocynthisagria, 185 (CLXXXV)
confirma, 60 (LX)
conize, 143 (CXLIII)
cotiledon, 44 (XLIV)
crision, 70 (LXX)
cucumeris siluatica, 115 (CXV)
cynoglossa, 98 (XCVIII)
cynosbatus, 170 (CLXX)

delfinion, 160 (CLX)
dictamnus, 63 (LXIII)

ebulus, 93 (XCIII)
eleborum album, 159 (CLIX)
eliotropus, 137 (CXXXVII)
elleborus albus, 140 (CXL)
erifion, 127 (CXXVII)
eringius, 173 (CLXXIII)
erinion, 109 (CIX)
erusti, 89 (LXXXIX)

felix, 78 (LXXVIII)
feniculus, 126 (CXXVI)
fraga, 38 (XXXVIII)

gallicrus, 45 (XLV)
gallitricus, 48 (XLVIII)
gentiana, 17 (XVII)
gladiolus, 80 (LXXX)
glycyrida, 145 (CXLV)
gorgonion, 182 (CLXXXII)
gramen, 79 (LXXIX)
gryas, 51 (LI)

Old English plant name

INDEX OF MEDICAL COMPLAINTS

The numbers refer to the chapters and subchapters of the *Herbarium* where the complaint is mentioned. The index is fairly complete but not exhaustive.

GENERAL INDEX

Note: Endnotes are indicated by the page number followed by "n" and the note number e.g., 51n20 refers to note 51 on page 20.

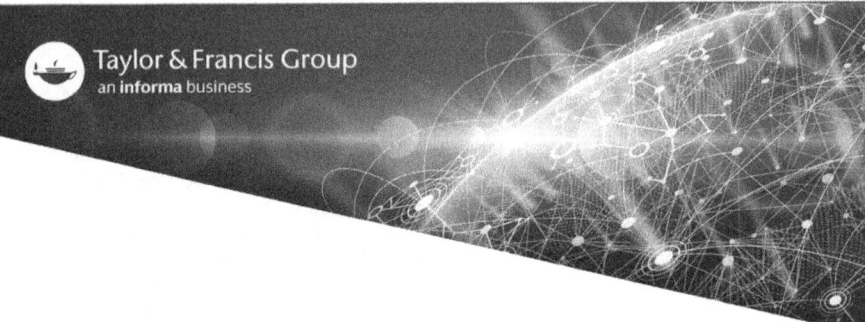
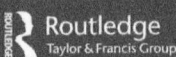
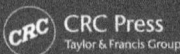